Culture, communication, and cognition: Vygotskian perspectives

Culture, communication, and cognition: Vygotskian perspectives

Edited by

JAMES V. WERTSCH

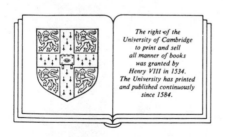

The right of the
University of Cambridge
to print and sell
all manner of books
was granted by
Henry VIII in 1534.
The University has printed
and published continuously
since 1584.

CAMBRIDGE UNIVERSITY PRESS

Cambridge
New York   Port Chester
Melbourne   Sydney

Published by the Press Syndicate of the University of Cambridge
The Pitt Building, Trumpington Street, Cambridge, CB2 1RP
40 West 20th Street, New York, NY 10011 USA
10 Stamford Road, Oakleigh, Melbourne 3166, Australia

© Cambridge University Press 1985

First published 1985
Reprinted 1985
First paperback edition 1986
Reprinted 1987, 1988, 1989

Printed in the United States of America

Library of Congress Cataloging in Publication Data

Main entry under title:
Culture, communication, and cognition.
Includes index.
1. Cognition and culture.   2. Vygotskiĭ, Lev
Semenovich, 1896–1934.   4. Psycholinguistics.
5. Cognition in children.   6. Interpersonal
communication.   I. Wertsch, James V.
BF311.C84   1984   302.2   83-14444

ISBN 0 521 33830 1 paperback

Contents

v

Foreword

This volume grows out of a conference held in Chicago in 1980 on the ideas of the Soviet psychologist and semiotician Lev Semenovich Vygotsky. This conference was one of a series sponsored by the Center for Psychosocial Studies to examine major issues in the social sciences and humanities. Previous meetings dealt with issues such as the social foundations of language and thought[1] and the concept of self. [2]

Vygotsky's work has had a major impact on the research of the Center. Our interest in his ideas stems from a general concern with the nature of human consciousness and the forces that play a role in its formation. In examining these issues over the course of a decade we have drawn on a variety of disciplines (e.g., philosophy, anthropology, psychoanalysis, history, psychology), but during the past few years the science of signs – semiotics – has come to play a particularly important role in our thinking. Our decision to use a semiotic approach was based on the realization that it may provide the key to a variety of interrelated social science problems. The approach we mapped out called on us to begin by examining the principles that underlie human sign systems, especially language, and then to use this knowledge to examine the role of these sign systems in the organization of psychological, communicative, and sociocultural processes.

If this sounds like a Vygotskian enterprise, it is; much in our basic line of reasoning stems from his ideas. In addition, we have tried to utilize advances in semiotic research from other quarters, especially the ideas of the American pragmatist C. S. Peirce and the research of Prague School linguists such as Roman Jakobson. As we have studied the writings of these figures at the Center we have become convinced that they represent traditions whose potential for constructing an integrated account of human social and psychological processes has been overlooked.

A major virtue of Vygotsky's sociohistorical approach to consciousness is that it provides an overarching theoretical framework in which these and other issues can be examined and interrelated. The chapters in this volume

vii

demonstrate the power and scope of his ingenious approach. The fact that a diversity of issues can be addressed and integrated within a single theoretical perspective reflects a strength that is all too often missing in today's academic world of fragmented disciplines and subdisciplines.

In addition to any intellectual progress that may ensue from our conference and from this volume, we hope that our efforts can play some role on another front, namely international understanding. At first glance, it seems as if there should be something ironic about the fact that the group attending the first international conference on a Soviet scholar was composed primarily of enthusiastic Westerners. However, the irony quickly dissipates when one considers the kind of issues Vygotsky addressed; they are issues that are just as pressing for contemporary Western societies as they were for the Soviet society in which Vygotsky lived and worked. In this sense Vygotsky was truly an international intellectual figure.

On a more personal level, the understanding and cooperation at our conference were greatly enhanced by the encouragement we received from friends and colleagues from the Soviet Union. Perhaps the best way to sum up our feelings on this point is to express our deep appreciation for the following telegram that arrived on October 20, 1980, the eve of the conference:

From the Vygotsky family.
We thank the organizers of your symposium and wish all of its participants success in their work and well-being.

Vygotsky's daughter, Gita Vygotskaya

Bernard Weissbourd
Center for Psychosocial Studies
Chicago, Illinois

[1]   M. Hickmann (Ed.), *Proceedings of a Working Conference on the Social Foundations of Language and Thought*, Center for Psychological Studies, Chicago, 1980

[2]   Benjamin Lee (Ed.), *Psychosocial Theories of the Self*, Plenum Press, New York, 1982; Benjamin Lee and Gil Noam (Eds.), *Developmental Approaches to the Self*, Plenum Press, New York, 1983.

Contributors

ANN L. BROWN Center for the Study of Reading, University of Illinois, Champaign, Illinois

JEROME BRUNER New School for Social Research, New York, New York

COURTNEY B. CAZDEN Graduate School of Education, Harvard University, Cambridge, Massachusetts

MICHAEL COLE Laboratory of Comparative Human Cognition, University of California, La Jolla, California

V.V. DAVYDOV Institute of General and Pedagogical Psychology, Academy of Pedagogical Sciences, Moscow, USSR

ROBERTA A. FERRARA Center for the Study of Reading, University of Illinois, Champaign, Illinois

ELLICE A. FORMAN Program on Learning Disabilities, Northwestern University, Evanston, Illinois

MAYA E. HICKMANN Max-Planck Institut für Psycholinguistik, Nijmegen, Holland (also Center for Psychosocial Studies, Chicago, Illinois)

KARSTEN HUNDEIDE Institute of Psychology, University of Oslo, Oslo, Norway

VERA JOHN-STEINER Educational Foundations Department, University of New Mexico, Albuquerque, New Mexico

BENJAMIN LEE Center for Psychosocial Studies, Chicago, Illinois (also Department of Anthropology, University of Chicago, Chicago, Illinois)

DAVID MCNEILL Committee on Cognition and Communication, University of Chicago, Illinois

L.A. RADZIKHOVSKII Institute of General and Pedagogical Psychology, Academy of Pedagogical Sciences, Moscow, USSR

RAGNAR ROMMETVEIT Institute of Psychology, University of Oslo, Oslo, Norway

SYLVIA SCRIBNER Developmental Psychology Program, City University of New York, New York, New York

MICHAEL SILVERSTEIN Department of Anthropology, University of Chicago, Chicago, Illinois

C. ADDISON STONE Program on Learning Disabilities, Northwestern University, Evanston, Illinois

JAMES V. WERTSCH Department of Linguistics, Northwestern University, Evanston, Illinois (also Center for Psychosocial Studies, Chicago, Illinois)

V.P. ZINCHENKO Department of Psychology, Moscow State University, Moscow, USSR

Introduction

JAMES V. WERTSCH

Lev Semenovich Vygotsky is one of those figures in intellectual history who might have never been. Had he lived in another time or place, it is unlikely that he would have developed his theoretical approach to psychology. The milieu that proved so supportive was provided by the intellectual and social ferment following the 1917 Revolution. This setting provided Vygotsky and other young scholars with opportunities and challenges that remain unparalleled in the twentieth century. They were asked to reformulate entire disciplines in accordance with Marxist philosophical principles, and they were asked to create sciences that could assist in the construction of a new socialist society. As numerous observers have pointed out, the period of intellectual excitement and freedom that followed the Revolution was destined to last only two decades or so. However, it provided enough time for Vygotsky to lay the theoretical foundation for an approach that has had a powerful impact on Soviet psychology and has recently began to be understood and utilized in the West.

Vygotsky was born in 1896, a "vintage year" for the social sciences and humanities considering that it was also a year that saw the birth of Roman Jakobson and Jean Piaget. He began his life in provincial Belorussia, completing gymnasium in Gomel in 1913 with a gold medal. After graduating from Moscow University with a specialization in literature in 1917 he returned to Gomel to teach literature and psychology in a local school. While working there between 1917 and 1923, Vygotsky also directed theater in an adult education center and gave numerous lectures on literature, psychology, and science.

In his first intellectual endeavors Vygotsky focused on art and literary criticism, literary history, aesthetics, and the psychology of art. By 1915 he had completed the first version of his major work on *Hamlet*. In 1916, at the age of 20, he remarked on the "innumerable notes made over a long period of time while reading and rereading *Hamlet* and thinking about him for several years" (quoted in Ivanov, 1968). He continued to revise and

1

expand his original work on this topic and eventually published it as his first major volume, *The Psychology of Art* (1925).

This early period in Vygotsky's career was one of intense preparation for all the work that would follow. He was reading the works of figures as diverse as Aristotle, Bühler, Darwin, Dostoevsky, Engels, Freud, Goethe, Hegel, Marx, Potebnya, Tolstoy, and Wundt. He was also staying abreast of the rapidly changing intellectual scene of his time. Particularly important in this regard was the work of the Russian Formalists. Through his cousin David Vygodsky in Leningrad, he remained in contact with the ideas of scholars such as Eikhenbaum, Shklovski, Tomashevskii, and Yakubinskii. As is evident from his comments in *The Psychology of Art* and *Thinking and Speech* (1934), Vygotsky did not agree with many of the claims of this school. However, the Formalists established the questions about linguistic form and function that had to be addressed during this period of his career. In the course of dealing with these questions Vygotsky formulated his early ideas about the role of signs in regulating human activity. His ideas about educational psychology and defectology also began to emerge then. While in Gomel he founded a psychological laboratory in the teacher training institute where he worked, and he gave a series of lectures later to be published as *Pedagogical Psychology* (1926). Thus we see that the period between 1915 and 1924 was a very busy one in Vygotsky's life. He was already heavily involved in theoretical research and was beginning to carry out empirical studies.

However, the beginning of Vygotsky's major involvement in Soviet science is usually traced to the year 1924. On January 6 of that year he gave a presentation at the Second All-Russian Conference on Psychoneurology in Leningrad. This presentation, entitled "Methods of Reflexological Research Applied to the Study of Mind," marked Vygotsky's first efforts to create a new theoretical orientation for psychology. His students never tired of relating the electrifying effect this unknown young man from the provinces had on the conference. Over a half-century later Luria (1979) wrote:

> When Vygotsky got up to deliver his speech, he had no printed text from which to read, not even notes. Yet he spoke fluently, never seeming to stop and search his memory for the next idea. Even had the content of his speech been pedestrian, his performance would have been notable for the persuasiveness of his style. But his speech was by no means pedestrian. Instead of choosing a minor theme, as might befit a young man of twenty-eight speaking for the first time to a gathering of the graybeards of his profession, Vygotsky chose the difficult theme of the relation between conditioned reflexes and man's conscious behavior . . . . Although he failed to convince everyone of the correctness of his view, it was clear that this man from a small provincial town in western Russia was an intellectual force who would have to be listened to. (Pp. 38–39)

After this presentation, K. N. Kornilov invited Vygotsky to join the staff of the Institute of Psychology in Moscow. Kornilov had just replaced the prerevolutionary director of that institute, G. I. Chelpanov, and was striving to create the setting in which scholars would formulate a new Marxist psychology (for more details on this, see Cole, 1979). In the autumn of 1924 Vygotsky moved to Moscow to take up his new position in this institute as Staff Scientist, 2nd Class. It quickly became apparent to those around him that his performance at the Leningrad conference had been no accident. He established himself as a brilliant thinker who was driven by seemingly boundless energy.

In Moscow Vygotsky began to develop a following of devoted students and colleagues. The first figures to join him were A. N. Leont'ev and A. R. Luria, the other members of what came to be known as the "troika." Luria (1979) described the heady optimism and contagious enthusiasm of Vygotsky and his group during those years in the following terms:

> It is extremely difficult, after the passage of so much time, to recapture the enormous enthusiasm with which we carried out this work. The entire group gave almost all its waking hours to our grand plan for the reconstruction of psychology. When Vygotsky went on a trip, the students wrote poems in honor of his journey. When he gave a lecture in Moscow, everyone came to hear him. (P. 52)

In light of the enormity of the task and the inexperience of the group (all of its members were in their 20s), such optimism and enthusiasm were needed.

As outlined by authors such as Cole and Scribner (1978), Luria (1979), and Radzikhovskii (1979), the decade Vygotsky spent in Moscow before his death of tuberculosis in 1934 was a time of rapid development and change. During this period he founded the Institute of Defectology in Moscow, he collaborated with Luria on a cross-cultural research project (Vygotsky and Luria, 1930), he continued his studies of semiotics with Luria and Eisenshtein, he produced innumerable articles and volumes, and he generally played a leading role in the development of Soviet psychology.

The ideas formulated by Vygotsky during the last decade or so of his life provide the focus of this volume. The authors of the various chapters have reexamined and extended one or more of Vygotsky's basic theoretical constructs. With the hindsight of nearly a half-century, we can see that some of his claims are naïve or incorrect. For example, his claims about aphasia (Vygotsky, 1960) are quite uninformed by today's standards. However, many of his ideas are just as valuable today as they were in the 1920s and 1930s. In particular, his proposal for reformulating psychology as part of a unified social science takes on a special relevance in light of the contemporary trend toward disciplinary specialization and fragmentation.

There are several possible ways to present Vygotsky's approach. In this introduction I will do so by tracing a line of reasoning that can be seen as guiding Vygotsky's program of scientific inquiry. This line of reasoning begins with the assumption that the science of psychology as it existed in his day was confronted with a "crisis." The crisis had arisen because various authors' explanations of psychological phenomena were grounded in different theoretical assumptions. At best, these different assumptions resulted in a failure to interrelate various investigators' findings. At worst, findings and claims were contradictory. Borrowing from Brentano, Vygotsky (1956) wrote that "there exist many psychologies, but there does not exist a unfied psychology" (p. 57). He argued that the ramifications of such a state of affairs are quite serious:

The absence of a single scientific system that would embrace and combine all of our contemporary knowledge in psychology results in a situation in which every new factual discovery ... that is more than a simple accumulation of details *is forced* to create its own special theory and explanatory system. In order to understand facts and relationships investigators are forced to create their own psychology – one of many psychologies. (Pp. 57–58)

Of particular importance in this respect was the irreconcilable split between subjective idealism and reductionistic behaviorism. Many of the disputes over this issue centered on the status of the concept of consciousness. As noted by authors in this volume such as Bruner (Chapter 1) and Davydov and Radzikhovskii (Chapter 2), Vygotsky played a major role in the "struggle for consciousness" in Soviet psychology. In an introduction to Vygotsky's work, Leont'ev and Luria (1956) described this struggle as consisting of "freeing oneself on the one hand from vulgar behaviorism and, on the other, from the subjective understanding of mental phenomena as exclusively internal subjective states that can only be investigated through introspection" (p. 6). Bruner points out that Vygotsky's ingenious solution to this seemingly intractable dilemma was to use one of Pavlov's constructs to account for how the child is integrated into a social community. Specifically, he used the notion of the "Second Signal System" (a notion about which Pavlov actually said very little). Vygotsky interpreted the Second Signal System as "the world encoded in language: nature transformed by history and culture" (Bruner, Chapter 1, this volume).

With this we begin to see the outlines of Vygotsky's proposal for reformulating psychology. If the impetus for this reformulation was his observation that the psychology of his day was incapable of producing a coherent account of human psychological processes, his first positive claim was that there are a few specific pillars on which one could construct such a reformulation. Specifically, he assumed that it could be based on ideas from psychology, Marxist philosophy, and semiotic theory. His integration of ideas from these three sources produced the approach that is examined in this volume.

With regard to psychology, it is important to note that although Vygotsky saw the weaknesses of existing approaches, he did not reject or ignore what this discipline had to offer. Because of Vygotsky's emphasis on criticizing and reformulating psychology, this fact is often overlooked. However, as several authors in this volume point out, much in Vygotsky's approach can be understood only if one recognizes the influences of the psychological theory of his day. Bruner (Chapter 1) notes the influence of Pavlov in this regard, and Wertsch and Stone (Chapter 7) note that Vygotsky formulated some of his claims in response to the ideas of Janet (1926–1927, 1928) and Piaget (1926). Finally, Davydov and Radzikhovskii (Chapter 2) make the general point that like several other Soviet psychologists in the 1920s, Vygotsky built his system by using "on the one hand, the ideas of Marxist philosophy and, on the other, the facts and conceptual schemes that existed in various psychological theories."

Once Vygotsky's debt to other psychologists is recognized, we must turn to the issue of how he proposed to recast their ideas. As I noted above, it seems to me that the key to answering this can be traced to two other major sources of Vygotsky's ideas: Marxist philosophy and semiotics. Various aspects of the first of these influences, Marxist philosophy, are examined by several authors in this volume. In many respects all of these authors are concerned with answering the question "What is Marxist about Vygotsky's approach?" It turns out that this is a complex matter. Vygotsky did not address many of the issues that immediately come to mind when one thinks of a Marxist psychology. For example, he did not deal with class consciousness or the psychology of fetishism and alienation. In this respect he is quite different from authors who have attempted to create a psychology that deals with specific issues raised by Marx. For example, authors such as Seve (1978) have examined specific Marxist socioeconomic processes and categories and their impact on the individual. In contrast, Vygotsky's approach is Marxist in more subtle but no less fundamental ways. I will outline here three areas in which Vygotsky borrowed from Marx: his method, his claims about the nature of human activity, and his claims about the social origins of psychological processes.

First, with regard to *method* Vygotsky's debt to Marx runs deeper than is commonly recognized. The method at issue here is what I have elsewhere (Wertsch, 1981a, b, 1983) termed Vygotsky's "genetic explanation." This method is built on the assumption that psychological phenomena can be understood only by examining *the genesis of complete living units of functioning*. Both the notion of genesis and the notion of a complete living unit are essential to it. To be sure, Vygotsky was influenced by figures other than Marx in formulating this method. For example, the ideas of the Russian psychologist Blonskii (1921) on development clearly had an influence. However, Marx's ideas seem to have played a central role in leading him to *combine* the notion of genesis and the notion of unit. Vygotsky readily acknowledged this debt to Marx:

I don't want to discover the nature of mind by patching together a lot of quotations. I want to find out how science has to be built, to approach the study of mind having learned the whole of Marx's *method* . . . . In order to create such an enabling theory-method in the generally accepted scientific manner, it is necessary to discover the essence of the given area of phenomena, the laws according to which they change, their qualitative and quantitative characteristics, their causes. It is necessary to formulate the categories and concepts that are specifically relevant to them – in other words, to create one's own *Capital.*

The whole of *Capital* is written according to the following method: Marx analyzes a single living "cell" of capitalist society – for example the nature of value. Within this cell he discovers the structure of the entire system and all of its economic institutions. He says that to a layman this analysis may seem a murky tangle of tiny details. Indeed, there may be tiny details, but they are exactly those which are essential to "microanatomy." Anyone who could discover what a "psychological" cell is – the mechanism producing even a single response – would thereby find the key to psychology as a whole. (Vygotsky's unpublished notebooks, quoted in Cole and Scribner, 1978, p. 8).

Several authors in this volume examine Vygotsky's ideas about processes of development and the complete living units (or "cells") that are involved. Lee (Chapter 3) and Scribner (Chapter 5) have broadened this examination by searching for the origins of his ideas in the writings of Marx. Both of these authors take up the issue of how Marx's mode of reasoning about change in phylogenesis and social history is utilized by Vygotsky to fashion an account of ontogenesis. Lee's detailed comparative analysis of the writings of Vygotsky and Marx leaves little doubt about the former's debt to the latter. Scribner examines this question by focusing on the relationship among three specific domains to which genetic explanation has been applied: general history, ontogeny, and higher psychological functions. Both Lee and Scribner conclude that Vygotsky's debt to Marx is to be found primarily in the area of method. In particular, they show how several points in Vygotsky's explanation of ontogenetic transition can be understood only if one appreciates their origins in the writings of Marx.

In his chapter Lee also touches on the role of functional explanation in Vygotsky's approach. He argues that functional reorganization is a key construct in Vygotsky's genetic explanation. The discussion of this construct in turn leads to the issue of *units* of analysis, since units are what undergo functional reorganization. The definition of the unit of psychological analysis involved in Vygotsky's approach is the topic for several other chapters in this volume as well.

Zinchenko, (Chapter 4) begins his analysis by pointing out that any psychological theory involves assumptions about units of mental functioning. Regardless of whether these assumptions are explicit or implicit, they impose powerful constraints on all other aspects of the theory. Zinchenko then goes on to outline several criteria inherent in Vygotsky's notion of a unit for the analysis of mind. Among the seven that he lists, several are concerned with the claim that a unit must be a functionally integrated whole while simultaneously allowing for the internal contradictions and "heterogeneity" that is the catalyst of development. This kind of claim provides a further specification of Lee's argument about Vygotsky's notion of functional reorganization.

As noted by several authors (e.g., Zinchenko, Chapter 4; Wertsch and Stone, Chapter 7; Silverstein, Chapter 9), the specific unit on which Vygotsky based his analyses was word meaning. He saw it as a "microcosm of human consciousness" (1956, p. 384). While not disagreeing with Vygotsky on the need for identifying some holistic unit, several authors in this volume question this particular choice. Some of these objections are concerned with the notion of word meaning itself. For example, Silverstein points out that with the development of grammatical analyses in the twentieth century, Vygotsky's interpretation of word meaning is no longer adequate. Other authors raise additional objections to Vygotsky's selection of the word as a unit of analysis. Of particular interest in this regard are criticisms that focus on the inability of word meaning to play a constructive role in Vygotsky's account of the relationship between the "natural" (or "elementary") and "higher" (or "cultural") lines of development in ontogenesis. (See Cole, Chapter 6, this volume, for comments on the history of this theoretical distinction.) In Vygotsky's view the elementary mental functions (e.g., involuntary attention, eidetic memory) result from the natural line of development and are transformed into higher mental functions (e.g., voluntary memory, logical memory) through the child's social interaction with more experienced members of a culture.

The very essence of cultural development is in the collision of mature cultural forms of behavior with the primitive [i.e., natural] forms that characterize the child's behavior. (Vygotsky, 1981, p. 151)

At several points in his theoretical writings Vygotsky argued that this collision of forces from the two lines of development is what leads to higher mental functions. His argument was that the "products" of the natural line of development are *transformed* by virtue of coming into contact with the forces of the social line. However, Vygotsky's concrete empirical studies failed to specify the exact role of the natural line in this process. His studies really focused on how the child masters sociocultural modes of mediation and said almost nothing about the elementary mental functions that are transformed. Indeed, authors such as Rubenshtein (1957) have argued that Vygotsky's actual studies ignore this line altogether.

Part of this problem can be traced to Vygotsky's choice of word meaning as the "living cell" to be examined in his analysis. Word meaning led him to focus almost exclusively on the cultural line of development and to ignore the natural line. As Zinchenko (Chapter 4, this volume) points out, the focus on this unit was almost certain to lead to difficulties because it is not a "genetically primary unit for the analysis of mind." Motivated by such observations several of Vygotsky's followers have sought to extend his theory by proposing a new unit of analysis. In this volume Zinchenko traces the history of this effort in Soviet psychology and outlines his own notion of the appropriate unit for a Vygotskian approach, the "tool-mediated action." He begins with the observation (grounded in the work of Davydov, 1972) that "the genetically primary 'cell' or 'the undeveloped beginnings of the fully developed whole' as a unit of analysis . . . must have an actual sensuous–contemplative form." That is, the original form of the unit of mental analysis must be practical or sensorimotor (to use the Piagetian term) action. Zinchenko argues that the research of scholars such as Zaporozhets (1959) and Bernshtein (1966) provides the foundation for an approach that integrates the early practical action of the natural line of development with the social forces of the cultural line of development. Zinchenko argues that the Bernshteinian cybernetic model of human movement contrasts with the Pavlovian approach used by Vygotsky (see Davydov and Radzikhovskii, Chapter 2, this volume, for details on the latter) at the very points that are crucial for linking the natural and cultural lines of development.

McNeill (Chapter 11, this volume) takes this argument a step further in connection with the specific issues raised by speech. Building on the ideas of Bernshtein and of Zinchenko (Chapter 4, this volume), he outlines a unit of speech action (the "syntagma") that can be used in efforts to integrate speech and nonspeech action in a psychological theory. A major point in McNeill's argument that will be of interest to those concerned with the relation between language and thought is the criticism of linguistic theories that "objectify" language. He argues that such theories cannot provide the foundation for understanding this relation and proposes instead that units of language as action must be used.

To summarize, the first way that Vygotsky incorporated Marxist ideas into his approach is in his method. As authors in this volume such as Lee, Scribner, Zinchenko, and McNeill point out, the issue is one of how to analyze the *genesis* of *wholistic living units*. The precise nature of these units is still a matter of debate.

The second point at which one can provide an answer to the question "What is Marxist about Vygotsky's approach?" concerns the notion of human activity. As I have noted elsewhere (Wertsch, 1981 a,b), the notion of activity (*deyatel'nost'*) is the most fundamental working concept in Soviet psychology. This applies to the Vygotskian school as well as to others. Indeed, while I did not point it out earlier in this introduction, the notion of activity has already been involved in my discussion. Zinchenko's notion of action (*deistvie*) is derived from one of the levels of analysis in the "Vygotsky–Leont'ev–Luria" theory of activity. But the chapter in this volume that deals the most with this issue is that by Davydov and Radzikhovskii (Chapter 2). Like Zinchenko, they point out that Vygotsky's ultimate concern was human consciousness. However, they note that it is only by using certain Marxist philosophical concepts that were not available in his lifetime that Vygotsky could have been able to answer some of the very questions he raised about consciousness. Davydov and Radzikhovskii argue that in order to understand how he would have answered such questions, it is necessary to distinguish between "Vygotsky the methodologist" (i.e., theoretician of psychology and metapsychology) and "Vygotsky the psychologist." In their opinion many of his most insightful and lasting contributions come from his work in the first category.

Davydov and Radzikhovskii conduct a thorough examination of Vygotsky's methodological assumptions about consciousness. In particular, they review his concern over whether consciousness is a substance or an attribute (categories of Spinoza, his "favorite philosopher"). On the basis of a review of the early writings of Vygotsky (1925, 1926), they argue that he outlined a position in which consciousness has a new "methodological status." Specifically, they outlined some of his "normative requirements" that a Marxist theory of consciousness would have to meet. Among these is the dual claim that human consciousness derives from external material reality and that no simple unidirectional link can account for this process. Rather, his methodological system called for psychology to "search for the reality that intervenes between the "external" world and the human mind." Davydov and Radzikhovskii argue that this link is activity and that Vygotsky himself recognized at least some of the implications of such a claim.

The cornerstone for the theory of activity that was to be developed after Vygotsky's death is Marx's First Thesis on Feuerbach. As Leont'ev (1981) was to note:

The importance of this category [i.e., activity] hardly needs to be emphasized. We need only recall Marx's famous theses on Feuerbach, in which he said that the chief defect of earlier metaphysical materialism was that it viewed sensuousness only as a form of contemplation, not as human activity or practice. Therefore, the active aspect of sensuousness was developed by idealism, the opposite of materialism. Idealism, however, understood it abstractly, not as the real sense activity of man. (P. 41)

Soviet psychologists such as Leont'ev have spent the last several decades developing the implications of this thesis for their discipline. [It is interesting to note that Western scholars such as Bourdieu (1977) have recently proposed similar arguments for other social science disciplines.] Among other things, the concept of activity in Soviet psychology has led to a new account of the process of internalization. As Leont'ev (1981), Davydov and Radzikhovskii (Chapter 2, this volume), and Zinchenko (Chapter 4, this volume) argue, an essential aspect of this interpretation is that it specifies the properties of external and internal forms of activity that make possible the genetic transitions between them. Wertsch and Stone (Chapter 7, this volume) base their examination of Vygotsky's notion of internalization on this theoretical framework.

Davydov and Radzikhovskii argue that Vygotsky anticipated the need to use activity as a fundamental theoretical construct in psychology. In support of this claim they cite his comments on practical and labor activity. There is currently an ongoing debate in the USSR over whether the theory of activity was already inherent in Vygotsky's ideas or whether it constitutes an extension of them. At least some scholars such as Davydov and Radzikhovskii see the category of activity as an essential point where Vygotsky's ideas are inspired by the writings of Marx. It is in this connection that I see the second answer one could provide to the question "What is Marxist about Vygotsky's approach?"

The third way that one could answer this question has to do with Vygotsky's claims about the social origins of individual mental processes. In this connection, Vygotsky drew on Marx's Sixth Thesis on Feuerbach to formulate the following basic assumption of his work:

To paraphrase a well-known position of Marx's we could say that humans' psychological nature represents the aggregate of internalized social relations that have become functions for the individual and forms of his/her structure. We do not want to say that this is the meaning of Marx's position, but we see in this position the fullest expression of that toward which the history of cultural development leads us. (1981, p. 164)

In this statement we see evidence of Vygotsky's concern for creating a psychology that would be compatible with Marx's basic claims about the social origins of human consciousness. Again, Vygotsky did not address specific Marxian issues such as class consciousness, but he was quite clear about his claim that "the first problem [of psychology] is to show how the individual response emerges from the forms of collective life" (1981, p. 165).

The way Vygotsky developed this basic claim is the topic for several of the authors' discussions in this volume. In one way or another, these discussions revolve around what he formulated as the "general genetic law of cultural development."

Any function in the child's cultural development appears twice, or on two planes. First it appears on the social plane, and then on the psychological plane. First it appears between people as an interpsychological category, and then within the child as an intrapsychological category. This is equally true with regard to voluntary attention, logical memory, the formation of concepts, and the development of volition. (1981, p. 163)

Various authors in this volume focus on different aspects of Vygotsky's formulation of this relation between social and individual functioning. For example, Cole (Chapter 6) examines Vygotsky's ideas with an eye toward overcoming the artificial separation of social science disciplines, whereas Wertsch and Stone (Chapter 7) review it in connection with Vygotsky's account of internalization.

Among the many specific issues raised by the general genetic law of cultural development, one stands out in importance in this volume. This is the notion of the "zone of proximal development." Vygotsky developed this notion in order to examine two major practices in education: instruction and psychological testing. Forman and Cazden (Chapter 14, this volume) point out that in the Vygotsky tradition educational practices take on special theoretical importance since they provide some of the social settings most crucial for children's development. In this connection these authors cite the statement by Leont'ev and Luria (1968) that "the assimilation of general human experience in the teaching process is the most important specifically human form of mental development in ontogenesis" (p. 365).

Vygotsky (1978) defined the zone of proximal development as *"the distance between the actual developmental level as determined by independent problem solving and the level of potential development as determined through problem solving under adult guidance or in collaboration with more capable peers"* (p. 86). This notion, which he originally formulated around 1930, has only recently come to be appreciated in the West. As Bruner points out in this volume (Chapter 1), the zone of proximal development was mentioned in the 1962 English translation of *Thinking and Speech* (1934). This provided the foundation for the notion of "scaffolding" that he and his colleagues subsequently developed (e.g., Bruner, 1976; Wood, Bruner, and Ross, 1976). For many researchers, however, it was not until Cole, John-Steiner, Scribner, and Souberman edited and published Vygotsky's *Mind in Society* (1978) that the implications of Vygotsky's claims about the zone of proximal development became apparent.

It quickly became apparent to those concerned with this issue that while

Vygotsky's ingenious insights had opened a whole new frontier, they needed to be clarified and extended. Authors in this volume such as Bruner, Cole, Brown and Ferrara, Hundeide, Forman and Cazden, and John-Steiner (Chapters 1, 6, 12, 13, 14, and 15, respectively) have undertaken this task.

One of the first problems that arises in this connection is how to specify ways in which a child can perform "under adult guidance or in collaboration with more capable peers" (1978, p. 86). Vygotsky (1978) made a few comments on this point, suggesting that various forms of demonstration and hints could be used by the adult or more capable peer, but such comments leave many questions unanswered. Brown and Ferrara examine this issue in connection with testing procedures. After reviewing the static nature of most IQ tests (tests that attempt to measure the "actual developmental level"), they examine some results from their studies of how the "level of potential development" can be incorporated into psychological testing. Specifically, they review the method of using "graduated aids in uncovering the 'readiness' of children to perform competently in any task domain." Included in this argument is a task analysis, something that authors such as Brown (1978) and Campione and Brown (1978) have been developing for the past several years.

Bruner (Chapter 1, this volume) outlines some of the ways that he has examined the issue of the zone of proximal development in his studies of scaffolding. In particular, he focuses on the forms of semiotic mediation that are involved in collaborative and individual problem-solving activity. This leads him to examine how such mediation can be abbreviated to form overt and internalized forms of self-regulative speech.

In Chapter 13, Hundeide examines the issues of perspective and perspective taking in communication. He outlines a general formulation of these issues and shows how they can be incorporated into a Vygotskian approach that avoids some of the confusions and dead ends of contemporary developmental psychology. By specifying how perspectives are coordinated in communication, he confronts some of the difficult problems Vygotsky raised in connection with interpsychological functioning. This is the problem of how an adult and a child with quite different interpretations of a situation can interact.

Cole (Chapter 6) examines yet another set of questions in connection with the zone of proximal development. In contrast to Vygotsky, who examined this zone primarily in connection with formal educational settings, Cole argues that it must be viewed as a more general mechanism "where culture and cognition create each other." He is concerned with how this zone can be created in a variety of settings outside the school. Furthermore, he asks how interpsychological functioning in such settings is related to the instructional activity of formal education contexts.

This concern with types of interpsychological functioning that do not fall under the heading of formal instruction is also evidenced in Chapter 14 by Forman and Cazden. In contrast to Vygotsky, who focused primarily on adult–child interaction, they examine the "cognitive value of peer interaction." Their examination of child–child interpsychological functioning in a Piagetian task setting leads them to conclude that a unique form of scaffolding is involved in such cases. They argue that "peer (and cross-age) relationships can function as intermediate transforming contexts between social and external adult–child interactions and the individual child's inner speech." Again, this is an aspect of interpsychological functioning that Vygotsky mentioned in passing, but Forman and Cazden identify and examine some of the specific issues involved.

In her analysis in Chapter 15 of bilingualism and language learning, John-Steiner also touches on Vygotsky's concern with the social origins of individual psychological functioning. However, the focus of her analysis of social and individual processes differ from that of those authors in this volume concerned with the zone of proximal development. In contrast to those who are interested in the emergence of higher mental functions that are mediated by language, John-Steiner focuses on the language development itself (e.g., first- and second-language acquisition, the development of writing). Throughout her chapter she emphasizes the difference between early forms of development that involve little in the way of conscious reflection and later forms that do, an issue that played a major role in Vygotsky's theoretical approach.

Thus several chapters in this volume touch on issues that Vygotsky raised as part of his Marxist reformulation of psychology. Only a few of the authors explicitly address these Marxist origins of his approach, but when reexamining and extending Vygotsky's ideas, one necessarily touches on them. In summary, it seems to me that the chapters in this volume touch on three ways that one can respond to the question "What is Marxist about Vygotsky's psychology?" First, I would point to the similarities in method. Second, I would argue that Marx's First Thesis on Feuerbach provides the foundation of activity as a basic concept in psychological theory. And third, I would note Vygotsky's use of Marx's Sixth Thesis on Feuerbach to formulate an account of the social origins of individual psychological functioning.

This leaves us with the third major source of Vygotsky's ideas: his study of literature and the semiotics of art. As I noted above, Vygotsky's early writings were concerned primarily with these topics. They stand in contrast to the writings he produced after he moved to Moscow in 1924 and began his career in academic psychology. From that time on he produced only a few additional writings on literary analysis. This does not mean, however, that he no longer had an active interest in the issues he had begun to explore in *The Psychology of Art* (1925).

This lifelong interest in the nature of signs and their impact on the organization of human activity is responsible for many of the most interesting aspects of Vygotsky's approach. This is not to say that his aproach is the product of semiotic analysis alone. It is no more accurate to say this than it is to say that it is the product solely of the psychological theory of his day or of Marxist theory. Rather, it is the unique integration of these three strands that produced his approach.

Several chapters in this volume examine Vygotsky's semiotic analysis and its role in his theoretical framework. In his review of the origins of Vygotsky's ideas, Lee (Chapter 3) points out the important role played by the American linguist Edward Sapir. On the basis of a comparative analysis of texts, Lee argues that essential aspects of Vygotsky's approach are best understood as an attempt to combine Marxists tenets with semiotic and linguistic theory. This combination yielded the particular form of instrumentalism noted by Bruner (Chapter 1, this volume). Indeed, this instrumentalism is an issue that reflects all three of the major sources of Vygotsky's ideas. It is based on a notion of tool mediation that can be traced to the writings of Marx and Engels. However, Vygotsky extended the notion of mediation to signs in general and language in particular. As Lee notes, he recognized that this extension must take into account the unique properties of signs. Thus his distinction between signs and tools. For Vygotsky, one of the inherent properties of humans' semiotic activity is that it involves categorization, a point that he credits to Sapir (1921). In developing this claim, he also drew on the third major source of his ideas, the psychological theory of his time. For example, he developed his notion of the sign in conjunction with an analysis of the Pavlovian distinction between signalization and signification. Hence, in this case (as well as others) we see a unique integration of theoretical sources: Marxist concepts, psychological theory, and semiotic analysis.

In addition to identifying the sources of Vygotsky's semiotic analysis, several authors examine its role in his approach. For example, Wertsch and Stone (Chapter 7) argue that Vygotsky's account of internalization rests squarely on his semiotic analysis. In his approach, the internal plane of consciousness comes into existence through "the emergence of control over external sign forms." One of Vygotsky's most important insights was that the uses of such external forms are based on semiotic principles such as the distinction between "meaning" and "object reference" and the primacy of the "indicatory function" of language. It is these principles that create the semiotic environment that is gradually mastered by the child. On the basis of this understanding of semiotic processes, Vygotsky constructed his account of word meaning and self-regulative speech.

Silverstein (Chapter 9, this volume) advances this argument by outlining a comprehensive account of the semiotic processes that seem to lie at the heart of Vygotsky's approach. He outlines several realms in the functional analysis of language and argues that Vygotsky's writings suggest a way to intergrate them in an ontogenetic account. In developing this line of reasoning Silverstein criticizes the very powerful unifunctional view of language that underlies so much of the contemporary research in linguistics and psycholinguistics.

In the course of his analysis Silverstein also identifies some points in Vygotsky's approach that are in need of revision in light of recent developments in linguistic and semiotic theory. For example, advances in grammatical theory, which provides the description of the "referential function" in Silverstein's analysis, create the need for revising Vygotsky's notion of word meaning.

A major concern in Silverstein's analysis is the use of language to talk about language. The "metapragmatic" and "metasemantic" functions of language play a crucial role in his account of how the various levels in his structure of functions are integrated into a system. For example, it is by drawing on the referential function to speak of the pragmatic function that the metapragmatic function of language exists. Silverstein proposes that a model of the structure of functions can provide the foundation for an account of the differentiation and integration of language functions. This is an issue that stands at the heart of Vygotsky's account of the ontogenesis of self-regulative speech.

In Chapter 10 Hickmann outlines empirical evidence for some of these claims. In particular, she focuses on the issues of functional differentiation and the ontogenesis of the pragmatic and metapragmatic functions of language. On the basis of a study of children's and adults' performance on a story retelling task, Hickmann reveals some of the complexities involved and shows that these uses of languages are mastered only at a late stage of childhood. For example, she examines the development of the ability to create and maintain reference through linguistic means alone, an ability that rests on the recognition that language can serve as its own context. With this development, a new form of linguistically created context can begin to serve along with the earlier forms of extralinguistic context as the foundation for interpreting utterances in human communication. Hickmann also mentions some of the complexities of using metapragmatic verbs (e.g., "said," "warned") that, as Silverstein points out, "regiment" our description and understanding of human speech events. Here again the use of language to operate on language is seen as the key to understanding ontogenetic change.

It seems to me that Hickmann and Silverstein have begun to provide an account of a missing link in Vygotsky's account of the ontogenesis of semiotic functioning. If we consider his account of concept development, we can see that they have specified the mechanisms that connect early linguistic activity that is inextricably tied to the concrete extralinguistic environment and later linguistic activity involving abstract definitions. That is, they have specified how the semiotic system motivates the many transitions involved between the early indicatory function of speech and the mastery of genuine concepts.

In Chapter 8 Rommetveit takes a somewhat different approach to the problem of linguistic mediation in ontogenesis. He begins with a review of the issues of intersubjectivity and dialogicality that have been overlooked in so much of the recent research on language and communication. Then he proceeds to examine some of the problems of interpsychological functioning in a Vygotskian framework. In particular, he focuses on the problems of instantiating and maintaining symbolic control over joint and individual human behavior, the central issue in Vygotsky's account of semiotic mediation. It is precisely by examining the type of interpsychological processes presented by Rommetveit that we can hope to attain increased understanding of intrapsychological forms of semiotic mediation.

Thus we see that the authors in this volume touch on a wide range of issues in Vygotsky's theoretical system. By introducing the contributions to his volume in terms of three major sources of Vygotsky's ideas, I have used only one of several possible interpretive frameworks. Indeed, another one is used to organize the chapters in this volume. In the table of contents I have divided up the chapters simply on the basis of whether they serve (1) to explicate a point in Vygotsky's own writings, or (2) to extend his ideas. Under the latter heading I have made the further distinction between chapters that focus on his semiotic theory and those that examine other issues, especially issues in education. This organization also glosses over several points, but it might be more helpful to readers who have not read my introduction. Of course, the interpretive framework I have used in this introduction has forced me to neglect at least a few of the points raised in any single chapter.

We are just beginning to decipher the breadth and depth of the ideas of Vygotsky, a figure who is truly one of the "titans" of modern psychology [to use Bruner's (1981) term]. Indeed, I hesitate to call Vygotsky a psychologist (or a pedagogue, or literary scholar, or semiotician, for that matter) inasmuch as he made such an effort to overcome the disciplinary boundaries of the social sciences, humanities, and historical sciences. He worked in a time and place that challenged scholars to unite the findings of many disciplines and to unite theory and practice. His response to this challenge remains unique and inspiring today, nearly a half-century after his death. It is a response that is worth reconsidering and emulating perhaps now more than ever before.

REFERENCES

Bernshtein, N. A. 1966. *Ocherki po fiziologii dvizhenii i fiziologii aktivnosti*. [Essays on the physiology of movements and the physiology of activation.] Moscow: Izdatel'stvo Meditsina.

Blonskii, P. P. 1921. *Ocherk nauchnoi psikhologii*. [An essay on scientific psychology.] Moscow: Gosizdat.

Bourdieu, P. 1977. *Outline of a theory of practice*. Cambridge: Cambridge University Press.

Brown, A. L. 1978. Knowing when, where, and how to remember: A problem of metacognition. In R. Glaser (Ed.), *Advances in instructional psychology*. Hillsdale, N.J.: Erlbaum.

Bruner, J. S. 1976. Early social interaction and language acquisition. In H. R. Schaffer (Ed.), *Studies in mother-infant interaction*. London: Academic Press.

Bruner, J. S. 1981. Concepts of the child. Invited address, American Psychological Association Annual Convention. Los Angeles, September.

Campione, J. C. and Brown, A. L. 1978. Toward a theory of intelligence: Contributions from research with retarded children. *Intelligence*, 2, 279–304.

Cole, M. 1979. Epilogue: A portrait of Luria. In A. R. Luria, *The making of mind: A personal account of Soviet psychology*. Cambridge: Harvard University Press.

Cole, M. and Scribner, S. 1978. Introduction to L. S. Vygotsky, *Mind in Society: The development of higher psychological processes*. Cambridge: Harvard University Press.

Davydov, V. V. 1972. *Vidy obobshcheniya v obuchenii*. [Forms of generalization in instruction.] Moscow: Pedagogika.

Ivanov, V.V. 1968. Commentary of Vygotsky's book: *Psikhologiya iskusstva*. [The psychology of art.] In L. S. Vygotsky, *Psikhologiya iskusstva*. Moscow: Iskusstva. (Translated as Commentary by V. V. Ivanov in L. S. Vygotsky, *The psychology of art*. Cambridge: MIT Press, 1971.)

Ivanov, V. V. 1976. *Ocherki po istorii semiotiki v SSSR*. [Essays on the history of semiotics in the USSR.] Moscow: Nauka.

Janet, P. 1926–1927. La pensée intérieure et ses troubles. Course given at the College de France.

Janet, P. 1928. *De l'angoisse à l'extase: Etudes sur les croyances et les sentiments*. Vol. 2 *Les sentiments fondamentaux*. Paris: Libraire Felix Alcan.

Leont'ev, A. N. 1981. The problem of activity in psychology. In J. V. Wertsch (Ed.), *The concept of activity in Soviet psychology*. Armonk, N.Y.: Sharpe.

Leont'ev, A. N. and Luria, A. R. 1956. *Psikhologicheskie vozzreniya L. S. Vygotskogo*. [The psychological views of L. S. Vygotsky.] In L. S. Vygotsky, *Izbrannye*

18   JAMES V. WERTSCH

psikhologicheskie issledovaniya. [Selected psychological investigations.] Moscow: Izdetel'stvo Akademii Pedagogicheskikh Nauk RSFSR.

Leont'ev, A. N. and Luria, A. R. 1968. The psychological ideas of L. S. Vygotsky. In B. B. Wolman (Ed.), *Historical roots of contemporary psychology*. New York: Harper & Row.

Luria, A. R. 1979. *The making of mind: A personal account of Soviet psychology*. Cambridge: Harvard University Press. [Edited by M. Cole and S. Cole.]

Piaget, J. 1926. *The language and thought of the child*. New York: Harcourt, Brace, and World.

Radzikhovskii, L. A. 1979. Analiz tvorchestva L. S. Vygotskogo sovetskimi psikhologami. [The analysis of L. S. Vygotsky's work by Soviet psychologists.] *Voprosy Psikhologii* [Problems in psychology], *6*, 58–67.

Rubenshtein, S. L. 1957. *Bytie i soznanie*. [Being and consciousness.] Moscow: Izdatel'stvo Akademii Nauk SSSR.

Sapir, E. 1921. *Language*. New York: Harcourt, Brace and World.

Seve, L. 1978. *Man in Marxist theory and the psychology of personality*. Sussex: Harvester Press.

Vygotsky, L. S. 1925. *Psikhologiya iskusstva*. [The psychology of art.] Moscow: Izdatel'stvo Moskovskogo Iskusstva (2nd ed., 1968). (Translated as L. S. Vygotsky, *The psychology of art*. Cambridge: MIT Press, 1971.)

Vygotsky, L S. 1926. *Pedagogicheskaya psikhologiya: Kratkii kurs*. [Pedagogical psychology: A short course.] Moscow: Izdatel'stvo Rabotnik Prosveshcheniya.

Vygotsky, L S. 1934. *Myshlenie i rech'*. [Thinking and speech.] Moscow: Sozekgiz. (Translated as L. S. Vygotsky, *Thought and language*. Cambridge: MIT Press, 1962.)

Vygotsky, L. S. 1956. *Izbrannye psikhologicheskie issledovaniya*. [Selected psychological research.] Moscow: Izdatel'stvo Akademii Pedagogicheskikh Nauk RSFSR.

Vygotsky, L. S. 1960. *Razvitie vysshikh psikhicheskikh functii*. [The development of higher mental functions.] Moscow: Izdatel'stvo Akademii Pedagogicheskikh Nauk.

Vygotsky, L. S. 1978. *Mind in society: The development of higher psychological processes* (edited by M. Cole, J. Scribner, V. John-Steiner, and E. Souberman). Cambridge: Harvard University Press.

Vygotsky, L. S. 1981. The genesis of higher mental functions. In J. V. Wertsch (Ed.), *The concept of activity in Soviet psychology*. Armonk, N.Y.: Sharpe.

Vygotsky, L. S. and Luria, A. R. 1930. *Etyudy po istorii povedeniya*. [Studies in the history of behavior.] Moscow–Leningrad: Gosudarstvennoe Izdatel'stvo.

Wertsch, J. V. 1981a. *The concept of activity in Soviet psychology*. Armonk, N.Y.: Sharpe.

Wertsch, J. V. 1981b. Trends in Soviet cognitive psychology. *Storia e critica della psicologia*, *2*(2), 219–295.

Wertsch, J. V. 1983. The role of semiosis in L. S. Vygotsky's theory of human cognition. In B. Bain (Ed.), *The sociogenesis of language and human conduct*. New York: Plenum.

Wood, D., Bruner, J. S., and Ross, G. 1976. The role of tutoring in problem solving. *Journal of Child Psychology and Psychiatry*, *66*, 181–191.

Zaporozhets, A. V. 1959. *Razvitie proizvol'nykh dvizhenii*. [The development of voluntary movements.] Moscow: Izdatel'stvo Akademii Pedagogicheskikh Nauk RSFSR.

PART I

Explicating Vygotsky's approach

1

Vygotsky: a historical and conceptual perspective

JEROME BRUNER

It might be appropriate for me to begin with some historical, indeed autobiographical, notes. For quite by chance, I lived through some of the events that may have led to Vygotsky having an impact on psychology in America. He is, I believe, going through a second cycle now. But we can come to that later.

Let me tell you of a distinction I used to make, half jokingly, between paleo- and neo-Pavlovian psychology. Like most Westerners before 1956, I knew only the former. It was about conditioned reflexes in the classic mold. As an undergraduate I had assisted Karl Zener in his conditioning experiments. They were, at least technically and on the surface, in the paleo-Pavlovian tradition: The salivary response of dogs was conditioned to the usual array of bells and buzzers. But Karl Zener was no paleo-Pavlovian in spirit. He had gone as a postdoctoral fellow to study at the Kaiser Wilhelm Institute in Berlin with Wolfgang Köhler and Kurt Lewin and Pavlov's connectionism was anathema to this young Harvard-trained Gestaltist. His particular bogeyman was the stimulus-substitution theory of conditioning, that an old response remains intact and is simply captured by a new stimulus that takes over the triggering functioning of the old. For Zener, the central idea was "action in a field": When a response becomes conditioned, it is not simply "transferred" to the control of a new stimulus. Rather, the context changes and with it the nature of the task and of the signaling properties of the stimuli and the response as well. Isolated responses and isolated stimuli were rejected in this view, their place taken by means-end structures that changed in the course of conditioning. And he proved his point, as I shall presently relate.

It was 1936. I was not yet old enough to vote. But I was old enough to take sides. I thought Karl Zener admirable for using the classical Pavlovian conditioning situation as the battlefield on which to defeat the old "switchboard theory." I even did my part by learning the surgery needed to turn the parotid salivary duct of the dog outward to the cheek so that its salivary flow could be measured through a capillary system attached to the dog's cheek by a drilled silver dollar glued there by a mix of bee's wax and sealing wax applied hot and soft and allowed to cool hard and adhesive. We needed that tough adhesive joint, for Zener's dogs did not just stand there at the tray awaiting food delivery (as they had in Moscow). When the buzzer sounded, they had to cross from another table, around the barrier of a whirring fan, and then position themselves at the tray. A dog conditioned in the classical Pavlovian task just standing there and waiting in the old harness would have no difficulty transferring to the new obstacle course. He didn't have to be taught when to start salivating: not when the buzzer sounded, but after you got round the obstacle. The whole response pattern was reorganized. Surely this was no simple matter of a response being transferred from one stimulus to another. With hardly a qualm, I became a thorough and mocking revisionist. Little did I know that the fates were preparing me to become an ally to the psychologists in Russia who were reacting in much the same way toward simplistic Pavlovianism.

I began to learn about all of this in a more first-hand way when I attended the International Congress of Psychology in Montreal in 1954. There was a Russian delegation. Their presented papers characteristically started with a genuflection to Pavlov, followed quickly by some rather interesting studies of attention or problem solving or whatever that had little to do with the Pavlov I had read. They seemed to represent some other interest whose nature I could not quite discern. And then there was a classically Russian reception toward the end of the week, replete with vodka and a barrel of caviar. It was at that reception (and at an informal party afterward at Wilder Penfield's) that I first encountered talk of Vygotsky, of the role of language in development, of the "zone of proximal development," and (of all things) a Second Signal System attributed to Pavlov. The Second Signal System was the world encoded in language: Nature transformed by history and culture. Vygotsky's work, I learned that evening, was widely circulated though it was officially banned. The Second Signal System, I thought, was a splendid way of getting beyond Pavlov while still maintaining a posture of high respect.

Vygotsky's *Thought and Language* appeared in 1934, shortly after his death of tuberculosis at the age of thirty-seven. It so deeply disturbed the guardians of proper Marxist interpretation that it was suppressed two years later, in 1936, the year of my engagement with the Pavlovian dogs in the obstacle course. As Luria and Leont'ev said of the book years later (1956), "The primary and fundamental task of that time [the late 1920s and 1930s when the 'battle for consciousness' raged] consisted of freeing oneself on the one hand from vulgar behaviorism and, on the other, from the subjective understanding of mental phenomena as exclusively internal subjective states that can only be investigated through introspection" (p. 6). It was not for another twenty years that the book could appear openly in Russian. It was republished in 1956. It was the same year that another volume on thought appeared, *A Study of Thinking,* by Bruner, Goodnow, and Austin (1956). It is a year, 1956, that has recently become a popular candidate as the year of birth of the cognitive sciences. Something was going on in the intellectual atmosphere.

Vygotsky's book finally appeared in English in 1962. I was asked to write an introduction to it. By then I had learned enough about Vygotsky from accounts of his work by Alexander Romanovich Luria, with whom I had become close friends, so that I welcomed this added goad to close study. And I read the book not only with meticulous care, but with growing astonishment. For Vygotsky was plainly a genius. Yet it was an elusive form of genius, his. Unlike, say, Pavlov or Piaget, there was nothing massive or glacial about the corpus of his thought and its development. Rather, it was like the later Wittgenstein: at times aphoristic, often sketchy, vivid in its illuminations.

To begin with, I liked his instrumentalism. That is to say, I admired his way of interpreting thought and speech as instruments for the planning and carrying out of action. Or as he puts it in an early essay, "Children solve practical tasks with the help of their speech, as well as with their eyes and hands. This unity of perception, speech and action, which ultimately produces internalization of the visual field, constitutes the central subject matter for any analysis of the origin of uniquely human forms of behavior" (1978, p. 26). Language is (in Vygotsky's sense as in Dewey's) a way of sorting out one's thoughts about things. Thought is a mode of organizing perception and action. But all of them, each in their way, also reflect the tools and aids available for use in carrying out action. Or to take his epigraph from Francis Bacon, "Nec manus, nisi intellectus, sibi permissus, multam valent; instrumentis et auxilibus res perficitur." But what a curious epigraph: Neither the hand nor the mind alone, left to themselves, would amount to much. And what are these prosthetic devices that perfect them (if you will allow me a modern gloss on "instrumentis et auxilibus")?

Well, for one thing, it would seem that there are concepts and ideas and theories that permit one to get to higher ground. Take the following quotation: "The new higher concepts in turn transform the meaning of the lower. The adolescent who has mastered algebraic concepts has gained a vantage point from which he sees arithmetic concepts in a broader perspective" (1934, p. 115). There seems, then, to be some interesting way in which it becomes possible to turn around upon one's thoughts, to see them in a new light. This is, of course, mind reflecting on itself. It is not very surprising that, given the plodding, *lumpen* nature of Marxist criticism and interpretation in those days, Vygotsky should have been banned for 20 years. Yet again there is something sibylline about this pronouncement too. It seems to be about consciousness and, indeed, about what today we call metacognition. So let us pursue the matter a step further.

About consciousness he says: "consciousness and control appear only at a late stage in the development of a function, after it has been used and practiced unconsciously and spontaneously. In order to subject a function to intellectual control, we must first possess it" (1934, p. 90). This suggests that prior to the development of self-directed, conscious control, action is, so to speak, governed by a more direct mode of responding to environmental events. This again is a rather dark way of talking about the issue. It suggests that consciousness or (in the classical sense) reflection is a way of buffering immediate response so that the situation can be better appraised from higher ground. And how is that achieved?

This brings us, then, to the heart of the matter: to Vygotsky's ideas about the famous zone of proximal development. It has to do with the manner in which we arrange the environment such that the child can reach higher or more abstract ground from which to reflect, ground on which he is enabled to be more conscious. Or to use his words, the zone of proximal development is *the distance between the actual developmental level as determined by independent problem solving and the level of potential development as determined through problem solving under adult guidance or in collaboration with more capable peers*" (1978, p. 86). Or to put it even more concretely, he says: "Human learning presupposes a specific social nature and a process by which children grow into the intellectual life of those around them" (1978, p. 88). And one final leap: "Thus the notion of a zone of proximal development," he says, "enables us to propound a new formula, namely that the only 'good learning' is that which is in advance of development" (1978, p. 89).

Now, if one takes this quite literally, there is a contradiction in Vygotsky's proposal. On the one hand the zone of proximal development has to do with achieving "consciousness and control." But consciousness and control come only after one has already got a function well and spontaneously mastered. So how could "good learning" be that which is in advance of development and, as it were, bound initially to be unconscious since unmastered? I have puzzled about this matter for many years, and I think I understand what Vygotsky might have meant. Or at least, I understand the matter somewhat as follows, and it is this point that I will want to develop. If the child is enabled to advance by being under the tutelage of an adult or a more competent peer, then the tutor or the aiding peer serves the learner as a vicarious form of consciousness until such a time as the learner is able to master his own action through his own consciousness and control. When the child achieves that conscious control over a new function or conceptual system, it is then that he is able to use it as a tool. Up to that point, the tutor in effect performs the critical function of "scaffolding" the learning task to make it possible for the child, in Vygotsky's word, to internalize external knowledge and convert it into a tool for conscious control.

Vygotsky then comments that the acquisition of language provides the paradigm case for what he is talking about. It is mastered at first in collaboration with an adult or a more competent peer solely with the objective of communicating. Once mastered sufficiently in this way, it can then become internalized and serve under conscious control as a means of carrying out inner speech dialogues. I quite agree with Vygotsky that language acquisition may provide an interesting paradigm case and, like him, I will presently consider some parallels and disanalogies between language acquisition and the way in which we enable children, by our calculated aid, to get ahead of their present levels of development into a new zone.

Before I do that, however, I would like to comment in passing on one point that has usually been overlooked or given second billing in our own achievement-orientated Western culture. It is inherent in his conviction that passing on knowledge is like passing on language – his basic belief that social transaction is the fundamental vehicle of education and not, so to speak, solo performance. But alas, he did not live long enough to develop his ideas about the subject. I believe that it was his eventual hope to delineate the transactional nature of learning, particularly since learning for him involved entry into a culture via induction by more skilled members. But though he did not live long enough to carry out this program, it seems to me that it remains an important one to pursue. Too often, human learning has been depicted in the paradigm of a lone organism pitted against nature – whether in the model of the behaviorist's organism shaping up responses to fit the geometries and probabilities of the world of stimuli, or in the Piagetian model where a lone child struggles single-handed to strike some equilibrium between assimilating the world to himself or himself to the world. Vygotsky was struck, rather, with how much learning is quintessentially assisted and vicarious and about social conventions and intellectual prostheses in the manner of Popper's World Three.

There are, I think, three kinds of concepts that would be needed in order to carry out a Vygotskian project on "learning by transaction," and there is enough extant in his writings to suggest how he would pose them. One has to do with "props" and "instruments" that make it possible for the child to go beyond his present "level of development" to achieve higher ground and, eventually, new consciousness. The second is some specification of the kinds of processes that make the child sensitive or receptive to vicarious or transactional learning. The third has to do with procedures that the more proficient partner in a transaction uses in order to ease the way for the intending (or even the initially unintending) learner. It takes no particular imagination to see that the three, props, processes, and procedures, are at the heart of what we ordinarily think of as education – curriculum, learning, and teaching. For Vygotsky, they were matters that grew out of his theory of development. I shall touch on these in passing and come back to them at the end.

Let me now return to the perspective of language, where Vygotsky felt we should begin. For all that there is a great deal of disagreement on how language acquisition occurs – and we need not review the contending views here – there are certain points on which there is consensus. I think we would all agree now that the input of speech to the language-acquiring child is highly tailored by adults to match the child's level of speech development and that it is altered systematically to stay matched with the child's progress. There are certain conventional and/or natural ways in which this fine-tuning is accomplished, and the result is the baby talk (BT) register or "motherese" – exaggerated stress, simpler segmentation, reduced syntactic complexity, and so forth. It is difficult to imagine that it is all merely conventional, since 4-year-olds use BT in speaking to 2-year-olds, and that seems a rather early age for acquiring so subtle a convention. Let me quickly add that there is no agreement (and little evidence) as to whether the existence of fine-tuning matters much or little in helping the child master the language. What we certainly do know is that language must be acquired across a wide range of variation in the degree of tunedness of adult tutors. This has led some to believe that language is not taught, only learned. A more correct inference would be that *learning to know* a language must be possible with a minimum instantiation of its constructive rules. That is, linguistic competence in the old sense of the word is not any obvious product of any obvious teaching.

What is altogether less clear is whether *learning to use* a language can be mastered with exposure to only scanty or degenerate input of instances. It would, I suppose, be impossible to master such things as the conditions on speech acts, how to handle the given–new contract in discourse, how to fulfill adjacency requirements, even how to appreciate deictic shifters like *me–you* and *here–there* without having entered into a considerable amount of contingent communication with a more expert speaker of the language who had in mind some pedagogical aims. I think that with the exception of some old-fashioned purists, most students of language acquisition would agree that the amount of explicit guidance or teaching in language transmission is probably inversely proportional to the formal structure of what has to be mastered. The loose rules and maxims of pragmatics – Grice's (1975) cooperative principles, Searle's (1969, 1975) speech acts, and so on – are worked over and negotiated in contingent discourse and at some length. Syntax, however, is hardly ever the object of explicit pedagogy or negotiation; phonology rarely. Semantics is the middling case. It would seem, then, that it is as a byproduct of learning to *use* language in discourse that the child masters its *structure*. As Roger Brown suggests in his discussion of BT (1977), there is indeed a point of the mother talking with her child in language that he has already mastered. It is not redundant. It keeps communication going in a way that assures the child will know how to *use* the new instrument in a variety of contexts with some effectiveness.

Indeed, there is even a continuity in pragmatic mastery that is quite uncharacteristic of the mastery of formal syntax. That is to say, the bulk of research – Halliday (1975), Bates and the Rome group (1976, 1979), Dore (1974, 1975, 1977a), Bruner (1981, 1983) – suggests that there is a slow acretion of skill in carrying out such elementary functions as referring, requesting, and offering. It begins before the onset of lexicogrammatical speech by the use of gesture, intonation, and so on, and as the child learns the structures of language, these are used to further the child's efforts "to do things with words." But before he has words, he does his things with gestures and babbles and stylized intonation contours. Communicative intent seems to be present from the start or very near the start. And intent of this kind uses whatever props are available. It is almost always in the interest of fulfilling his communicative intentions that the child recognizes and picks up new structural tricks relating to language. Only late in the day do the new tricks suggest new functions – like Michael Halliday's (1975) more elaborated mathetic functions or John Searle's (1979) commissives like promising.

One last point about language acquisition that will be crucial to the argument I want finally to make. A great deal of it occurs in highly framed or formated situations: familiar and routinized settings in which the two members of the pair are operating in a highly known microcosm, with fairly easily recognized intentions, and where the adult can most easily calibrate his or her hypotheses about what the child means. Michael Silverstein has suggested that these microcosms are often so tiny that they deserve to be called "nanocosms." A good example of such a developing format is provided by Ninio and Bruner (1978) for the mastery of labeling and simple topic–comment structures. Its main procedural characteristic is that the adult maintains a very constant routine over time to which the child responds with increasing skill and decreasing variability. In the Ninio–Bruner case, the adult has a standard way of requesting of the child the names of objects in picture books and the like and manages it in such a way that the child learns the names of things and how to comment on things named without ever making an error. The only errors recognized or responded to by the mother are regressions or backslidings that she knows the child knows he can correct if challenged. I would liken the procedure in such formats to the constructing of scaffolds. In effect, the child is permitted to do as much as he can spontaneously do; whatever he cannot do is filled in or "held up" by the mother's scaffolding activities. When he cannot respond to her request for a label save by uttering an extended babble, she accepts what he has on offer and then provides the word – until such a time as he can produce a lexeme-length babble, at which point she will no longer accept extended babbles in response to her stylized *What's that, Jonathan?* Formats of this kind are very characteristic of the settings in which errorless learning occurs in many indigenous societies. Such "errorless learning" has been notably well described by Fortes (1938) in a remarkable monograph on education among the Tale of West Africa.

The last thing to say about language acquisition of this formated, pragmatically paced kind is that it is governed by a rule of "voluntary hand-over and willing receipt." Anything the child masters is his to use and there is no question about whether, how, or why it should be used in speech. All such decisions are left to the learner. There are astonishingly few cases on record suggesting normal resistance to learning. When resistance occurs, it seems to accompany profound pathology. I have never heard anybody say, even in the most deeply anti-intellectual times, "What a waste of time learning to speak." The only exception to this general case are to be found in matters of truth, sincerity, and felicity, all of which are negotiable in terms of criteria that are inherently extralinguistic.

All that I have said thus far about language acquisition has led me to conclude that there is a Language Acquisition Support System (LASS) that is at least partly innate. I see it as a counterpart to some sort of Language Acquisition Device (LAD). LAD is what makes it possible for the child to master the constitutive rules of his native language without a sufficient sample of instances to support his inductive leaps. Without it we would be sunk, for there is no unique grammar that can be logically induced from any finite sample of utterances in any language. The function of LASS is to assure that input will be a form acceptable to the recognition routines of LAD, however those recognition routines may eventually be described. Although I think there are enormous differences between the way a language is acquired and the way other forms of knowledge and skill are acquired, I agree with Vygotsky that there is a deep parallel in all forms of knowledge acquisition – precisely the existence of a crucial match between a *support system* in the social environment and an *acquisition process* in the learner. I think it is this match that makes possible the transmission of the culture, first as a set of connected ways of acting, perceiving, and talking, and then finally as a generative system of taking conscious thought, using the instruments of reflection that the culture "stores" as theories, scenarios, plots, prototypes, maxims, and so on. The fact that we learn the culture as readily and effectively as we do must give us pause – considering how poorly we do at certain artificial, "madeup" subjects that we teach in schools and whose use is *not* imbedded in any established cultural practice.

I can only sketch roughly some examples of the match I have in mind. Let me take first a study of 3- and 5-year-old children being "tutored" in the task of putting together sets of interlocking wooden blocks, a study by Wood, Bruner, and Ross (1976) that I am only beginning to understand. We were exactly in the position of most schools that set out to teach a subject without the advice or consent of the pupils involved and without the task having any contextualization in the children's lives. The task was to build a pyramid out of interlocking wooden blocks that could, of course, have been used for any number of other, perhaps more engaging activities – like building castles or radar installations. The subjects were 3s and 5s, and they were in the hands of a tutor who was to help them build a pyramid. The tutor, I must report, was genuinely fascinated by what children did in such tasks, was highly sophisticated about both problem solving and children, and in general radiated interest and responsive goodwill. The details are not important, but there are some generalities worth noting about the ways in which the tutor had to behave in order to do her job. Let me spell out some of these inevitabilities of acting as a support system for the child's foray into the zone of proximal development.

After the child is induced into taking on the task – even 3-year-olds follow the universal rule of doing what people ask of them, particularly if the people are the likes of Gail Ross – the main tasks of the tutor are these. First is to model the task, to establish that something is possible and interesting. In this case, it consisted of constructing the pyramid slowly, with conspicuous marking of the subassemblies that the child will need later. At that moment, the tutor has a monopoly on foresight. She is consciousness for two. The child, somehow, is induced to try. That is surely a crucial part of what the more experienced do for the less experienced, and let us not confuse ourselves with words like *identification* or whatever: It is very obscure how an adult gets a child to venture into the zone. I think it is easiest when the venture is seen as play, but that is too large a topic (see Bruner, Jolly, and Sylva, 1976). It relates to minimizing the cost, indeed the possibility, of error. Once the child is willing to try, the tutor's general task is that of scaffolding – reducing the number of degrees of freedom that the child must manage in the task. She does it by segmenting the task and ritualizing it: creating a format, a nanocosm. Like the adults in the Fortes study in Taleland, she sees to it that the child does only what he can do and then she fills in the rest – as in slipping the pegs of certain blocks into the holes of others to which they are mated, the child having brought them next to each other. She limits the complexity of the task to the level that the child can just manage, even to the point of shielding his limited attention from distractors.

Recall what Vygotsky said about leading the child on ahead of his development. This is done with some prudence by the tutor. Once the child has mastered some routine that was modular to the task, putting together a subassembly of blocks for example, the tutor then tempted the child to use his skill to build a higher-order assembly. That, of course, was structurally built into the nature of the blocks as we had constructed them. Yet it is often enough observed, this "raising the ante," whatever the nature of the materials of a task (including language), that it merits being considered as a candidate for a principle. Curiously, it is what keeps the child "in the zone" and, at the same time, what keeps him from getting bored.

Now, after all this has been accomplished, then and only then do the child and the tutor interact in a way that fits the title "instruction." Instruction – telling the child what to do or what he might try next or what he is doing that is getting in his way, and the like – instruction in words comes only after the child knows how to do the problem. Vygotsky somewhere notes that at first language and action are fused and it is for this reason that the child talks to himself while carrying out a task. Eventually, language and action become separated, and the latter (the task) can be represented in the medium of the former (words). It is when that stage is reached that one can incorporate what one knows into words, and thereby into the process of dialogue.

There are only a few studies on the role of dialogue in problem solving although there are many claims to the effect that thought is internalized dialogue – claims by writers as various as Vygotsky, George Herbert Mead, and many contemporary hermaneuticists who believe in the negotiated nature of meaning and are therefore bound to abide by a social definition of the thought processes. We do not know what dialogue about a problem does during problem solving, before problem solving, or after – although there are some tempting clues in the literature such as it is [see Zivin (1979) for a review and evaluation of this literature]. I want to present a hypothesis about the internalization that is based on a reinterpretation of Vygotsky presented by Wertsch (1979).

Once dialogue is made possible by the child now being able to represent linguistically the aspects and elements of the operations he has mastered that he can share with an assisting adult, a powerful discourse device becomes available. It is a device that permits the taking for granted what is known and shared between speaker and listener and going beyond it to what is a comment on what is shared and known. This is sometimes called the topic-comment structure of language and it has most recently been revitalized by the linguist Chafe (1974, 1976) and the psycholinguists Clark and Haviland (1977) under the interesting rubric the "given–new contract." It is a rather old idea that was originally formulated by the Prague School of linguists to embody a discourse-sensitive version of the subject–predicate distinction. In their functional view, a subject (or topic) is that which is shared in the consciousness (or intersubjectivity, to use the more fashionable term) of speaker and listener. A predicate is that which introduces something new, a comment upon the topic or subject that is in joint consciousness. The given in discourse is the unstressed, the unmarked, the easily pronominalized, the background. The new is the stressed, the marked, the fully nominalized, the foregrounded. It is the means whereby language permits (even encourages) the adult to lure the child into the zone of proximal development, and of course, it likewise permits the child to put questions of his own to the adult about what is beyond the information given. It is obviously a reciprocal process for adult and child, as we know from a recent study by Tizard and her colleagues (Tizard, Griffiths, and Atkinson, 1980) that shows that the children (3 to 5) who ask the most searching questions are the ones whose parents are most likely to answer them fully and, of course, the parents who are most likely to answer are the ones with children most likely to ask!

So what does this tell us about the internalization of dialogue? How can the child internalize a procedure for distinguishing what is shared consciousness and what is asymmetric with respect to an addressee? Let me go back for a moment to a comment I made in passing earlier: that at the earliest stage of inducting a cild into a new activity, the adult serves almost as the vicarious consciousness of the child in the sense of being the only one who knows the goal of the activity the two of them are engaged in. When the child masters a new task, he masters its means–end structure: he too now knows the goal, although at any moment he may be unclear about how to get there. It seems to me to be the case (and I cannot yet put it more strongly than that) that the given–new discourse pattern becomes converted when internalized into a system for distinguishing the givens and the knowns of a situation from that which is problematic, new, and uncertain. It becomes the medium for the sort of task analysis that all who are concerned with metacognition brood about – from Feuerstein and Jensen (in press) and Edward deBono (in press) at one side, such artificial intelligence people as Hays (in press) at the other, with Ann Brown (in press) and Courtney Cazden (1981) in the middle.

You will know, of course, that Vygotsky had some very evocative, rather puzzling things to say about the structure of inner speech. It was he that commented upon the fact that inner speech was principally predicative, that the subject dropped out. Along with Wertsch (and with Roman Jokobson who first introduced me to the idea) I think Vygotsky was using subject—predicate in the Prague sense of given and new rather than in the strictly syntactic or the derived case grammatical sense. Inner speech, on this view, so exaggerates the unmarked–unstressed–backgrounded versus marked–stressed–foregrounded distinction of the given–new as to ban the former altogether. It becomes, if you will forgive me a weakness for nautical metaphors, an ideal navigational instrument for operating in the zone of proximal development, beyond the information given. Who needs a navigational instrument that tells you that you are where you already know you are? Wertsch puts it well:

In the case of private speech, given information is that knowledge that is in the speaker's consciousness at the time of the utterance. So-called new information is what is being introduced into the speaker's consciousness as a result of the action he is carrying out. (1979, p. 95)

And he means by action, of course, intended action where there is some representation of a goal and a set of alternative means for getting to it.

Let me conclude with a few final remarks about where things stand. As you can see, I have been attempting to follow the spirit of the Vygotskian project to find the manner in which aspirant members of a culture learn from their tutors, the vicars of their culture, how to understand the world. That world is a symbolic world in the sense that it consists of conceptually organized, rule-bound belief systems about what exists, about how to get to goals, about what is to be valued. There is no way, none, in which a human being could possibly master that world without the aid and assistance of others for, in fact, that world *is* others. The culture stores an extraordinarily rich file of concepts, techniques, and other prosthetic devices that are available (often in a highly biased way, for the file constitutes one of the sources of wealth in any society and most societies do not share their wealth equally among all). The prosthetic devices require for their use certain fundamental skills, notable among them the ability to use the language as an instrument of thought – natural language, and eventually such artificial languages as mathematics, Polish logic, Fortran, sprung rhythms, and especially written language. As Vygotsky said, it is a matter of using whatever one has learned before to get to higher ground next. What is obvious and, perhaps, "given" in this account is that there must needs be at any given stage of voyaging into the zone of proximal development a support system that helps learners get there. If tutors are seen not as partners in advancement, but, as reported in some recent research (Hood, McDermott and Cole, 1980), as sources of punishment, then it may have disastrous consequences for the candidate learner. That problem has not been at the center of my attention, although I know how desperately important it is. Rather, I have tried to address myself to the issue of how we learn from others and I have chosen Vygotsky as my model because he was the first to look. I hope I have convinced the reader that his project is still worth pursuing.

REFERENCES

Bates, E. 1976. *Language and context: The acquisition of pragmatics.* New York: Academic Press.
Bates, E. 1979. *The emergence of symbols: Cognition and communication in infancy.* New York: Academic Press.
Brown, A.L. In press. The importance of diagnosis in cognitive skills instruction. In S. Chipman, J. W. Segal, and R. Glaser (Eds.), *Thinking and learning skills: Current research and open questions.* (Vol. 2.) Hillsdale, N.J.: Erlbaum.
Brown, R. 1977. Introduction. In C. E. Snow and C. A. Ferguson (Eds.), *Talking to children: Language input and acquisition.* Cambridge: Cambridge University Press.
Bruner, J. 1981. Interaction and language acquisition. In W. Deutsch (Ed.), *The child's construction of language.* New York: Academic Press.
Bruner, J. 1983. *Child's talk.* New York: Norton.
Bruner, J., Goodnow, J., and Austin, G. 1956. *A study of thinking.* New York: Wiley.
Bruner, J. S., Jolly, A., and Sylva, K. (Eds.) 1976. *Play: Its role in evolution and development.* London: Penguin.
Cazden, C. 1981. Performance before competence: Assistance to child discourse in the zone of proximal development. *Quarterly Newsletter of the Laboratory of Comparative Human Cognition, 3,* (1), 5–8.
Chafe, W. L. 1974. Language and consciousness. *Language. 50,* 111–113.
Chafe, W. L. 1976. Giveness, contrastiveness, definiteness, subjects, topics, and point of view. In C. N. Li (Ed.), *Subject and topic.* New York: Academic Press.
Clark, H. H., and Haviland, S. E. 1977. Comprehension and the given-new contract. In R. Freedle (Ed.), *Discourse production and comprehension.* Norwood, N.J.: Ablex.
DeBono, E. In press. The Cort thinking program. In J. W. Segal, S. Chipman, and R. Glaser (Eds.), *Thinking and learning skills: Current research and open questions* (Vol. 1.) Hillsdale, N.J.: Erlbaum.
Dore, J. 1974. A pragmatic description of early language development. *Journal of Psycholinguistic Research, 3,* 343–350.
Dore, J. 1975. Holophrases, speech acts, and language universals. *Journal of Child Language, 2,* 21–40.
Dore, J. 1977. "Oh them sheriff": A pragmatic analysis of children's responses to questions. In S. Ervin-Tripp and C. Mitchell-Kernen (Eds.), *Child Discourse.* New York: Academic Press.
Feuerstein, R., and Jensen, M. In press. Instrumental enrichment: An intervention program for low-functioning adolescents. In J. W. Segal, S. Chipman, and R. Glaser (Eds.), *Thinking and learning skills: Relating instruction to basic research* (Vol. 1.) Hillsdale, N.J.: Erlbaum.

Fortes, M. 1938. "Social and psychological aspects of education in Taleland." *Africa.* *11*(4), Supplement. International Institute of African Languages and Cultures, Memorandum 7.

Grice, H. P. 1975. Logic and conversation. In P. Cole and J. Morgan (Eds.), *Syntax and Semantics* (Vol. 3.) New York: Academic Press.

Halliday, M. A. K. 1975. *Learning how to mean: Explorations in the development of language.* London: Edward Arnold.

Hays, J. R. In press. Three problems in teaching general skills. In S. Chipman, J. W. Segal, and R. Glaser (Eds.), *Thinking and learning skills: Current research and open questions* (Vol. 2.) Hillsdale, N.J.: Erlbaum.

Hood, L., McDermott, R., and Cole, M. 1980. "Let's try to make it a good day" – Some not so simple ways. *Discourse Processes, 3,* 155–168.

Luria, A. R., and Leont'ev, A. N. 1956. Introduction to L. S. Vygotsky, *Izbrannie psikhologicheskie issledovaniya.* [Selected psychological research]. Moscow: Izdatel'stvo Akademii Pedagogicheskikh Nauk.

Ninio, A., and Bruner, J. S. 1978. The achievement and antecedents of labelling. *Journal of Child Language. 5,* 1–16.

Searle, J. R. 1969. *Speech acts: An essay in the philosophy of language.* Cambridge: Cambridge University Press.

Searle, J. R. 1975. Indirect speech acts. In P. Cole and J. L. Morgan (Eds.), *Syntax and Semantics,* (Vol. 3.) New York: Academic Press.

Searle, J. R. 1979. *Expression and meaning: Studies in the history of speech acts.* Cambridge: Cambridge University Press.

Tizard, B., Griffiths, B., and Atkinson, M. 1980. Children's questions and parents' answers. Paper presented at the annual meeting of the Psychology Section, British Association, Salcombe, England.

Vygotsky, L. S. 1934. *Myshlenie i rech'.* [Thinking and speech.] Moscow: Sotsekriz. (English translation: *Thought and language.,* Cambridge: MIT Press, 1962.)

Vygotsky, L. S. 1956. *Izbrannie psikhologicheskie issledovaniya.* [Selected psychological research.] Moscow: Izdatel'stvo Akademii Pedagogicheskikh Nauk.

Vygotsky. L. S. 1978. *Mind in society: The development of higher psychological processes.* Cambridge: Harvard University Press.

Wertsch, J. V. 1979. The regulation of human action and the given-new organization of private speech. In G. Zivin (Ed.), *The development of self-regulation through private speech.* New York: Wiley.

Wood, D., Bruner, J. S., and Ross, G. 1976. The role of tutoring in problem solving. *Journal of Child Psychology and Psychiatry, 17,* 89–100.

Zivin, G. (Ed.) 1979. *The development of self-regulation through private speech.* New York: Wiley.

2

Vygotsky's theory and the activity-oriented approach in psychology

V. V. DAVYDOV and L. A. RADZIKHOVSKII

The problem formulated in the title of this chapter has recently attracted the intense interest of Soviet psychologists. We will attempt to reveal the significance of this problem and the principles in Soviet psychology for resolving it. We will also attempt to present Vygotsky (1896–1934) as a founder of a psychological theory based on the concept of activity.

Problems and principles in analyzing Vygotsky's work

The relationship between Vygotsky's theory and the activity-oriented approach in psychology has been at the center of all analyses of his work from the 1930s through the 1970s. This is particularly clear in the writings of members of his school who have elaborated the so-called theory of activity in Soviet psychology (see Radzikhovskii, 1979b). The changing analyses of Vygotsky's work over almost 50 years reflect definite stages in the formation of this theory.

Briefly, the development of the theory of activity in Soviet psychology, or, more precisely, the development of the school most closely connected with Vygotsky (i.e., the "Vygotsky–Leont'ev–Luria school"), can be outlined as follows. It came into being during the early 1930s within the sphere of Vygotsky's "cultural–historical theory." During the 1930s, the main problems, conceptual apparatus, and so forth of the theory of activity were defined. In the 1940s, the conceptual apparatus of this theory was developed to the point where one can speak of several essential elements. These have been preserved from the 1940s up to the 1970s. During the 1950s and 1960s, the explanatory and structural schemes of the theory of activity were extended into new fields (e.g., the psychology of sensory and cognitive processes). In the 1970s, this extension of the theory of activity continued (e.g., in the field of the psychology of personality). But the main point is that, beginning in the late 1970s, a period of intense methodological debate on the fundamental principles of the theory of activity began. This is a critical period, a turning point in the development of the theory (e.g., Davydov, 1979).

At each of these stages, the theory of activity has been related to Vygotsky's theory, but it has been related for quite different purposes. Thus, in the 1930s, the work of Vygotsky's students (e.g., Leont'ev, 1934) was guided by the research of their teacher. Subsequently, they were concerned with establishing the specifics of their approach independently of him, in particular, independently of his cultural–historical theory (e.g., Zinchenko, 1939). Beginning in the 1950s, when the theory of activity (separated from Vygotsky's work by 20 years or more) appeared in a more or less developed form, the problem of a strictly *historical analysis* of his work arose (e.g., Leont'ev and Luria, 1956).

Notwithstanding the differences among these various phases and various tasks, Vygotsky's students have always considered his work from the perspective of the theory of activity that they were developing. Vygotsky's works were viewed as one of its early stages. His work was reconstructed proceeding from the theory of activity, and the valuable characteristics of Vygotsky's work were inevitably formulated in this context (e.g., Leont'ev, 1967; Leont'ev and Luria, 1956). In its time this approach turned out to be justified. But such an approach to analyzing Vygotsky's work has exhausted its possibilities. The current state of the theory of activity allows one to begin to search for other ways to analyze it.

Of course, one should not forget the merits of earlier analyses. These analyses permitted the reconstruction of many of Vygotsky's basic ideas. It also revealed the general inspiration of his approach, bringing it into the theory of activity. The critical nature of this problem is reflected by the fact that even though this analysis, within the sphere of the theory of activity, was carried out in the 1930s, it became known among psychologists only in the 1960s. But even today, many deny Vygotsky's connection with the activity-oriented approach in philosophy and psychology. (We will not be concerned here with those works in which his ideas are related to non–activity-oriented approaches.)

Let us now turn to our more general problem of how one can study the history of this theoretical research. Like all cultural phenomena, Vygotsky's work is not amenable to being studied outside of its historical context, that is, as a "thing in itself." But it is possible to outline a twofold approach to the study of his ideas by taking the historical context into account. One can begin with the contemporary state of science and attempt to identify aspects of Vygotsky's approach that do or do not share similarities with various theories. On the basis of this one can then express a preference for one or another alternative. This can be done, for example, to specify the extent to which it is possible to reduce Vygotsky's ideas to those of modern theory or, in contrast, to clarify the extent to which modern theory can be reduced to Vygotsky's ideas. But a second approach is also possible. It is possible to follow a fundamentally different course. It is possible to evaluate Vygotsky's works on the basis of their internal logic.

It seems to us that the second point of departure is more relevant to the current problems of the theory of activity. These problems require the explication of Vygotsky's implicit philosophical–methodological premises. This kind of explication presupposes, above all, an analysis of his methodology.[1] By doing this we reveal a critical factor that has remained concealed in many previous Soviet analyses of Vygotsky's work. It is well known that Vygotsky was a distinguished methodologist of psychology and, more broadly, of human sciences in general. However, in the analyses mentioned above, this fact has simply been asserted rather than discussed in detail. This resulted from the orientation of those analyzing Vygotsky's work. In their analyses, they did not go beyond the bounds defined in the existing theory of activity. But this theory, in itself, was not adequate for examining Vygotsky's methodology. If one views Vygotsky simply as a founder of a concrete psychological theory, then he can be evaluated only as a psychologist. Vygotsky's role as a methodologist is either ignored or simply mentioned. The disparity between methodology and psychology in his words disappears, and his methodological ideas remain beyond the limits of the analysis.

However, the critical point is that the internal bond of methodology and psychology constitutes the very foundation of all Vygotsky's work. In this connection we come upon an interesting problem. Nearly all researchers have noted some contradiction in his works. This contradiction has taken many forms. For Gal'perin (1970), it appeared as a contradiction between Vygotsky's interest in the emotions and the rationalist position in psychology that he took up in the last years of his life. For El'konin (1966) the contradiction was between Vygotsky's historical method and his opposition of "cultural" and "natural" mental functions. In the most profound analysis of this problem, Leont'ev (1975; see also Leont'ev and Luria, 1956) identified the contradiction between Vygotsky's initial concepts and their concrete realization in works based on them. Leont'ev's analysis reveals some of the limitations of the internal logic of Vygotsky's approach from the position of the psychological theory of activity. If we go beyond the limits of this position, this "contradictory nature" of Vygotsky's work can be examined as the interaction of the two strata of his work – the methodological and the psychological.

Vygotsky's work is far from homogeneous. As a psychologist he did not use all of the possibilities presented by Vygotsky the methodologist. Similarly, not all of Vygotsky's ideas as a psychologist were motivated by his own methodological foundations. It is also necessary to take into consideration the fact that his methodological and psychological notions were constantly evolving and not always in parallel. Vygotsky reacted to these varied methodological ideas with varying degrees of clarity. As a result, a very complex picture of the interaction of his methodological and psychological ideas presents itself to those concerned with their analysis.

Vygotsky: a methodologist of psychology

Since we cannot examine all of Vygotsky's methodological works in a single chapter, we will focus on a few of them that were written in a characteristic manner and give a notion of the range of problems reflected in his psychological theory.

Vygotsky began somewhat earlier as a methodologist of psychology than as a psychologist concerned with developing concrete theory. When the 28-year-old Vygotsky came to scientific psychology, he was deeply concerned with the philosophical problems of the humanities. He had not decided on a specific course for investigating the mind. But from the very beginning he sought to establish normative methodological requirements for psychology.

His 1925 article "Consciousness as a Problem in the Psychology of Behavior" is of great interest in this context. At first glance, it seems to involve nothing more than the declaration that the traditional introspectionist psychology of consciousness is invalid. But Vygotsky argued that by ignoring the problem of consciousness, representatives of the new objective psychology and reflexology were also following an incorrect path. In reality, the problem of consciousness exists as a very real problem. Vygotsky (1925) considered consciousness, first, as a "reflex of reflexes" [it being clarified that he had in mind something like a reflex arc with reverse connections (p. 198)], second, as the "problem of the structure of behavior" (p. 181), and third, as an issue in human labor activity (p. 197).

This kind of article may appear to be concerned solely with concrete science. Various theories of consciousness were proposed and there were constant appeals to psychological reality and concrete methods for studying it. Moreover, it inevitably appears as eclectic as well as logically contradictory. Three different theories of consciousness were proposed, being brought together without a detailed study of their interrelationships. Finally, there is little that is original in it. A comparison with other works [in particular, the works of the leading Soviet psychologist of those years, Kornilov (1926)] reveals immediately that both the charge of introspectionism and the corresponding positive programs were to a large extent commonplace in those times.

However, beneath the external simplicity of Vygotsky's formulations is hidden a subtext with profound implications. In order to analyze the specifics of Vygotsky's ideas one must follow an indirect path, beginning with the general context of Soviet psychology of that time.

In this connection, one must keep in mind the following characteristics of Vygotsky's work. First, one constantly encounters terminological carelessness and imprecision. This involves the use of terms alien to the internal logic of his system, something that reflected the impossibility of expressing his ideas through "his" words (we will consider several examples of this below). This is explained, first, by the circumstances of Vygotsky's biography and by his personality. According to his students, some "carelessness of genius" distinguished Vygotsky generally. In addition, he was in a great hurry. He produced all his basic work (over 160 titles) between two outbreaks of tuberculosis (in 1926 and in 1934), clearly sensing his doom. Second, Vygotsky was frequently unable to borrow existing terminology adequate for his ideas because, in general, it simply did not exist in the 1920s.

To a certain extent, Vygotsky was ahead of his time. Many of his basic ideas could be more adequately formulated only by using the mechanisms developed by Soviet Marxist philosophers and methodologists in the 1960s and 1970s. It is possible that many of Vygotsky's ideas will find still more adequate formulation only with the future development of philosophy and methodology.

But there is a more subtle aspect of this issue. Up to this point, we have considered instances of imprecision, carelessness, and contradiction in Vygotsky's texts. We have some reason to believe that he recognized and criticized these himself. However, just as introspection is no longer accepted as the *sole* method of studying the mind, one can say that the scientific self-reflection of a creator of a theory cannot serve as the *only* source of information *about his work "as a whole."* Therefore, in many cases where there is no information about Vygotsky's self-reflection one can "decipher" the implicit sense of his statements (in particular, consider them as "inexact" or "contradictory") by proceeding from the internal structure of his system and from the logic of the development of the specific scientific tradition to which he was objectively related and to which he subjectively attached himself.

As is well known, during the 1920s Soviet psychologists were involved in the intense and rapid demolition of the traditional subjective–empirical psychology that had dominated Russian psychology up to the Revolution. It was also a period of impatient attempts to replace this psychology with a new Marxist, materialist, and objective psychology. In this connection, psychologists experienced strong pressure from the physiology of higher nervous activity which represented itself as the model of an objective and materialist scientific approach. At the beginning of the 1920s, the success of this school inevitably had an influence on all scholars. In addition, ideas about a direct sociological explanation of mental processes had a tremendous influence on the Soviet psychologists of that time. In a situation where the essence of Marxist philosophy was still not interpreted or mastered in sufficient depth by Soviet scholars of human sciences, these ideas were frequently perceived as particularly "Marxist." (Ideas of this type had a strong influence not only in psychology, but in a number of the social sciences, such as history. It also surfaced in the literature and art of the 1920s.) Finally, of the genuinely psychological schools, behaviorism had the greatest influence on Soviet psychology, attracting interest because it was seen as an objective and materialist approach.

A motley picture resulted from the influence of these and other circumstances in psychology. Some scholars defined psychology as "the science of behavior" (Borovskii, Blonskii), others as the science "of reflexes" (Behkterev), others as the science "of reactions" (Kornilov), and still others as the science "of systems of social reflexes" (Reisner), and so on.[2]

Notwithstanding the crucial differences that separate these approaches, historians of psychology have identified something that was common to them all. Their common inspiration was clearly the tendency to argue against the conception of psychology as "the science of the spirit" and to make psychology objective. In practice, this objectivization was purchased at the cost of abandoning the consideration of all subjective features of the human mind. The mind was reduced to a system of behavioral responses, to the combination of conditioned reflexes, or to a collection of what modern researchers call "social positions," "social roles," and so on.

What significance did this have for the problem of consciousness? In the 1920s many prominent Soviet psychologists (e.g., Blonskii, Borovskii) practically ignored this problem. Since it was considered to be impossible to examine it by using objective scientific methods, they considered it to be unrelated to the domain of scientific psychology. In contrast, another group of psychologists headed by Kornilov considered consciousness to be a very important object of psychology and asserted that it had to be studied. For this reason, Kornilov (1925) did not renounce the introspective method. Moreover, he concluded that "the coming system of Marxist psychology will be "a synthesis of two . . . trends: . . . a subjective trend and . . . the psychology of behavior" (1925, p. 9). Finally, a group of psychologists (true, only a small group) maintained the position of the traditional subjective–empirical psychology of consciousness (as is known, Chelpanov was the ideological leader of the group in those years).

Thus, in Soviet psychology of the 1920s there were three perspectives on the problem of consciousness. It was argued that (1) psychology must ignore consciousness as an issue insoluble by research based on objective methods; (2) consciousness is the basic object of psychology; and (3) it is necessary to unify the first and second extreme points of view, that is, unify objective and subjective methods. It was as if these three positions exhausted the possible solutions to the problem of consciousness in psychology. However, in his 1925 article, Vygotsky was able to reject all three positions. As a result, he broke out of the circle that they formed, the circle that dominated Soviet psychology in those years.

Although Vygotsky clearly and concisely stated his position at the very beginning of his article, it is not easy to understand. He wrote: "But what is most important is that the exclusion of consciousness from the domain of scientific psychology [by "scientific psychology" he meant the "psychology of behavior" that was dominant in Soviet psychology] preserves. . .all the dualism and spiritualism of earlier subjective psychology" (1925, p. 178).

Because it was "inside" the circle noted above, it is possible to understand this statement only as a critique of the psychologists who completely ignored the problem of consciousness (it is no accident that in the next sentence Vygotsky began a polemic with Bekhterev's reflexology). In such a case, Vygotsky's statement would seem to represent his solidarity with Kornilov's position. But the comments about the "dualism and spiritualism of earlier subjective psychology" then cannot play a particularly meaningful role in relation to the problem of consciousness. They must be viewed simply as a tribute to the good relations customary in Soviet psychology of those years. Analogously, speaking of the necessity of analyzing consciousness, Kornilov was not able to offer anything other than a return to a subjective–empirical psychology of consciousness (though in a somewhat less radical form). But such an interpretation of Vygotsky's work is completely incorrect because in the case of all three of the programs for analyzing consciousness he not only avoided any mention of a return to a traditional "psychology of consciousness," but argued against this kind of psychology.

Thus, Vygotsky actually came out against all three approaches. How is this possible when these approaches would seem to exhaust the list of possible solutions? In reality, the answer is already contained in the formulation Vygotsky introduced. He condemned the psychology of behavior for the fact that it ignored the problem of consciousness. He considered this to be a critical problem in psychology. The actual historical situation was such that whereas the psychology of behavior ignored the problem of consciousness, this problem remained in the forefront of subjective–empirical psychology, and Vygotsky was not satisfied with how the latter approach dealt with this problem.[3]

It is precisely here that Vygotsky broke out of that circle in which, unbeknownst to themselves, all Soviet psychologists of those years moved. This circle arose as a consequence of a single premise that, in practice, was silently accepted by everyone. The essence of this premise is that *one can study consciousness in psychology only as this was done in the subjective–empirical psychology of consciousness.*

Beyond this, one finds only purely evaluative differences. Psychologists either attached themselves to subjective–empirical research and considered consciousness to be the object of science, or they completely rejected such a psychology and ignored the problem of consciousness, or, finally, they accepted some compromise position. A new, powerful tradition in the analysis of consciousness within psychology had been born. The foundations were amassed for a strong critique of subjective–empirical psychology on this question. Vygotsky was able to make an important contribution toward the development of the problem of consciousness. This contribution reflected the development of early twentieth-century psychology. He was also able to take up his special place, primarily because he approached the problem of the analysis of consciousness as a methodological problem.

We will analyze this point further since, in addition to its objective importance, one can trace its influence on Vygotsky's work. The 1925 article by Vygotsky (as well as several other of his works on the problem of consciousness written in those same years) is related to his well-known works. But it has always been read (both by Vygotsky's contemporaries and by historians) from a strictly *psychological* position. Accordingly, it has generally been viewed only in terms of the minor argument that Vygotsky made against ignoring the problem of consciousness in the psychology of behavior and so forth. Thus, Vygotsky became something like Kornilov's imitator. The contradiction that such an interpretation evokes is either unnoticed or ignored.

If one considers Vygotsky's article as a strictly psychological article, no other interpretation is possible. Leont'ev (1967) has examined this article primarily as a methodological rather than a psychological piece. This allowed him to reveal several new strata in it (1967, p. 27). But Leont'ev's general theoretical analysis was flawed by his tendency to judge Vygotsky from the perspective of the psychological theory of activity that Leont'ev himself was developing. He used this as a reference point for analyzing all activity-oriented trends in twentieth-century psychology.

In order to understand the essence of Vygotsky's methodological position (and how it is distinct from the position of most psychologists) it is above all necessary to investigate his reason for condemning the traditional subjective–empirical psychology of consciousness. When he writes of its "dualism and spiritualism," he was properly concerned first with the inherent division of all reality into Nature and Spirit (consciousness being related to the latter). Second, he was concerned with the fact that the domain of the latter phenomenon is located outside the sphere of scientific determination.

But, in addition, it is necessary in this context to note one peculiarity of Vygotsky's position. The issue arises as to what is to be understood by "scientific determination." The representatives of subjective–empirical psychology considered their research to be completely scientific (as Chelpanov wrote in the 1920s). They simply thought that the concept of "scientific determination," when applied to psychology, did not coincide with the notions of "natural science determination" accepted in a number of sciences (in particular, in physiology) at the beginning of the twentieth-century. (Incidentally, this same perspective was held by Pavlov.)

The representatives of the psychology of behavior maintained the opposite position. For them, "scientific" and "natural scientific" determination were synonyms. From this perspective, they rejected subjective–empirical psychology as unscientific. (Actually, they were forced to reach a compromise with it, since they wanted to keep the problem of consciousness in psychology.)

The unique feature of Vygotsky's position consisted of the fact that while arguing that conciousness in traditional subjective–empirical psychology was outside the sphere of scientific determination, he never equated *scientific and natural scientific* determination (in the sense used at the beginning of the twentieth century). In Vygotsky's work, it is not difficult to find numerous *declarations* in which there is an identification of the concepts "scientific" and "natural scientific" for psychology. But, as we noted previously, if one judges not by declarations (which were closely linked to the specific situation), but in accordance with the actual internal structure of his system (that is, in accordance with the manner in which Vygotsky actually posed and resolved the problem in his methodological and strictly psychological works), then the answer becomes very clear. In his actual work, Vygotsky never equated "scientific" and "natural scientific." Such a practice would have contradicted the very spirit of this work.

Where was the weakness of subjective–empirical psychology for Vygotsky, and how did he contemplate the course of introducing consciousness into the domain of scientific determination? In 1925, Vygotsky was not able to answer these questions directly. The necessary terminology and apparatus were still not developed. But his thought is sufficiently clear. First, we will consider the three programs that Vygotsky formulated: (1)

"consciousness is a reflex of reflexes," (2) "consciousness is the problem of the structure of behavior," and (3) "consciousness is a feature of human labor activity." Their differences are so apparent that the question automatically arises as to whether it is possible that Vygotsky himself did not see these differences. And if he saw them, what caused him to conflate them? Why did he not even raise the question of their compatibility?

In our opinion, no answer is possible if one considers the article as a psychological article and Vygotsky as a psychologist. (More accurately, one must arrive at an aswer that is not compatible with Vygotsky's notion. One is brought to suggestions of eclecticism, logical confusion, and so on.) Therefore, this question has not been raised previously in the analysis of this article.

A different picture is revealed if one considers this article as a methodological work. The suggestion then arises that Vygotsky did not raise the question of the compatibility of these programs simply because the question was not critical to him. These programs did not serve as part of the content of this methodological article. Rather, they served as an illustration. He described them in order to point out possible alternatives to the subjective–empirical treatment of consciousness. The alternatives were strictly methodological and concerned one major point.

In order to articulate this point more clearly, it is necessary to turn to another feature in that article. At the end of the article, Vygotsky (1925) pointed out "the coincidence in conclusions that exists between the notions developed here and the ingenious analysis of consciousness conducted by James" (p. 11). Further, he introduced a quotation from the Russian translation of James's article, "Does Consciousness Exist?": "Thoughts . . . are made of the same matter as things" (1913, p. 126). It is clear that this idea of James was directed against dualism. Characteristic of it is its similarity to the position of Vygotsky's favorite philosopher, Spinoza, who wrote that thinking and extension are not two different substances, but two attributes of one and the same substance. However, in what manner does James propose to remove the dualistic approach and, consequently, to subject consciousness to a completely scientific determination?

As is known, James was the author of the conception of the "stream of consciousness." However, it is impossible to identify any trace of its influence on Vygotsky. On the other hand, there is one very important aspect of James's thought in the article "Does Consciousness Exist?" that seems to us to provide the key to Vygotsky's methodological quest and his admiration for James.

James (1913) wrote: "It has already been 20 years since I have come to doubt the existence of the essence that we call 'consciousness.' . . . It seems to me that the time has come when all will openly renounce it" (p. 120). But

James, of course, "denies" consciousness in a completely different sense than did the reflexologists of Vygotsky's time. For Vygotsky, this difference is a critical matter. James (1913) went on to write: "I intend only to disclaim the sense of this word [consciousness], as an essence or substance, but I will insist on its significance as a *function*" (p. 120); (emphasis added). We will not examine the place of this formula in the work of James, but it is indisputable that, for Vygotsky, this opposition between essence and function had enormous significance.

In the thought of James we have a clear-cut indication of the semifunctionality of the concept of "consciousness" in a system of psychology. To define such semifunctionality was impossible. It remained only as a part of the psychological analysis of the problem. In any empirical research based, for example, on introspection, consciousness emerged as "equal to it itself"; it apparently emerged only from the point of view of its essence and not from any other perspective. The semifunctionality of consciousness did not appear even in the critique of traditional subjective–emperical psychology by behavioral psychology. This was so even though behavioral psychology rejected introspection and set the goal of identifying behavioral reactions through objective methods. At the same time, the problem of consciousness was removed from the agenda of scientific psychology.

This type of semifunctionality could only have arisen in the *methodological* account of consciousness, since it appealed not to psychological reality itself but to the categories used in psychological theories. It was precisely this type of position, emerging from the ideas of James, that Vygotsky takes up in the article "Consciousness as a Problem in the Psychology of Behavior."

What could Vygotsky derive from this statement on the semifunctionality of the concept of "consciousness"? This type of statement, with the "denial of consciousness as an essence" (or more precisely – with the denial of the possibility for the psychologist to accept such an approach to consciousness) integrated many of the methodological ideas of twentieth-century psychology.

Vygotsky understood this issue very well, and it had a great influence on his work. For Vygotsky, the concepts of "essence" and "function" emerge as somewhat analogous to what the modern methodologist of psychology would call the "general explanatory principle" and the "object of independent research."

In connection with another of Vygotsky's works we will later show how he understood the problem of the relationship between the "explanatory principle" and the "object of independent research." Here we will only note the role that the elaboration of these two categories played in his analysis of the problem of consciousness. For the methodologist, the recognition of this type of distinction leads to addressing the psychological problem of consciousness in a completely new manner. In order to be able to study the essence of consciousness (its genesis, structure, determinants, etc.), one must accept this type of methodological position in order for consciousness to appear as an object of independent study. But for this, in turn, a somewhat more general explanatory principle is necessary. This is a category in the conceptual system of psychology that reflects a specific stratum of reality. Consequently, it is necessary to search for this statum of reality, a stratum whose *function* is consciousness. In this manner, one can study the essence of consciousness only when consciousness appears as a function. It is impossible to study the essence of consciousness if consciousness itself emerges as an explanatory principle. (This is precisely how the matter stood in the traditional "psychology of consciousness." Consciousness was automatically reflected in the definition of consciousness as a "stage," as the "general keeper of mental functions," and so on.) It is only possible to describe various phenomena that are related to consciousness.

It was precisely this methodological mistake (e.g., the pretense of studying the essence of consciousness from a position that makes this impossible in principle) that led to the concept of "consciousness" based on semifunctionality. From Vygotsky's perspective, this mistake represented the basic defect of the traditional subjective–empirical approaches to consciousness. With this in mind his position in the article "Consciousness as a Problem in the Psychology of Behavior" becomes transparent. Its inspiration emerges quite clearly.

In this article Vygotsky was one of the first in Soviet science to examine the problem of consciousness on the methodological plane. This permitted him to reveal the basic, concealed weakness of the traditional subjective–empirical psychology of consciousness. As a result, it also permitted him to reject all three proposals for resolving the problem of consciousness that were available to Soviet psychology in those years. They all proceeded from identifying the problem of consciousness with the specific mode of its resolution in empirical psychology. They failed to see a real alternative to it (except for the liquidation of the problem itself).

Such an alternative emerged for Vygotsky. As he already saw then, it is necessary to give consciousness a different methodological status. It is necessary to place it in the position of an object of independent study (we purposefully use the terms of the 1960s and 1970s, since this kind of "modernization" clarifies the essence of Vygotsky's thought for which no adequate expressions existed in the 1920s). For this, in turn, it was necessary to find a new explanatory principle in psychology. In other words, it was necessary to identify a stratum of reality that determines consciousness. This involved beginning with a *nonreductionistic* reconstruction of consciousness. Such is the main task that Vygotsky broached as a result of his analyses of the problem of consciousness, and this was also the main result of that analysis. The resolution of this problem became one of the basic tasks in all of Vygotsky's scientific work. Of course it is necessary to explore this question beyond the limits of the present chapter. But this chapter does provide some material for thought along these lines.

As we have already said, Vygotsky placed all three of his positive programs on a methodological plane. Their purpose was to illustrate several strata of reality that are capable of determining consciousness. Therefore, one factor is common to all Vygotsky's programs. They all lead the analysis of consciousness beyond the bounds of consciousness itself. Through them Vygotsky proposed three variants for resolving one and the same methodological problem. This is the problem of searching for strata of reality that could fulfill the role of an intermediate link between objective reality (the external world) and consciousness. Through the analysis of this link, it is possible to include consciousness (not separate phenomena, but the essence of consciousness) within the domain of phenomena that can be described by the laws of scientific determination.

Although stating the necessity for this search was of great importance for Vygotsky, his proposals for how the search should proceed arc also very interesting. Let us consider Vygotsky's first formula, that is, "Consciousness is a reflex of reflexes" (1925, p. 198). This is an extreme expression of the formulas common at the time. It comes from Vygotsky's first well-known presentation (January 6, 1924) at the Second All-Russian Conference on Psychoneurology. The title of this presentation was "Methods of Reflexological Research Applied to the Study of Mind" (Vygotsky, 1926, p. 42). This formula was proclaimed by Vygotsky not with methodological but with concrete psychological goals and methods in mind. It served him as an expression for a specific position. This reflected a very short period (one that had little lasting influence on Vygotsky) during which he was captivated by physiological reductionism. In this connection he called himself "more of a reflexologist than Pavlov himself" (1926, p. 42).

After a year-and-a-half, Vygotsky shifted to a completely different position. The basic meaning of the formula that consciousness is a reflex of reflexes was lost, but the formula itself was mechanically tranferred to the article "Consciousness as a Problem in the Psychology of Behavior." Vygotsky had already moved so far away from this formula that after expressing it he immediately reduced it to nothing. He subjected it to a sharp criticism. For example, he wrote: "It is necessary to change our view of human behavior as a mechanism that is completely revealed by the conditioned reflex" (1925, p. 181) and "It is necessary to study not reflexes, but behavior – its mechanisms, its composition, and its structure" (1925, p. 180).

Thus, Vygotsky's reflexological program was not original, and Vygotsky himself evaluated it, at best, ambivalently. An analysis of his subsequent work shows that the notion that consciousness is a reflex of reflexes did not actually play any important role. This is completely natural. Such a program that sees the determination of consciousness in the physiology of the brain is incompatible with the profound methodological analysis that Vygotsky carried out in his later years.

Vygotsky did not clarify the second formula: "Consciousness is the problem of the structure of behavior" (1925, p. 181). He clearly said only that behavior "is not explained by the conditioned reflex." It is difficult to understand how this program is related to behaviorism, reactology, and other approaches, but there is an idea here that points to his transition to the third program. It is possible to approach the analysis of consciousness through the analysis of behavior. If this is so, then the difference in the behavior of animals and humans must have great significance. Namely, this difference is connected with the appearance of consciousness, something that exists only in humans. The unique nature of human behavior, according to Vygotsky (1925, pp. 175, 197), is linked to labor activity in humans (here, he was relying directly on Marx's ideas in *Kapital*).

Thus, in Vygotsky's third program, which in essence was an extension of the second, consciousness emerged as an aspect of the structure of labor activity. This program was the most significant one. First it was original and expressed the specific character of Vygotsky's ideas most precisely. It is true that he only searched for it and did not even have adequate means to formulate it clearly. Second, this program was not directly linked with concrete methods (reflexological, behaviorist, and so on), but emerged on a solid methodological and philosophical foundation. Finally, and most importantly, its underlying significance becomes apparent only in Vygotsky's subsequent methodological and psychological work. In this work this third program (in contrast to the first two) had decisive significance.

The next level in the analysis of these problems that were posed in the article "Consciousness as a Problem in the Psychology of Behavior" can be found in Vygotsky's large 1926 manuscript "The Historical Significance of the Crisis in Psychology" (1982). The continuity between these two works is indisputable. However, in this latter work questions were raised that were not raised in the first. Vygotsky clearly wrote this manuscript from a methodological position. Its purpose, as Vygotsky himself revealed, was to conduct a historical, logical, and philosophical analysis of psychology in order to formulate several normative methodological requirements. In a certain sense, this work contains the sum of Vygotsky's activity as a methodologist of psychology. He continued his methodological studies up to his last days, but he seldom again touched on such a broad range of problems. The formulation and resolution of these problems in this manuscript remained unchanged. To a certain extent, these contributions to the resolution of these problems comprised all of Vygotsky's work on this issue.[4] Our purpose here is not to examine all of the questions discussed in this manuscript. We will only consider a few key issues.

The goal of this work was to formulate normative methodological requirements for a future system of Marxist psychology, that is, for a general psychological theory based on Marxist philosophical principles. As Vygotsky pointed out, what is required is the creation of a psychological analogue of *Kapital*. If *Kapital* had the subtitle "A Critique of Political Economy," then a methodological critique of scientific psychology is necessary as well.

There was no shortage of this kind of statement in the 1920s. Almost every Soviet theoretician of psychology in one form or another declared the necessity of developing a Marxist psychology and stated that his proposal could serve as the basis for it. Much was said and written in connection with this, as well as in reference to the necessity of combining methodological, philosophical, and other work.

In practice, however, enormous difficulties were encountered. As a result, fundamental doubts arose about the potential for resolving such a problem and about its constructiveness. Opponents of Marxist psychology, such as Chelpanov (1925), clearly said that there is no such "Marxist psychology" and that there would not be one. They stated that this was only a "play on words." The crux of the matter was as follows. It was apparent that in the construction of a Marxist psychology it was necessary to utilize, on the one hand, the ideas of Marxist philosophy and, on the other the facts and conceptual schemes that existed in various psychological theories. And this is exactly how matters proceeded. The general ideas of dialectical and historical materialism ("the mind is a property of highly organized material," "matter is primary, consciousness secondary," etc.), as well as combinations of various ideas taken from behaviorism, reflexology, Freudianism, and so forth were utilized. The combination of these was tested in accordance with the formal–logical criteria of coherence. Subsequently, this combination was declared "Marxist psychology."

But critics subsequently noticed that in such constructions there exists not a formal–logical contradiction, but an incompatibility of content. The ideas of dialectical materialism exist independently of the ideas of the various psychological theories. No real synthesis resulted from the fact that they were combined by means of the conjunction "and." But psychologists did not see a more radical solution to the problem.

What did Vygotsky introduce here that was new? Method. According to Vygotsky's analysis of the problem of consciousness, the old idea of explanatory principle and object of independent study was already at work.

However, it had not been made explicit. In "The Historical Significance of the Crisis in Psychology," Vygotsky raised this idea to the rank of a general methodological law.

He argued that a central feature of any psychological theory is the presence of a general explanatory principle that he clearly separated from the object of study. Vygotsky saw in this principle that critical point of danger in the methodological analysis of theory. "The idea remains an explanatory principle until it goes beyond the boundaries of a basic concept [a concept of the theory under study]: as we saw after all, to explain also means to go beyond boundaries in search of external causes" (1982, p. 21).[5] He examined in detail, for example, the problem of the relationship between the category of an *explanatory principle* and that of an *object of a study* in the well-known psychological theories of that time (reflexology, behaviorism, Freudianism, and so forth).

Thus, Vygotsky's first principle as a methodologist was as follows: It is necessary to identify the explanatory principle that defines the boundaries and structure of a theory. Along with this he identified still another important feature that must be observed in developing a typology of scientific theories. We refer to the units of analysis (Vygotsky, 1982, p. 208).

The fact that Vygotsky attached great significance to identifying the units of psychological analysis is noted by almost everyone who has written about him. However, this usually leads only to Vygotsky's statement that it is impossible to study the chemical characteristics of water by decomposing it into its constituent elements, that is, into the atoms of hydrogen and oxygen (analysis into elements). It is necessary to search for the minimal unit that preserves the properties of the whole – the molecule (analysis into units). One should search for the adequate units of mental life in a similar way. The significance of this example, an example that Vygotsky (1934, 1960a) loved to use, is usually seen only in Vygotsky's rejection of analysis into elements and in his search for intact formations, and so forth. However, such a reading produces only a trivial declaration. In the 1920s the attention of psychologists was strongly attracted to the problem of the units of the analysis of mind [for a survey of the views of Soviet scholars in this regard see Tkachenko (1980)]. There was a great deal of talk at that time about the necessity of utilizing analysis of units. [Vygotsky's own example was borrowed from Müller-Freienfels (1922).] However, Vygosky did not focus on this feature by accident. Those who have studied his work have correctly sensed that this example was especially significant for Vygotsky.

Vygotsky's ideas about the necessity of "analysis by units" acquires a completely different significance if it is considered from within his general methodological system. If one proceeds from Vygotsky's methodological premise that psychological theory is outlined and structured by a general, frequently implicit, explanatory principle, then it is clear that this explanatory principle assigns quantitative size to the unit of psychological analysis. The unit of analysis is one of the most clearly established features in any psychological theory. Thus Vygotsky attempted to utilize the unit of analysis as one of the indicators of a theory's latent explanatory principle.

We have now elucidated the means by which Vygotsky, as a methodologist, proposed to study psychological theory (and further, on the basis of this, how Vygotsky as a psychologist attempted to elaborate his own conceptual system). Vygotsky was faced not with a static and one-sided picture of theory, but with a picture that included a dynamic relationship between "explanatory principles" and the "object of study." This was the dynamic involved in developing an explanatory principle.

However, this picture is incomplete as long as we do not address the question of the origin of the explanatory principle. This is a concept (as a rule semifunctional) that reflects a certain reality that, in turn, determines mental phenomena and makes possible their reconstruction. Vygotsky believed that explanatory principles that are relevant for psychology are philosophical conceptions that have been further developed. They are borrowed from philosophy by psychologists.

But the introduction of explanatory principles into psychology is frequently carried out without the support of the philosophical standard of thought. The basic problem of the methodologist is to monitor this work. In the course of their transplantation to psychology, philosophical concepts must undergo a process of concretization relevant to the logic of the philosophical tradition in which they were conceived (see Vygotsky, 1982, p. 224).

Thus, according to Vygotsky, methodological analysis in psychology involves a twofold process. First, it begins with an existing theoretical apparatus (in particular, with units of analysis). Then it develops an explanatory principle and defines its place in a philosophical tradition. Then, conversely, Vygotsky envisioned the verification from the perspective of the logic of this philosophical tradition, a verification of the application of the philosophical concept as an explanatory principle in psychological theory and its development on the basis of the given explanatory principle. Vygotsky (1982, p. 55) himself called this the "logical–historical" method, in contrast to the "formal–logical–semantic" method.

What sorts of *results* did Vygotsky's method provide on the problem he raised, that is, about the elaboration of the methodological foundations of Marxist psychology? The method provided exactly what a methodology must provide when constructing a theory. Without predetermining the specifics of this construction, it provided a general system of normative requirements and a mode of verification of the results.

This method led to the necessity of a multistage construction of psychological theory as an organic system. This system had its own philosophical premises, and it identified and described each stage (including several that most psychologists did not notice). The fact that multiple stages were involved was closely connected with another very important feature. This was the unwillingness to accept simple, direct determination and reduction. Instead, it argued that mediating links, interconnected by complex (especially genetic) relations, are necessary.

This approach to the problem of constructing a Marxist, materialist psychology was manifested on various levels and had several consequences. Let us consider some of these.

First, from the very beginning the construction of a Marxist psychology proceeded by combining the positions of dialectical materialism with the content of specific psychological theories. Vygotsky demonstrated the necessity of elaborating the "intervening links" of such a synthesis. Proceeding from the internal logic of Marxism, it was necessary to build a corresponding methodology of psychology. Only then, having isolated the explanatory principle, could one elaborate concrete theories.

Second, this approach argued against the idea of a direct determination of mind by a concrete material vehicle (for example, the brain): It stimulated the search for the reality that intervenes between the "external" world and the human mind. The concept that expresses this reality can then appear as the explanatory principle in the categorical apparatus of a nonreductionistic psychological theory.

Third, Vygotsky's general approach influenced the question of units of analysis. It is understandable that the two-part schema "stimulus–response" that assumes a direct determination cannot create this. If we proceed from the fact that Vygotsky was forced to deal with this scheme in some way, then the methodological unity of this theory requires its tranformation because of the introduction of an intermediate link.

The requirements of this system led to an approach in which it was necessary to search for the reality that determines mind. Already in his article "Consciousness as a Problem in the Psychology of Behavior," Vygotsky considered consciousness in connection with *labor activity*. In the manuscript "The Historical Significance of the Crisis in Psychology," he wrote about the importance of analyzing humans' *practical activity* for psychology.

If one proceeds on the basis of the methodological requirements outlined above, then it is possible to conclude that for Vygotsky the category of practical human activity played *the role of a general explanatory category;* this category identified *the ability that determines mind.* Vygotsky did not explicate the nature of this category. One of the main reasons for this was the undeveloped state of Marxist philosophical literature of those years on the concept of activity itself. However, the true methodological significance of Vygotsky's work consists of the assertion that activity is the explanatory principle in psychological theory. Now we will turn to the question of how this idea is expressed in Vygotsky's psychological theory.

Vygotsky as creator of a psychological theory

Over the past half-century Vygotsky's psychological theory has been examined in great detail by Soviet and foreign authors (Radzikhovskii, 1979b, pp. 204–225). We will not attempt to add anything to this analysis from a factual perspective. Our purpose here is to clarify one additional aspect of how the *category of activity* fits into Vygotsky's work.

The starting point in Vygotsky's theory is considered to be his idea of the *mediation* of elementary (natural) mental functions by so called psychological tools (e.g., Leont'ev and Luria, 1956; Vygotsky, 1960b). Such an approach seems to us to be quite justified. The idea of the mediation of elementary mental functions by "psychological tools" has the following consequences:

1. One of Vygotsky's pivotal concepts was that explanatory psychology reduced the higher mental functions to the lower ones, and therefore could not adequately explain the specific character of the higher mental functions. Conceptual psychology, though maintaining the specific character of higher mental functions, severed the connections between them and the lower mental functions and renounced a casual explanation of higher mental functions. Vygotsky always considered it one of his main problems to overcome the division of psychology into two sciences. He always wanted to transform explanatory psychology so that it could be applied to the analysis of the higher mental functions. The hypothesis of psychological tools gave him the solution to this problem. If one thinks that higher mental functions arise on the foundation of lower ones (due to mediation by psychological tools), then it becomes possible through the analysis of psychological tools to begin explaining the specific properties of higher mental functions (properties that were inaccessible to explanatory psychology) and the connection of higher with "lower" functions (the latter being inaccessible to conceptual psychology).

2. This idea led directly to an integrated, historical approach to mental functions. This constituted one of the important aspects of Vygotsky's theory. On the one hand, the assumption of mediation led to an understanding of mental functions as integral formations in a complex structure. On the other hand, mental functions were examined from the point of view of their genesis (both ontogenesis and phylogenesis), in which the process

of mediation emerges. Integration and historicism were inextricably bound together. They appeared as the projection of one idea, the idea of mediation.

3. This idea led Vygotsky immediately to the problem of *internalization,* something that is considered central to his psychological work. At the same time it served as a means for concretely having the sociocultural determination of the human mind. According to Vygotsky, all the "tools" that are developed artificially by humanity are the elements of culture. This was not a simple assertion, but a concrete proposal for the scientific analysis of the sociohistorical determination of mind. Initially, "psychological tools" were directed "externally," toward a partner. Subsequently they turn in "on themselves," that is, they become a means of controlling one's own mental process. Furthermore, they become internal (i.e., they "go underground"). Mental functions are then mediated "from within." The necessity for using external stimulus–means disappears. Vygotsky (1928) referred to this entire process as the complete circle of cultural–historical development of mental functions in ontogenesis. It provides the key to explicating the process of internalization.

4. It is well known that Vygotsky saw *signs* as fulfilling the role of psychological tools. He understood something very specific by the notion of sign. His notion differed from that of the reflexologist (where the sign was viewed as a conditioned stimulus in a system of conditioned reflexes), and it was unlike the notion used by representatives of depth psychology (who viewed the sign as a visual symbol, the vehicle of unconscious inclinations). For Vygotsky, a sign is a symbol with a definite meaning that has evolved in the history of a culture. This interpretation of symbol came from Vygotsky's early work on the psychology of art and from his training in humanities and philology. In this connection it is possible to identify several ideas and schools of thought that had a strong influence on Vygotsky: the historical linguistics of Humboldt, Shteinthal, and Potebnya; the members of "Opoyaz"[6] and other related researchers, especially Bakhtin; symbolism in literature and art at the beginning of the twentieth century; ethnopsychology (Levy-Brühl, Thurnwald); and, possibly, the semiotic works of Saussure. The idea of the sign as a psychological tool in Vygotsky's theory is one of the most successful examples of the application of semiotic ideas in psychology. This is frequently seen as the basic merit and result of Vygotsky's research as a psychologist.[7]

5. The notion that the sign is a "psychological tool" made it possible for Vygotsky (1960a) to transform the two-part scheme for the analysis of mind accepted by behaviorism into a three-part scheme, introducing the "psychological tool" as an intervening link.

What is most important is the fact that the aspects of Vygotsky's approach mentioned so far (as well as several others) form a unified system of essentially *new constructs in psychology.* They point to a new level of psychological reality on which Vygotsky was able to conduct an objective scientific analysis by introducing the notion of "psychological tool." With this, special methods of research emerged (for example, the methods of double stimulation). These were the concrete embodiment of the idea of psychological tools. Also, the development of mental functions such as attention, memory, and thinking began to be predictable and understood as subordinated to a general law. This new discovery for psychology was the idea of psychological tools, the key idea in understanding Vygotsky's work.[8]

Thus, what sort of explanatory principle lay behind the idea of psychological tools and the psychological theory of Vygotsky's? By turning to this question, we encounter, even at first glance, an astonishing picture. Vygotsky (1960a) described the origins of the hypothesis about the role of "psychological tools" as follows: "In human behavior one encounters . . . many artificial devices for mastering mental processes. By analogy with technical means we may justifiably label these devices 'psychological tools'" (p. 5), inevitably, it seems strange that with the help of a rather tentative and arbitrary analogy a fundamental hypothesis was substantiated. In fact, one can draw an analogy between, say, a knot or a notch "for memory" (the well-known models of "psychological tools") and the tools of labor (for example, analysis). However, on the basis of this analogy, why did Vygotsky assign such an important role to "psychological tools"? Why did speech or the word become such a fundamental psychological tool?

There is a well-known paradox here. Many facts of the role of external means in memory were perfectly well known to psychologists before Vygotsky (the term "mnemotechnics" even existed). These facts indicated nothing more than the presence of some artificial mode of "simulation" that passes for memory. Vygotsky considered these same facts as capable of shedding light on the *basic patterns* of the ontogenesis of memory. Consequently, the main difference between Binet and Vygotsky is a difference in their initial theoretical positions. How was it possible for Vygotsky to develop a theoretical position on the basis of an analogy with the tools of labor?

The fact that tools play a central role in the process of labor has been noted by many thinkers, among whom one can name Bacon,[9] Franklin, and others. For Vygotsky, the position developed by Engels in the *Dialectics of Nature* was particularly important in this respect. However, an important question arises here. Given that the tools of labor play a decisive role in the structure and genesis of labor activity, why did Vygotsky propose that their analogues exist in the domain of the mind as so-called psychological tools? It is of course possible to search for these analogies, but even if they are found, on what basis is it possible to propose that psychological tools play such a decisive role in the structure of genesis of mental functions?

In our view, only one answer is possible. If one does not assume that the mind is determined by labor activity, then the introduction into psychology of psychological tools *as nothing more than an analogy with the processes of labor* can represent only a fortuitous step that is completely incompatible with Vygotsky's fundamental methodological search for an explanatory principle in his theory. If one considers the fact that, in Vygotsky's opinion, the mind is determined by labor activity, and the category of practical activity is the general explanatory principle of his theory, then his hypothesis becomes completely justified and logical.[10]

As noted earlier, Vygotsky always opposed the conception of direct, unmediated determination in psychology (and in methodology) as a kind of reductionism. This applies to the present case.[11] The hypothesis of the determination of mind through activity placed human practical activity and mental functions in a relationship of phylogentic continuity. For Vygotsky, this hypothesis proposed a resemblance between the structure of labor activity and the structure of mental processes.[12]

In the analysis of the determination of mind through practical activity, Vygotsky relied on a Marxist idea. He singled out the presence of tool mediation as the structurally and genetically central feature of labor activity. He proposed the possibility of an analogue to this in the structure and genesis of mental functions. Vygotsky *consciously* searched for psychological tools (he by no means accidentally discovered them through an arbitrary analogy) and gave them major significance.[13]

No less important is the question of why Vygotsky chose the sign as the concrete embodiment of psychological tools. This led to the fact that in the 1930s *meaning* became the unit of mental life for Vygotsky. Here again, one should follow the course of Vygotsky the methodologist: In analyzing the unit, it is necessary to specify the idea of an explanatory principle.

In Vygotsky's semiotic analysis it was no accident that the sign appeared as a psychological tool. It was the result of a conscious theoretical position. The fact that "stimuli–means" (the original designation of "psychological tools") having meaning (that is, they are *signs*) was "discovered" by Vygotsky in the course of experiments on generalization (Leont'ev and Luria, 1956). However, this can hardly be called a "discovery" in the empirical sense of the word. It was not a discovery but another step in the examination motivated by his general theoretical inclination.

It is indisputable that the semiotic ideas with which Vygotsky became acquainted beginning in 1910 influenced his formulation of this issue.

However, we are interested not in providing a detailed analysis of these influences, but in the question of the extent to which this type of semiotic interpretation of psychological tools conforms with the concept of activity as an explanatory principle in psychological theory. It is precisely in this respect that criticism of Vygotsky arose (including criticism from his students) for pursuing a non–activity-oriented approach and for the contradictory nature of his work.

In our opinion, the very idea of *sign meaning,* as an important concept in psychological theory, *does not contradict* the idea of activity as a general explanatory principle. On the contrary, the concept of sign creates one of the interesting paths for developing the explanatory principle of activity. Indeed, if one accepts as the basis of psychological theory the concept of historically evolving object-practical activity (carried out by humankind), and assumes that this activity determines the genesis, structure, and contents of the human mind, then communicative sign systems that emerge as a product of this activity can reasonably be considered as a specific form of this type of determination.

The idea of mediated determination rooted in activity that follows from Vygotsky's general methodological position corresponds with modern methodological notions. In the future it may be possible for a homogeneous theory to arise in which activity will function as an explanatory principle relevant to the sign system (the product of activity), while the sign system will function as the vehicle of determination that mediates mental functions. Of course, one should keep in mind that sign systems are not in any sense the sole vehicle of determination through activity.

The present position can be considered complete and self-evaluated in the activity oriented approach. It reveals one of the important boundaries of the category of activity in psychology. In this sense these notions do not introduce any contradiction into Vygotsky's work. Nor do they contradict the activity-oriented approach in any way. The fact that studies of the sign-mediated nature of mental functions have not been developed further in the activity-oriented approach can be considered as a weakness that needs to be overcome in the near future.

However, this question has another aspect as well. Up to this point we have spoken only about the researcher's initial methodological inclination. To what extent was this initial position present in Vygotsky's work? It seems to us that Vygotsky's understanding of the problem of "sign and meaning" in his concrete works went considerably beyond his initial methodological program, particularly in the later stages of his work. In Vygotsky's last works, the problem of meaning acquired an independent character, while the idea of activity as an explanatory principle and the idea of determination through activity (even if indirectly) was not represented as logically necessary. However, it was implicit in all his works. Precisely in this connection, several authors (e.g. Gal'perin, 1970; Leont'ev and Luria, 1956) have repeatedly noted the internal contradictions in the later works of Vygotsky. This is a contradiction between the basic methodological–philosophical position and its realization. It is important to understand the causes of this contradiction (not only for historical purposes, but also when considering prospects for further research).

It is possible to understand these causes if one utilizes the method of analyzing scientific theories developed by Vygotsky. Vygotsky created the explanatory principle of activity in the Marxist philosophical tradition. He called for analyzing psychological theory in a reverse sequence, from the philosophical tradition to concrete scientific formulations, at every stage checking the logic of the formulation of the theory with the logic of the original philosophical tradition. The more monolithic and organic a psychological theory becomes, the nearer the logic of the two domains coincides.

In this context, Vygotsky encountered a difficulty that was unknown to him, but practically insurmountable. We have already spoken about the fact that the Marxist theory of activity had not been reconstructed in any detail by philosophers and psychologists in the 1920s. Therefore, Vygotsky was not able to rely on it to any degree.[14] Even the *dialectical logic* of Marxism had not been sufficiently elaborated.

In this time Lenin (1969) wrote: "If Marx did not leave 'Logic' (writ large), then he left the *logic* of *Capital*" (p. 301). But it was necessary to reconstruct this dialectical logic of Marxism. Soviet philosophy attained outstanding successes in this, above all in the works of Rozental' (1960), Kedrov (1969), and especially Il'enkov (1960). But this occurred 25–30 years after Vygotsky's death. Vygotsky himself, despite the dialectics inherent in his thinking, was not able to solve this problem.

This problem has a wider and more fundamental character. In essence, the analogy between "processes of labor" and "mental processes" or between "tools of labor" and "psychological tools" is more formal than dialectical. It must be viewed as a first attempt to solve the problem, rather than a finished element in the organic system of Marxist psychology. Apparently, Vygotsky himself viewed the situation in this way. It is no coincidence that he did not call his theory a complete system of Marxist psychology.

The "gap" between the basic Marxist orientation and concrete psychological results was too great to be overcome by a single investigator under these conditions. The actual situation concerning Vygotsky's ideas was such that it is only today, on the basis of a reconstructed Marxist philosophical theory of activity and dialectical logic, that we are able to attempt to answer the question posed by Vygotsky. That is, we are able to develop the activity-oriented approach in psychology, relying on a dialectical logic adequate for the problem.

To summarize our analysis we emphasize the following points:

1. In Vygotsky's work one must separate two aspects, the methodological and the psychological. They form a logical rather than a chronological sequence. Vygotsky the methodologist formulated the normative requirements for the construction and analysis of psychological theories. Vygotsky the psychologist sought to realize this methodological program and attained results in the form of the creation of a concrete psychological theory.

2. Among the basic ideas of Vygotsky the methodologist, one must include the following:

a. The development in psychological theories of: (i) the category of an "explanatory principle" that reflects a reality and on the basis of which the totality of mental processes is explained; (ii) the category of an "object of study" (based on the example of various psychological theories); and (iii) an analysis of the dynamics of the relations between these categories.

b. The conception of the philosophical origin of explanatory principles, the demand for the elaboration and corresponding analyses of psychological theories as organic systems, proceeding from their philosophical premises to their concrete scientific conclusions; at every stage the logic of analysis must correspond to the logic of the philosophical tradition from which it arose;

c. Antisubstantionalism and antireductionism; the understanding of determination not as direct, substantial, and reductionistic, but as mediated, functional, and genetic;

d. The conception of object-practical activity (in its Marxist interpretation) as the reality that determines the mind, and the conception of the category of activity as the explanatory principle of psychological theory.

3. The basic contradiction in Vygotsky's work is connected with the contradiction between his methodological and psychological works. In the 1920s, the Marxist theory of activity was not sufficiently reconstructed by psychologists, and dialectical logic was not elaborated by philosophers. Therefore, Vygotsky was not able to realize his methodological program. His concrete psychological theory did not completely reflect his own normative requirements for psychological theories.

4. Nonetheless, in accordance with its goal Vygotsky's psychological theory can be considered an extremely valuable contribution to the activity-oriented approach. The basic ideas here were the following:

a. Mental processes (their genesis and structure) are determined by humanity's historically developed, object-practical activity that incorporates tools;

b. This determination proposes an analogy between the structure of external (labor) activity and mental functions (the hypothesis of "psychological tools");

c. The conception of determination as the mediating mechanism in ontogenesis and phylogenesis; the vehicles of determination; the "psychological tools" including such products of the historical activity of humanity as signs and communicative systems (this presented the opportunity for applying semiotic ideas in psychology).

The problems we have considered clearly have a practical as well as historical significance for the activity-oriented approach in Soviet psychology (and more broadly, for Soviet psychology in general). This is because of the fact that neither Vygotsky's general methodological position nor the unified system of psychological ideas he was developing has been sufficiently reconstructed in psychology after this death. We will summarize several of the best known examples.

1. After Vygotsky's death, his students provided a detailed elaboration of the basic line of his work, that is, the activity-oriented approach in psychology (true, the activity-oriented approach of Vygotsky himself was insufficiently analyzed). Following Vygotsky, they saw in object activity the general explanatory principle of psychological theory. It was precisely in this context that the well-known three-part scheme, "activity–action–operation," was developed. But subsequently, this scheme was more and more frequently accepted as the object of study. Thus there was a merging of two methodological functions. There was a confusion on the explanatory principle and the object of study. In addition, this confusion was neither identified nor realized. [This feature was first noted only in the 1970s by Yudin (1978).] The possibility in principle of this type of methodological inaccuracy was analyzed by Vygotsky in the 1920s in connection with the origins of the theory of activity (moreover, as indicated above, he elaborated the category of activity as an explanatory principle precisely in order to overcome this type of methodological mistake).

2. The idea of the sign systems was not assimilated by the approach that dominated the activity-oriented approach to psychology after Vygotsky. The roots of this idea in the theory of activity were not recognized. The idea was considered to be contradictory to the activity-oriented approach. Its renunciation was seen as a step forward in comparison with Vygotsky. But if the polemic with concrete works of Vygotsky on the problem of the sign was necessary and natural, the removal of this problematic – in principle – led only to a substantial "narrowing" of the theory of activity. The cause of this narrowing lies in the fact that one of the basic features of Vygotsky's scientific world view was not identified. We refer specifically to his constant appeal to the search for mediated rather than direct determination in psy-

chology at all levels, as well as his well-known strong repudiation of the "postulate of immediacy," which he raised to the rank of a basic philosophical and methodological principle. Every determination in psychology (in particular the determination of historically developed activity) of the genesis and structure of the human mind, according to Vygotsky, must be of a mediated nature. He attempted to outline one of the possible mechanisms of such mediation in his idea of the sign.

3. In psychology, formal logic prevailed both before and after Vygotsky's time. This is apparent both in analogies with natural sciences and in the very approach to the resolution of concrete psychological problems. A vivid example here is instructional psychology. The idea of mastering knowledge through generalization from the concrete to the abstract is a typical case of the formal–logical and empirical approach to psychology. In the 1930s, Vygotsky, in a work on the formation of generalizations, demolished that approach. He showed its inadequacy relative to the actual psychological processes of the formation of abstractions, and indicated the solution is in an appeal to dialectic logic (see Davydov, 1966). However, this approach began to be elaborated only in the 1960s under direct influence of Vygotsky's ideas. It was elaborated from the very point where it was left off in the 1930s, on the basis of the newly developed apparatus of dialectic logic (see Davydov, 1972).

The example of instructional psychology is characteristic. It seems to us that many branches of psychology (first and foremost general psychology and psychological methodology) are in the same position as instructional psychology at the beginning of the 1960s. Precisely as a result of this the 1980s can become the years of the Vygotsky "renaissance." Psychology (above all the theory of activity of Vygotsky, Leont'ev, and Luria) has reached the point in its development when it is experiencing the necessity, and has the potential, to assimilate the methodological standard of Vygotsky and to develop his concrete ideas on the basis of modern methodology and logic.

NOTES

1 Here, as in Soviet psychology in general, application of the terms "methodology," and "methodologist" is not restricted to problems of designing and conducting empirical research. Rather, these terms are used to refer to the study of general theoretical and metatheoretical issues that underlie any investigation of psychological phenomena. [J.V.W.]

2 We will not evaluate these schools from the point of view of their role in the development of psychology in the Soviet Union or throughout the world. Analyses of this problem have already been carried out by historians of Soviet

psychology (e.g., Budilova, 1972; Petrovskii, 1967; Smirnov, 1975). We touch on these schools only in order to outline the situation in which Vygotsky worked. If they are not taken into consideration, it is impossible to understand his work.

3   It is not difficult to find many other statements by Vygotsky on this issue. In 1933 he said, "Psychology defined itself as the science of consciousness [here he was dealing with a subjective–empirical psychology of consciousness], but psychology says almost nothing about consciousness" (1968a, p. 182). What Vygotsky saw as the defect of previous psychological research was not the paucity of factual knowledge, but false beginning positions and a misguided search for such factual knowledge. This is reflected in an even stronger statement by Leont'ev. He wrote, "Vygotsky will say that psychology *called* itself the science of consciousness, but *it never was such a science*" (Leont'ev, 1959, p. 16).

4   The fate of this manuscript is interesting. It has been well known to a wide circle of Soviet psychologists since the late 1920s and early 1930s (many references, although not always accurate, to "Vygotsky's manuscript on the crisis in psychology" as well as various sections of it can be found in the works of Leont'ev, Luria, and others). However, it was not actually analyzed until the 1970s. The first attempts to examine this work were undertaken by Yaroshevskii and Gurgenidze (1977). Without going into detail on their interesting interpretation we can simply point out the basic fact that they concluded that Vygotsky was an outstanding methodologist of science and one of the predecessors of contemporary scientific inquiry. This manuscript appeared in 1982 in the first volume of a six-volume collection of Vygotsky's work.

5   Once again, we would point out that this formula in essence is a generalization and explication of Vygotsky's analysis of consciousness. Indeed, the main methodological mistake of traditional psychological treatments of consciousness is that instead of going beyond the boundaries of its basic concept (the object of study) the explanatory principle coincides with it.

6   "Opoyaz" (an abbreviation for Obshchestvo izucheniya poeticheskogo yazyka [Society for the Study of Poetic Language]) was one of the leading discussion groups in Russian Formalism. It began meeting in 1915–16 in Leningrad. Among its active members were Yakubinskii, Polivanov, Shklovskii, and Eikhenbaum. As Radzikhovskii (1979b) notes, Vygotsky's cousin, David Vygodsky, was in close contact with membrs of Opoyaz, a fact that indicates that Vygotsky was at least kept up to date on its discussions. Vygotsky's disagreements with members of Opoyaz are formulated in the first volume he wrote (Vygotsky, 1968b). [J.V.W.]

7   For a more detailed account of this issue see Ivanov (1968, 1976).

8   It is therefore no accident that the evolution of Vygotsky's approach to psychology is usually described as the evolution of his ideas about "psychological tools." It is this that is seen as the center and unique point in his theory. Vygotsky (1968a) himself made this point. He divided his work into two periods: before and after he began to consider "psychological tools" (signs) as having meaning.

9   One of Bacon's insightful formulae was especially close to Vygotsky's ideas. Vygotsky used it as an epigraph for his "Studies in the History of Behavior" and in general cited it quite often. This formula is: "Neither the hand by itself nor reason in and of itself has any great power. This issue is one of tools and aids" (Bacon, 1978, p. 12).

10   This idea has already been proposed in the literature on the history of psychology, especially by Yaroshevskii (1976).
11   It was precisely this that Vygotsky's critics [Talankin (1931) and others] did not understand in the 1930s. They accused him of proposing non-Marxist views. In particular, they accused him of not recognizing how labor activity determines mental processes. In their own way they were correct. Vygotsky indeed never recognized determination in the form that they did, in the form of direct and simple dependency. He did not recognize determination as a simple reduction of mind to labor activity. On the basis of such notions of determination these critics of Vygotsky tried to develop several original conceptualizations (e.g., Talankin's "historical labor" theory).
12   Thus it was here that Vygotsky identified the proximity between the structure of external activity and mental functions. This had an influence on the analogous ideas developed later by Leont'ev (1975).
13   Vygotsky clearly evaluated the importance for his theory of the claim that an activity-based determination of mind played a central role. We are not considering his declarations and self-evaluations that are based on a single standard, although they undoubtedly are of interest. We will introduce only one of many statements. "It is impossible to assume that labor is not tied to a change in the type of human behavior if we agree with Engels that 'the tool implies specific human activity, the transforming reaction of man on nature, production.' Is it possible that in the psychology of the human nothing corresponds to the distinction in nature that separates humans from animals?" (Vygotsky, 1960b, pp. 80–81).
14   In recent years the development of a theory of sign systems in the theory of activity (e.g., Shchedrovitskii, 1964) has made considerable progress.

REFERENCES

Bacon, F. 1978. [New organon.] In F. Bacon, *Sochineniya v 2-kh tomakh.* [Essays in two volumes.] Moscow: Mysl'.

Binet, A. 1922. *L'étude expérimentale de l'intelligence.* Paris: Costes.

Budilova, E. A. 1972. *Filosofskie problemy v sovetskoi psikhologii.* [Philosophical problems in Soviet psychology.] Moscow: Nauka.

Chelpanov, G. I. 1925. *Psikhologiya i marksizm.* [Psychology and Marxism.] Moscow: Russkii Knizhnik.

Davydov, V. V. 1966. [The problem of generalization in the works of L. S. Vygotsky.] *Voprosy Psikhologii* [Problems in psychology], *6,* 42–45.

Davydov, V. V. 1972. *Vidy obobshcheniya v obuchenii.* [Forms of generalization in instruction.] Moscow: Pedagogika.

Davydov, V. V. 1979. [The category of activity in mental reflection in A. N. Leont'ev's theory.] *Vestnik MGU. Psikhologiya* [Reports of MGU: Psychology], *4,* 25–41.

El'konin, D. B. 1966. [The problem of instruction and development in Vygotsky's works.] *Voprosy Psikhologii* [Problems in psychology], pp. 33–42.

Gal'perin, P. Ya. 1970. [Introduction to Vygotsky's article: Spinoza and his doctrine of the passions in light of modern psychoneurology.] *Voprosy Filosofii* [Problems in philosophy], *6,* 119–120.

Il'enkov, E. V. 1960. *Dialektika abstraktnogo i konkretnogo v "Kapitale" Marksa.* [The dialectics of the abstract and concrete in Marx's *Kapital.*] Moscow: Izdatel'stvo Akademii Nauk SSSR.

Ivanov, V. V. 1968. [Commentary on Vygotsky's ьook: *1ne psychology of art.*] in L. S. Vygotsky, *Psikhologiya iskusstva.* [The psychology of art.] Moscow: Iskusstvo. (Translated as Commentary by V. V. Ivanov in L. S. Vygotsky, *The psychology of art.* Cambridge: MIT Press, 1971.)

Ivanov, V. V. 1976. *Ocherki po istorii semiotiki v SSSR.* [Essays on the history of semiotics in the USSR.] Moscow: Nauka.

James, W. 1913. [Does consciousness exist?] In *Novye idei v filosofii.* [New ideas in philosophy.] Petersburg: Saint-Petersburg, 4.

Kedrov, V. M. 1969. [Dialectical logic as a generalization of the history of natural science.] In *Ocherki istorii i teorii razvitiya nauki.* [Essays on the history and theory of the development of science.] Moscow: Nauka.

Kornilov, K. N. 1925. [Modern psychology and Marxism]. In K. N. Kornilov (Ed.), *Psikhologiya i marksizm.* [Psychology and Marxism.] Moscow–Leningrad: Gosizdat.

Kornilov, K. N. 1926. *Uchebnik psikhologii, izlozhennoi c tochki zreniya dialekticheskogo materializma.* [A textbook for psychology, presented from the perspective of dialectical materialism.] Leningrad: Gosizdat.

Lenin, V. I. 1969. *Polnye sobrannye sochineniya.* [Complete collected works (Vol. 29).] Moscow: Politizdat.

Leont'ev A. N. 1934. [L. S. Vygotsky.] *Sovetskaya Psikho-neurologiya* [Soviet psychoneurology], *6,* 187–190.

Leont'ev, A. N. 1959. *Problemy razvitiya psikhiki.* [Problems in the development of mind.] Moscow: Izdatel'stvo Akademii Pedagogicheskikh Nauk RSFSR. (Translated as A. N. Leont'ev, *Problems in the development of mind.* Moscow: Progress, 1981.)

Leont'ev, A. N. 1967. [The struggle for the problem of consciousness in the making of Soviet psychology.] *Voprosy Psikhologii* [Problems in psychology], *2,* 14–23.

Leont'ev, A. N. 1975. *Deyatel'nost', Soznanie, Lichnost'.* [Activity, Consciousness, Personality.] Moscow: Izdatel'stvo Politicheskoi Literatury. (Translated as A. N. Leont'ev, *Activity, consciousness, and personality,* Englewood Cliffs, N.J.: Prentice Hall, 1978.)

Leont'ev A. N. and Luria, A. R. 1956. [L. S. Vygotsky's view of psychology.] In L. S. Vygotsky, *Izbrannye psikhologicheskie issledovaniya.* [Selected psychological research.] Moscow: Izdatel'stvo Akademii Pedagogicheskikh Nauk RSFSR. (Translated as A. N. Leont'ev and A. R. Luria, The psychological ideas of L. S. Vygotskii. In B. B. Wolman (Ed.), *The historical roots of contemporary psychology,* New York: Harper & Row, 1968.)

Müller-Freienfels, R. 1922. *Psychologie der Kunst* (Vol. 1). Leipzig–Berlin: Teubner.

Petrovskii, A. V. 1967. *Istoriya sovetskoi psikhologii.* [The history of Soviet psychology.] Moscow: Prosveshchenie.

Radzikhovskii, L. A. 1979a. [The analysis of Vygotsky's work by Soviet psychologists.] *Voprosy Psikhologii* [Problems in psychology], *6,* 58–67.

Radzikhovskii, L. A. 1979b. [Fundamental stages in Vygotsky's scientific work.] State University (Moscow), doctoral (Kandidatskaya) dissertation.

Rozental', M. M. 1960. *Printsipy dialekticheskoi logiki.* [Principles of dialectical logic.] Moscow: Sotsekgiz.

Shchedrovitskii, G. P. 1964. *Problemy metodologii sistemnogo issledovaniya.* [Problems in the methodology of systems research.] Moscow: Znanie.

Smirnov, A. A. 1975. *Razvitie i sovremennoe sostoyanie psikhologicheskoi nauki v SSSR.* [The development and current state of psychology in the USSR.] Moscow: Pedagogika.

Talankin, A. A. 1931. [A turning point on the psychological front.] *Sovetskaya psikhoneurologiya* [Soviet psychoneurology], *2–3,* 8–23.

Tkachenko, A. N. 1980. [The problem of the initial unit in the analysis of mind in the history of Soviet psychology (1920 – 1940).] *Voprosy Psikhologii* [Problems in psychology], *3*, 155 – 159.

Vygotsky, L. S. 1925. [Consciousness as a problem in the psychology of behavior.] In K. N. Kornilov (Ed.), *Psikhologiya i marksizm.* [Psychology and Marxism.] Moscow–Leningrad: Gosizdat. [Translated as L. S. Vygotsky, Consciousness as a problem in the psychology of behavior, *Soviet psychology, 27*(4), 1979, 3–35.]

Vygotsky, L. S. 1926. [The method of reflexological and psychological research.] In K. N. Kornilov (Ed.), *Problemy sovremennoi psikhologii.* [Problems in contemporary psychology.] Leningrad: Gosizdat.

Vygotsky, L. S. 1928. [The problem of the cultural development of the child.] *Pedologiya, 1,* 58–77.

Vygotsky, L. S. 1934, *Myshlenie i rech'.* [Thinking and speech.] Moscow: Sozekgiz. (Translated as L. S. Vygotsky, *Thought and language.* Cambridge: MIT Press, 1962.)

Vygotsky, L. S. 1960a. [The instrumental method in psychology.] In L. S. Vygotsky, *Razvitie vysshikh psikhicheskikh funktsii.* [The development of higher mental functions.] Moscow: Izdatel'stvo Akademii Pedagogicheskikh Nauk RSFSR. [Translated as L. S. Vygotsky, The instrumental method in psychology, in J. V. Wertsch (Ed.), *The concept of activity in Soviet psychology.* Armonk, N.Y.: Sharpe, 1981.]

Vygotsky, L. S. 1960b. [The history of the development of higher mental functions.] In L. S. Vygotsky, *Razvitie vysshikh psikhicheskikh funktsii.* [The development of higher mental functions.] Moscow: Izdatel'stvo Akademii Pedagogicheskikh Nauk RSFSR.

Vygotsky, L. S. 1968a. [From unpublished materials. Vygotsky's presentations on a paper by A. R. Luria on December 5 and 9, 1933.] In A. A. Leont'ev (Ed.), *Psikhologiya Grammatiki.* [The psychology of grammar.] Moscow: Izdatel'stvo Moskovskogo Universiteta.

Vygotsky, L. S. 1968b. *Psikhologiya iskusstva.* [The psychology of art.] Moscow: Iskusstvo. (Translated as L. S. Vygotsky, *The psychology of art.* Cambridge: MIT Press, 1971.)

Vygotsky, L. S. 1982. *Istoricheskii smysl psikhologicheskogo krizisa.* [The historical significance of the crisis in psychology.] In L. S. Vygotsky *Sobranie sochinenii.* [Collected essays (Vol. 1.)] Moscow: Pedagogika.

Yaroshevskii, M. G. 1976. *Istoriya psikhologii.* [The history of psychology.] Moscow: Mysl'.

Yaroshevskii, M. G. and Gurgenidze, G. S. 1977. [Vygotsky: An investigator of problems in the methodology of science.] *Voprosy Filosofii* [Problems in philosophy], *8,* 91–106.

Yudin, E. G. 1978. *Sistemnyi podkhod i printsip deyatel'nosti.* [The systems approach and the principle of activity.] Moscow: Izdatel'stvo Moskovskogo Universiteta.

Zinchencko, P. I. 1939. [The problem of involuntary memory.] *Nauchnie zapiski Khar'kovskogo gosudarstvennogo pedagogicheskogo instituta inostrannykh yazykov.* [The scientific record of the Khar'kov State Pedagogical Institute of Foreign Languages (Vol. 1).] Khar'kov.

3

Intellectual origins of Vygotsky's semiotic analysis

BENJAMIN LEE

Vygotsky was a polymath; his intellectual interests included not only psychology, but also Marxism, neurophysiology, art (his first book is on the psychology of art), and literature. His intellectual influences range among such diverse figures as the Russian Formalists, Sergei Eisenstein, Husserl, Marx, Edward Sapir, and Pavlov. Borrowing a phrase from Bakhtin, Vygotsky was a "polyphonic" thinker who wove a subtle tapestry of ideas carefully chosen from the intellectual fabric of his times.

His life goal was to create a psychology that would be theoretically and methodologically adequate for the investigation of all aspects of human consciousness. Like many original and profound thinkers, his followers have tended to restrict themselves to one or another aspect of his thought. Soviet psychologists have, of course, emphasized the Marxist aspects of his work, and see him as the founder of a modern theory of activity. American researchers have focused on his work on language and thought and neglected his Marxist and functionalist side. By isolating the contributions of his work to one or another school of psychology, this division of research labor mislocates the contemporary significance of Vygotsky's ideas. His greatest importance probably lies neither in his Marxism nor in his psycholinguistic work, but rather in the profound and unique way he introduces a communicative dimension to Marxist conceptions of practical activity, thereby providing the foundation for a semiotic and functionalist psychology. This line of thought would situate his contributions not only among psychologists, but also with such semioticians as Charles Sanders Peirce, Roman Jakobson, Mikhail Bakhtin, and Benjamin Whorf.

Marx and Vygotsky

Vygotsky's life goal was to create a psychology that would be theoretically and methodologically adequate for the investigation of consciousness. Since the analysis of consciousness is also a critical point in Marxist theories, it is not surprising that Vygotsky uses many of Marx's ideas about the relationship between consciousness and practical activity at the societal level and then applies them to problems in the psychological analysis of consciousness.

I want to find out how science has to be built, to approach the study of the mind having learned the whole of Marx's method. . . .In order to create such an enabling theory-method in the generally accepted scientific manner, it is necessary to discover the essence of the given area of phenomena, the laws according to which they change, their qualitative and quantitative characteristics, their causes. It is necessary to formulate the categories and concepts that are specifically relevant to them – in other words to create one's own *Capital.* (Vygotsky 1978, p. 8)

Vygotsky and Marx share several basic assumptions about the relationships between consciousness and activity. First, they both insisted that the analysis of consciousness must start with practical activity. Consciousness is constructed through a subject's interactions with the world and is an attribute of the relationship between subject and object. Second, the basic components of an analysis of practical activity must be interpreted in a functional form. Third, consciousness changes as the organization of practical activity changes, entailing that an adequate study of consciousness must be historical or genetic. Finally, new levels of the organization of practical activity and consciousness presuppose different principles of organization and development.

Thesis 1: interactions

Marx saw his work as a critique of problems raised by the idealism of Hegel and materialism of Feuerbach.

The main shortcoming of all materialism . . . is that the object, the reality, sensibility, is conceived only in the form of the object or of perception, but not as sensuous human activity, practice, not subjectively. Hence the active side was developed abstractly in opposition to materialism by idealism, which naturally does not know the real, sensuous activity as such. Feuerbach urged the real distinction between sensuous activity and thought objects; but he does not conceive of human activity itself as an objective activity. (Marx, quoted in Avineri, 1968 pp 68–69)

Marx's solution was to develop an interactionist viewpoint of the relation between consciousness and activity. Man shapes, changes, and creates reality, and consciousness is an integral part of this process. Subject and object are created by their constant interaction in practical activity.

Men are the producers of their conceptions, ideas, etc. – real, active men, as they are conditioned by a definite development of their productive forces and of the intercourse corresponding to these, up to its furthest forms. Consciousness can never be anything else than conscious existence and the existence of men is their actual life process. (Marx, 1959, p. 247)

Vygotsky began his analysis of consciousness with a critique of the counterparts to materialism and idealism in the psychological theories of his day. He rejected the radical empiricist reductionism espoused by Bekhterev who insisted that all behavior could be analyzed as combinations of reflexes and therefore saw consciousness as an unnecessary concept. On the other hand, Vygotsky believed that the subjective–idealist approach was incapable of supporting a science of psychology because of its use of introspection as its main source of data. "Vulgar behaviorism" reduces consciousness to an attribute of the physical aspects of behavior, whereas subjective idealism reifies it into some form of mental substance. Both positions in some sense "objectify" consciousness by not seeing it as a relation between subject and object. Marx believed that various forms of social consciousness are attributes of and determined by the organization of the productive forces and relations of a given society at a given moment in history. Vygotsky's solution at the psychological level was like Marx's at the societal level: Consciousness is neither reducible to behavior nor separate from it, but is instead an attribute of the organization of practical activity.

Thesis 2: functionalism

According to Marx, different forms of social consciousness are attributes of and determined by the organization of the productive forces and relations of a given society at a given moment in history. At the level of society, practical activity is analyzed in terms of production.

This mode of production must not be considered simply as being the reproduction of the physical existence of the individuals. Rather it is a definite form of activity of these individuals, a definite form of expressing their life, a definite mode of life on their part. As individuals express their life, so they are. What they are, therefore, coincides with their production, both with what they produce and how they produce. The nature of individuals thus depends on the material conditions determining their production. (Marx, quoted in Avineri, 1968, p. 73)

Marx's analysis of production is functionalist and involves showing that production and consumption cannot be defined without showing the role each plays with respect to the other. Vygotsky used this form of definition in his idea of a functionalist psychology in which the definition of all psychological states and processes presuppose one another.

A functional analysis of a given item consists in showing what role or effect that item has in some system of which it is a part. Although many types of functional systems exist, the most interesting for Marx and Vygotsky would be those systems which are made up of interfunctinal connections among their various subsystems. Each such subsystem would depend upon the effect or relation it has with some other subsystems, and it is precisely because of these interconnections that each element exists. The various subsystems both presuppose and create each other. The overall system would be analyzed in terms of how its various subsystems were functionally interconnected.

Marx's analysis of production is functionalist in the above sense. Production consists of two mutually defining aspects – production consumption – each of which presupposes the other and provides some aspect that is logically necessary for the existence of the other portion of the cycle of production.

Production, then, is also immediately consumption, consumption is also immediately production. Each is immediately its opposite. But at the same time a mediating moment takes place between the two. Production mediates consumption; it creates the latter's material; without it, consumption would lack an object. But consumption also mediates production, in that it alone creates for the products the subject for whom they are products. (Marx, 1973, p. 91)

Marx points out that there are at least three levels of "identity" or interfunctional connection between production and consumption. First, every act of production "consumes" the means of production through wear and tear and also involves the expenditure of labor. On the other hand, every act of consumption involves production because it "produces human beings in some particular aspect" (Marx, 1973) in a manner similar to the way digestion "produces" the person.

Second, each one is mediated by the other, and they are therefore mutually dependent and presuppose each other, while preserving their independence as subsystems.

[There is] a movement which relates them to one another and makes them appear indispensable to one another but still leaves them external to one each other. Production creates the material, as external object, for consumption; consumption creates the need, as internal object, as aim, for production. Without production, no consumption; without consumption no production. (Marx, 1973, p. 93)

Finally, besides there being a mutual presupposition or dependency between production and consumption, each creates essential aspects of the other.

Each of them, apart from being immediately the other, and apart from mediating the other, in addition to this creates the other in completing itself, and creates itself as the other. Consumption accomplishes the act of production only in completing the product as product by dissolving it, by consuming its independently material form, by raising the inclination developed in the first act of production, through the need for repetition, to its finished form; it is thus not only the concluding act in which the product becomes product, but also that in which the producer becomes producer. On the other side, production produces consumption by creating the stimulus of consumption, the ability to consume, as a need. (Marx, 1973, p. 93)

Vygotsky similarly maintained that all psychological states are functionally interrelated by consciousness.

Memory necessarily presupposes the activity of attention, perception, and comprehension. Perception necessarily includes the function of attention, recognition or memory, and understanding. However, in previous as well as contemporary psychology, this obviously correct idea of the functional unity of consciousness and the indissoluble connection of the various forms of its activity has remained on the periphery. (Vygotsky, 1965, p. 243)

Consciousness is the process that organizes behavior. The investigator can observe how behavior is organized, how it changes according to the context in which it occurs, and how it is connected with other behavior. From this starting point he must not only make hypotheses about what psychological representations and processes are necessary to explain the behavior, but also how they are functionally organized with respect to one another.

Vygotsky recognized the implications of a functionalist psychology. He criticized much of the psychological research of his time for its "atomistic" and "piecemeal" analysis of psychological processes. Such work did not investigate the functional connections between psychological processes and states and thus completely bypassed the study of consciousness.

The atomistic and functional analysis that has dominated scientific psychology in recent decades has resulted in the examination of individual psychological functions in isolation. . . .The problem of the connections among these functions, the problem of their organization in the overall structure of consciousness has remained outside the field of investigators' attention. (Vygotsky, 1956, p. 43)

By "functional" Vygotsky was here referring to Thorndike's "faculty" psychology. Consciousness is not an attribute of any particular state or process such as attention or memory, but rather an attribute of the way in which such states are organized and functionally related both to behavior and each other. The atomistic study of psychological functions not only does not investigate consciousness, but it also fails to see that the very processes it studies depend upon the integrative characteristics of consciousness. Consciousness establishes the connections between the various processes, thereby giving them a certain unity and continuity – in organizing such processes, consciousness both creates them and transforms them.

The unity of consciousness and the interrelation of all psychological functions, were, it is true, accepted by all; the single functions were assumed to operate inseparably, in an uninterrupted connection with one another. But in the old psychology the unchallengeable premise of unity was combined with a set of tacit assumptions that nullified it for all practical purposes. It was taken for granted that the relation between two given functions never varied: that perception, for example, was always connected in an identical way with attention, memory with perception, thought with memory. As constants, these relationships could be, and were, factored out and ignored in the study of the separate functions. Because the relationships remained in fact inconsequential, the development of consciousness was seen as determined by the autonomous development of single functions. Yet all that is known about psychic development indicates that its very essence lies in the change of the interfunctional structure of consciousness. (Vygotsky, 1962, pp. 1–2)

Thesis 3: dialectical nature of consciousness

Marx also insisted that consciousness changes as the organization of productive forces and relations develops. This development involves the continuous reorganization of these forces and relations, their gradual negation, and eventual incorporation and transformation at a new level of economic and social organization. As new levels of the organization of productive forces and relations develop, new forms of consciousness emerge. Particular economic social structures exist as moments in the dialectical interplay between productive forces and relations. This dialectic is a process that takes place in "real" time, and both organizes and creates the particular types of productive forces and relations existing in a given society at a given time. Because these forces and relations in turn structure consciousness, the study of consciousness must be both dialectical and have a historical or genetic dimension. Vygotsky insisted that at the psychological level, psychological processes must be studied genetically. At the level of individual psychology, development consists of stages of growth and consolidation that also obey dialectical laws of negation, incorporation, and transformation. Furthermore, later stages of development represent new levels in the organization of consciousness.

Our concept of development implies a rejection of the frequently held view that cognitive development results from the gradual accumulation of separate changes. We believe that child development is a complex dialectical process characterized by periodicity, unevenness in the development of different functions, metamorphosis or qualitative transformation of one form into another, intertwining of external and internal factors, and adaptive processes which overcome impediments that the child encounters. (1978, p. 73)

Vygotsky viewed development as the gradual reorganization of consciousness. This implies that the study of child development should investigate changes in the interfunctional relationships between psychological processes that in turn obey certain dialectical principles. There is a

dialectical law that in the course of development causes and effects become interchanged. Once higher mental formations have emerged from certain dynamic preconditions, these formations themselves influence the processes that spawned them. . . .Above all the interfunctional connections and relationships among various processes, in particular intellect and affect, change. (1956, p. 467)

The development of the child is "a dialectical process in which the transition from one step to another is accomplished not by evolutionary, but by a revolutionary path" (1972, p. 121). Because consciousness develops dialectically, the only adequate approach must be genetic.

We need to concentrate not on the product of development, but on the very process by which higher forms are established. . . . To encompass in research the process of a given thing's development in all its phases and changes is to discover its nature, its essence, for "it is only in movement that a body shows what it is." Thus the historical study of behavior is not an auxiliary aspect of theoretical study, but rather forms its very base. (1978, pp. 64–65)

Thesis 4: nature versus culture

Finally, both Marx and Vygotsky believed that new levels of the organization of consciousness followed different principles of development, and these principles depend upon differentiating between the social nature of human practical activity and the "natural" activity of animals. Marx insisted that what distinguished men from animals was that human productive labor was necessarily social whereas animal production and consumption were only contingently social. Principles of Darwinian evolution were adequate to explain the development of animal social organization, but the structure of human productive labor required the introduction of new principles of development, namely those of dialectical materialism. The emergence of the social nature of humans requires a new mode of analysis.

Vygotsky took this Marxist thesis and applied it to child development. He distinguished between a natural line of development, which includes the tool activity of primates and probably corresponds to Piaget's sensorimotor period, and a social line of development that is heavily dependent upon the child's acquisition of language. Vygotsky believed that the processes underlying the natural line of development were mostly subject to physiological laws of development along with some relatively simple principles of learning. The child's social line of development follows principles based upon the structure of communication. It is at this point that Marx's and Vygotsky's approaches converge. As the child moves from a "natural" line of development to the "social" line, he also becomes part of a social system whose evolution is governed by the principles of dialectical materialism.

It is my belief, based upon a dialectical materialist approach to the analysis of human history, that human behavior differs qualitatively from animal behavior to the same extent that the adaptability and historical development of humans differ from the adaptability and development of animals. (1978, p. 60)

For Marx, the major differences between men and animals lie in the nature of human consciousness and labor. First, people are aware of their relations with their environment and others, whereas animals are not.

My relationship to my surroundings is my consciousness. . . .For the animal, its relation to others does not exist as a relation. Consciousness is therefore, from the very beginning a social product and remains so as long as men exist at all. (Quoted in Avineri, 1968, p. 71)

Second, human labor is self-sustaining.

[Humans] themselves begin to distinguish themselves from animals as soon as they begin to produce their means of subsistence, a step which is conditioned by their physical organization. By producing their means of subsistence men are indirectly producing their actual material life. (Quoted in Avineri, 1968, p. 73)

These two theses lead to the position that human production differs from animal production in presupposing a different level of awareness. Human productive labor includes subjects who are aware of their relationships to others and their activities, and it is this awareness that guides their production.

Labour is, in the first place, a process in which both men and Nature participate, and in which man of his own accord states, regulates and controls the material reactions between himself and Nature. . . .By thus acting on the external world and changing it, he at the same time changes his own nature. He develops his slumbering powers and compels them to act in obedience to his sway. We are not now dealing with those primitive instinctive forms of labour that remind us of the mere animal. . . .We presuppose labour in a form that stamps it as exclusively human. A spider conducts operations that resemble those of a weaver, and a bee puts to shame many an architect on the construction of her cells. But what distinguishes the worst architect from the best of bees is this, that the architect raises his structure in imagination before he erects it in reality. At the end of the labour-process, we get a result that already existed in the imagination of the labourer at its commencement. (Quoted in Avineri, 1968, p. 81)

Marx, as his desire to dedicate the second volume of *Kapital* to Darwin indicates, believed that the evolution of animal "society" could be explained by Darwinian principles. Human society evolves through the dialectical interplay of productive forces and relations, both of which presuppose a level of social awareness not shared with animals.

Vygotsky saw two lines of development in the child. The first, or "nature" line, corresponds to that of the early uses of tools by primates described by Bühler.

Bühler interpreted the manifestations of practical intelligence in children as being of exactly the same type as those we are familiar with in chimpanzees, indeed, there is a phase in the life of the child that Bühler designated the "chimpanzee age." At a certain point, the child crosses over to a social-historical line of development –

"the type of development itself has changed from biological to socio-historical." (Vygotsky, 1956, p. 146)

This line overrides and transforms the "natural" line:

The cultural development of the child is characterized first by the fact that it transpires under conditions of dynamic organic changes. Cultural development is superimposed on the processes of growth, maturation, and the organic development of the child. It forms a single whole with these processes. It is only through abstraction that we can separate one set of processes from the other.

The growth of the normal child into civilization usually involves a fusion with the processes of his/her organic maturation. Both planes of development – the natural and the cultural – coincide and mingle with one another. The two lines of changes interpenetrate and in essence form a single line of socio-biological formation of the child's personality. (Vygotsky, 1960, p. 47)

At this point, individual psychological development obeys sociohistorical principles of evolution, based upon learning principles derivable neither from biology, nor, more importantly, from the level of individual psychological functioning. All the "higher" (by this Vygotsky means both more abstract and more generalized) mental functions are social in origin.

For the first time in psychology, we are facing the extremely important problem of the relationship of external and internal mental functions . . .everything internal in higher forms was external, i.e., for others it was what it now is for onself. Any higher mental function necessarily goes through an external stage in its development because it is initially a social function. This is the center of the whole problem of internal and external behavior. . . .When we speak of a process, "external" means "social." Any higher mental function was external because it was social at some point before becoming an internal, truly mental function. (Vygotsky, 1981, p. 162)

The semiotic dimension

In applying Marxist principles to psychological development, Vygotsky had to face the problem of how higher mental functions involving abstract thought develop. Among his contemporaries much was being made of the primitive tool-using capabilities of chimpanzees and apes that indicated that tool use, the psychological counterpart to labor at the social level, was not a distinctly human characteristic. Something else had to occur to lift the essentially noninstitutional, ahistorical, and asocial nature of animal tool use into its human form. Vygotsky's great contribution to the formulation of a Marxist psychology was his proposal that it is the semiotic mediation of tool use that creates the truly human forms of labor activity.

Although practical intelligence and sign use can operate independently of each other in young children, the dialectical unity of these systems in the human adult is the very essence of complex human behavior. Our analysis accords symbolic activity a specific organizing function that penetrates the process of tool use and produces fundamentally new forms of behavior. (Vygotsky, 1978, p. 24)

The semiotic mediation of practical activity, primarily through speech, transforms humans and creates the possibility of human society. Human labor differs from animal tool use because humans are aware of and plan their actions using historically transmitted and socially created means of production. This awareness and planning ability is a form of generalization made possible only through speech.

The most significant moment in the course of intellectual development, which gives birth to the purely human forms of practical and abstract intelligence, occurs when speech and practical activity, two previously completely independent lines of development, converge. Although children's use of tools during their preverbal period is comparable to that of apes, as soon as speech and the use of signs are incorporated into any action, the action becomes transformed and organized along entirely new lines. The specifically human use of tools is thus realized, going beyond the more limited use of tools possible among the higher animals.

Prior to mastering his own behavior, the child begins to master his surroundings with the help of speech. This produces new relations with the environment in addition to the new organization of behavior itself. The creation of these uniquely human forms of behavior later produce the intellect and become the basis of productive work: the specifically human form of the use of tools. (Vygotsky, 1978, pp. 24–25)

Language, as a historically determined social institution, is the means through which society converts the principles of cognitive development from biological to social dialectical.

We can now formulate the main conclusions to be drawn from our analysis. If we compare the early development of speech and of intellect – which we have seen develop along separate lines in animals and in very young children – with the development of inner speech and of verbal thought, we must conclude that the later stage is not a simple continuation of the earlier. The nature of the development itself changes, from biological to sociohistorical. (Vygotsky, 1962, p. 51)

Vygotsky saw the incorporation of speech into human consciousness as the fundamental mechanism that transforms cognitive development along a completely new line. Earlier development is of the type Piaget would later call "sensorimotor," where the development of thought is governed primarily by biological factors and simple reflex learning. When the child learns to speak, however, he is acquiring a system of signs, which, like any social institution, develops according to sociohistorical principles of dialectical materialism. Vygotsky maintained that the planning aspect of human labor activity that is essential to Marx's conception of human nature is created through human acquisition of a social system of signs that itself shares the same dialectical foundation as does the organization of human productive forces.

Verbal thought is not an innate, natural form of behavior but is determined by a historical cultural process and has specific properties and laws that cannot be found in the natural forms of thought and speech. Once we acknowledge the historical character of verbal thought, we must consider it subject to all the premises of historical materialism, which are valid for any historical phenomenon in human society. It is only to be expected that on this level the development of behavior will be governed essentially by the general laws of the historical development of society. (Vygotsky, 1962, p. 51)

Vygotsky began with Marx's praxis–interactionist thesis: Consciousness develops through the organism's interaction with the world. The nature of practical activity determines consciousness. In particular, the nature of the means in a goal-directed activity transforms its user. Vygotsky thus introduced the category of "externally" mediated activity – actions that involve the use of some external means to reach some goal. There are two major types of "external" mediators – tools and signs. Tools (i.e., as used by infants or Köhler's apes) and signs differ fundamentally in their organization. A tool is externally oriented toward the goal, a mere instrument in the hands of its user who controls it. Signs, however, are inherently "reversible" – they feed back upon or control their users. A favorite example of Vygotsky's is a knot used as mnemonic device. An external sign is used to control its user – to help him remember.

Vygotsky focused upon language as a mediating device, rather than such isolated semiotic devices as the aforementioned knot used as mnemonic aids because language is a system of *reversible* signs organized in terms of principles of multifunctionality, communication, and generalization. Vygotsky saw consciousness as "the experiencing of experiences" (1979, p. 19), and to be conscious of one's own experiences "means nothing less than to possess them in object form (stimulus) for other experiences" (1979, p. 78). Speech is reversible because words can be both stimulus and response. "A heard word is the stimulus, and a word pronounced is a reflex producing the same stimulus" (1979, pp. 78–79). This property of signs allows their users to use signs to control their own behavior. If consciousness is the use of reversible signs to "experience experience," then consciousness is basically social since the linguistic signs are part of a system of signs, one of whose dominant structuring principles is social contact and communication.

The second property of language, its multifunctionality, lies in its ability to be used as a means in many types of goal-directed activity. According to Vygotsky, any action, whether it is carried out internally or externally, must be analyzed in terms of its goal(s) and the means whereby this goal is achieved. Since in any goal-directed system the means has the function of contributing to the goal of the action and is, at least in part, selected because of this effect, the multifunctionality of language derives from its use as a functional means in a variety of interactive situations such as getting someone to do something, providing information, or promising. In particular, Vygotsky believed that speech forms are regimented with respect to two major functions: communications or social contact, and representation. The former property links language to its roots in ongoing, contextualized social action. The latter function, that of representation (i.e., reference and predication) links language to its unique properties of encoding multiple levels of generality in its surface forms and self-reflexivity – language is the only sign system that can refer to itself.

Vygotsky drew upon the work of the American linguist Edward Sapir to articulate how these last two properties of language were related. He adopted three points of Sapir's about the relation between communication and generalization. First, words are symbols of concepts and "the single word expresses either a simple concept or a combination of concepts so interrelated as to form a psychological unity" (1979, p. 82). Second, although language, particularly in its grammatical aspects was organized in terms of levels of generality, conceptualization was only a latent potential in the structure of language. Third, language shaped thought. Vygotsky interpreted these premises developmentally and added to them his thesis of reversibility. The child developed higher forms of thought through his differentiating the various levels of generality and communication in his language.

In the first chapter of *Thought and Language*, Vygotsky presented the "overall problem and approach" and then used Sapir to substantiate that communication and thus language involve generalization.

First Vygotsky criticized an associationistic account of the origins of linguistic meaning as too simplistic.

It was assumed that the means of communication was the sign (the word of sound); that through simultaneous occurrence a sound could become associated with the content of any experience and then serve to convey the same content to other human beings. (Vygotsky, 1962, p. 6)

This account leaves out the generalized nature of linguistic meaning. The key is to see communication and generalization as inextricably linked.

Closer study of the development of understanding and communication in childhood, however, has led to the conclusion that real communication requires meaning – i.e., generalization – as much as signs. According to Edward Sapir's penetrating description, the world of experience must be greatly simplified and generalized before it can be translated into symbols. Only in this way does communication become possible, for the individual's experience resides only in his own consciousness and is, strictly speaking, not communicable. To become communicable, it must be included in a certain category which, by tacit convention, human society regards as a unit. (Vygotsky, 1962, pp. 6–7)

These passages of Vygotsky's are clearly paraphrases of points made in the first chapter of Sapir's *Language*. In this chapter, Sapir also pointed out that a purely associational account is inadequate. The connection between a word and what it stands for is "symbolic." The following passage of Sapir's is the basis for Vygotsky's linkage of generalization and communication.

The world of our experiences must be enormously simplified and generalized before it is possible to make a symbolic inventory of all our experiences of things and relations and this inventory is imperative before we can convey ideas. The elements of language, the symbols that ticket off experience, must therefore be associated with whole groups, delimited classes, of experience rather than with the single experiences themselves. Only so is communication possible, for the single experience lodges in an individual consciousness and is, strictly speaking, incommunicable. To be communicated it needs to be referred to a class which is tacitly accepted by the community as an identity. (Sapir, 1949, pp. 6–7)

However, even though language, especially its grammatical portions (for Sapir, a grammar is how language arranges concepts into propositional form), are organized around principles of generalization, this does not imply that "the use to which language is put is always or even mainly conceptual." In ordinary life, people are not "so much concerned with concepts as such as with concrete particularities and specific relations" (Sapir, 1949, p. 14).

Fully generalized thought is only a latent possibility in language. From the point of view of language, thought may be defined as the highest latent or potential content of speech, the content that is obtained by interpreting each of the elements in the flow of language as possessed of its very fullest conceptual value. From this it follows at once that language and thought are not strictly coterminous. At best language can but be the outward fact of thought on the highest, most generalized, level of symbolic expression. To put our viewpoint somewhat differently, language is primarily a pre-rational function. It humbly works up to the thought that is latent in, that may eventually be read into, its classification and its forms; it is not, as is generally but naively assumed, the final label put upon the finished thought. (Sapir, 1949, pp. 13–14)

Sapir then formulated the thesis that underlies *Thought and Language*.

Most people, asked if they can think without speech, would probably answer, "Yes, but it is not easy for me to do so. Still I know it can be done." Language is but a garment! But what if language is not so much a garment as a prepared road or groove? It is, indeed, in the highest degree likely that language is an instrument originally put to uses lower than the conceptual plane and that thought arises as a refined interpretation of its content. The product grows, in other words, with instrument, and thought may be no more conceivable in its genesis and daily practice, without speech than is mathematical reasoning practicable without the lever of an appropriate mathematical symbolism. (Sapir, 1949, p. 15)

Vygotsky "clothed" his response to Sapir's insight in a similar metaphor on the creative dialectic between thought and word.

The structure of speech does not simply mirror the structure of thought; that is why words cannot be put on by thought like a ready-made garment. Thought undergoes many changes as it turns into speech. It does not merely find expression in speech; it finds reality and form. (Vygotsky, 1962, p. 126)

For Sapir, language creates the possibility of abstract thinking, and language and thought grow in a dialectical fashion.

The point of view that we have developed does not by any means preclude the possibility of the growth of speech being in a high degree dependent on the development of thought. We may assume that language arose pre-rationally – just how and on what precise level of mental activity we do not know – but we must not imagine that a highly developed system of speech symbols worked itself out before the genesis of distinct concepts and of thinking, the handling of concepts. We must rather imagine that thought processes set in, as a kind of psychic overflow, almost at the beginning of linguistic expression; further, that the concept, once defined, necessarily reacted on the life of its linguistic symbol, encouraging further linguistic growth. We see this complex process of the interaction of language and thought actually taking place under our eyes. The instrument makes possible the product, the product refines the instrument. (Sapir, 1949, p. 17)

In *Mind and Society* Vygotsky self-admittedly sets out to write a *Kapital* for psychology. Vygotsky's starting point is the Marxist position that human tool use differs from animal instrumental activity in that humans plan their activities beforehand, creating in the mind a plan or rule to guide activity. These rules, of course, are produced in a given society according to processes of historical evolution governed by the laws of dialectical materialism. What Vygotsky added to Marx was to show how this planning ability develops through the linguistic mediation of action, and what he added to Sapir was a developmental account of how language mediates thought.

[The child] plans how to solve the problem through speech and then carries out the prepared solution through overt activity. Direct manipulation is replaced by a complex psychological process through which inner motivation and intentions, postponed in time, stimulate their own development and realization. This new kind of psychological structure is absent in apes, even in rudimentary form. (Vygotsky, 1978, p. 28)

The semiotic mediation of activity allows the child to plan his activities according to what will eventually be a socially created and transmitted set of rules.

When speech and thought begin to interweave in action, a dialectic is set up in which the reversible nature of signs allows the child to "bootstrap" himself up through the various levels of abstraction present in language. At first, the child is guided by these reversible semiotic signs without being aware of their effects. They are silent means in his goal-directed activity. Yet these very activities, because they involve the use of means structured along principles of reversibility and generalization create effects that later will become causes of the child's behavior. This reversal of cause and effect is one of Vygotsky's interpretations of Marx's dialectic and is a key genetic law in his psychology. Vygotsky viewed this process of differentiation through action and the child's becoming aware of that differentiation as a confirmation of Marx's dictum that individual consciousness is produced through the subject's becoming aware of the structures underlying social relations. His particular addition was to show how the structure of language as a multifunctional, communicative, and representational system allows it to mediate and represent action. This mediation and representation of practical activity forms the basis for the uniquely human forms of rule governed and plan guided human action.

According to Vygotsky, action and speech are, for the very young child, undifferentiated parts of the same psychological function that is directed to fulfilling some ongoing and context specific goal-directed activity. Speech is a mere component of the means to instrumental ends. Because speech and activity are initially undifferentiated in the context of ongoing activity and are thus part of the same overall perceptual field, the gradual differentiation and internalization of speech allow language to become a mediator for the perceptual field. This internalization of the perceptual field gives the child's operations a greater freedom from the concrete visual aspects of the situation. Speech mediates and supplants the immediacy of natural perception – the child perceives the world through his speech as well as through sensory perception. With the help of words, the child begins to master his attention, creating new structural centers in the perceived situation. By allowing the child to shift his attention from the ongoing situation, this shift in the relation between perception and attention makes it possible for the development of a new kind of motivation. Instead of a preoccupation with the outcome of an interaction, the emotional thrust can now be shifted to the nature of solution. The use of an auxiliary sign system such as language dissolves the fusion of the sensory and the motor system, making new kinds of behavior possible. The semiotic mediation of activity allows the planning function to develop by restructuring the decision-making process on a totally new basis.

[A] functional barrier is created between the initial and final moments of the choice process; the direct impulse is "shunted" by preliminary circuits. This change is a mandatory condition for the development of all uniquely human, higher psychological functions. The child who formerly solved the problem impulsively, now solves it through an internally established connection between the stimulus and the corresponding auxiliary sign; the movement which previously had been the choice now serves only as a system which fulfills the prepared operation. The system of symbols restructures the whole psychological process enabling the child to master his environment. (Vygotsky, 1978, p. 35)

The child uses artificially created external signs as the immediate causes of his behavior. The signs have the quality of reversibility. They can act upon the agent in the same way they act upon the environment or others.

In this new process the direct impulse to react is inhibited and an auxiliary stimulus which facilitates the completion of the operation by indirect means is incorporated. Careful studies demonstrate that this type of organization is basic to all higher psychological processes, although in much more sophisticated forms than that shown above. The intermediate link in this formula is not simply a method of improving and perfecting the previously existing operation. Because this auxiliary stimulus possesses the specific function of reverse action, it transfers the operation to higher and qualitatively new forms, permitting humans by the aid of outer stimuli to control their behavior from the outside. The use of signs leads humans to a completely new and specific structure of behavior, breaking away from the traditions of biological development and creating for the first time a new form of a culturally based psychological process. (Vygotsky, 1978, p. 40)

Vygotsky's account of the dialectical origin of the higher mental functions and the creation of the uniquely human forms of thought and motivation are clearest in his analyses of the development of scientific concepts, inner speech, and play. In both play and inner speech a new form of consciousness is created through the child's differentiation of the functional structures of a social institution, language, and the child's psychological processes take on the multifunctional, generalized, and dialectical properties of speech itself. When the child differentiates the representational function of speech from its other functions, he can use language to represent these other functions. In so doing, he both transforms these functions by "infusing" them with a new level of generality and creates new interfunctional connections through their mutual regimentation by the representational function.

In both play and inner speech, at first the child is not aware of the representational function of words. His system of communicative tools contains a potential level of consciousness that he will become aware of only through his interactions with others. In the case of his early speech, he uses signs which have the interpreted *effect* (from the adult viewpoint) of referring and predicating. In the case of play, he uses signs that represent social categories without his being aware of their social meaning. In both cases, when the child differentiates the representational function from other speech functions and uses it to represent them, meaning becomes a motivated *cause* of his actions, not just an effect. The same dialectical reversal of cause and effect that guides the development of scientific concepts, inner speech, and play, when applied to the other functions that language can serve, forms the basis for the growth of all the higher mental functions and the development of the uniquely human forms of rule governed and plan guided human action.

The development of scientific concepts and inner speech

The development of the higher mental functions can be understood only in conjunction with Vygotsky's overall theory of how speech creates new interfunctional connections among psychological processes, thereby radically restructuring consciousness. Vygotsky's work on concept development shows his conviction that language provides the foundation for abstract thought through its systematic interweaving of different levels of generality and reversibility. His work on inner speech shows the influence of language in mediating affect and motivation. Both trains of development depend upon the differentiation of the representational function of language during the development of egocentric speech. The development of scientific concepts depends upon the self-reflexive application of the representational function of language to its own representational properties, whereas the development of inner speech occurs through the child's representation of other goal-directed functions of language.

As pointed out earlier, Vygotsky believed that language eventually comes to serve two major well-differentiated functions for the adult. For adults, these two functions of social contact (communication) and representation are constantly intertwined. Ontogenetically, the representational function grows out of the social–communicative function that is primary. The major body of Vygotsky's work on language development focuses on showing the long and gradual differentiation between these two functions, then the use of the representational function to regiment both itself and other speech functions, and the consequent internalization of speech. This development takes the child from the earliest phases where speech, ongoing actions, and perceptions are completely fused, and the different functions of speech are completely undifferentiated, to the adult systems at which point speech is distinguished as a kind of action and is "internalized" and forms an inner system, allowing the adult to regulate and reflect internally on any action.

Thought and Language records the child's development of abstract scientific concepts and complex patterns of motivation from their origins in early child language. First the child uses speech to accomplish certain goals. Although he is interpreted by adults as referring and predicating along with accomplishing other speech acts, to the child speech and action are undifferentiated. Egocentric speech occurs when the child begins to differentiate the representational aspects of speech from its pragmatic communicative functions. When the child names things in order to guide his own action, he has thereby differentiated the referential function of speech from its goal-directed function and can use a representation of the world to guide his actions. When the child begins to separate this function, he can use language not only to get things done in the world, but also to represent it. As the referential function becomes differentiated, it can be used to represent anything, including language itself. Vygotsky's insight was to see that the use of language to represent functions would result in two dialectically related but contrasting "vectors" of development. Language used to represent or refer to the referential aspects of language use eventually results in the development of logic and abstract thought. Language used to represent the means–end and interpersonal aspects of communicative interactions leads to the development of "inner speech" and linguistically mediated motivation.

In the former vector, which leads to the development of abstract concepts, once the referential function is differentiated, the development of thinking in complexes is the child's gradual formation of stable denotational class criteria for word meanings. For example, a given word stands for some set of objects because they possess some perceptual property in common across referential uses of the word. At this early stage of cognitive development, these denotational equivalences are determined only by stable perceptual equivalences among the denotata themselves. Later on, the equivalences become less perceptual and more conceptual.

In his work on concept formation, Vygotsky introduced a distinction between "meaning" and "reference" that is similar to Frege's distinction between "sense" and "reference."[1] His theory of concept development shows how the child's grasp of the "meaning" or "mode of presentation" of words changes from purely perceptual criteria to purely conceptual or symbolic features. This distinction is critical for understanding how the levels of generality expressed by words contribute to the levels of generality expressed by a sentence. Frege's discovery of quantification theory was a way of showing how the truth value of sentences regimented into propositional form was a function of systematic relationships of "multiple generality." In order to make clearer some of the epistemological implications of his work, Frege distinguished between the "sense" and "reference" of words and sentences. This distinction hinges upon the relationship between equivalence and generality. Frege's classic example is that of the two names 'the evening star' and 'the morning star' that both refer to the the planet Venus. The names have the same referent, but different modes of presentation or "senses" are associated with each name. The sense of 'the evening star' is something like 'the brightest starlike object visible after the sun sets' and that of 'the morning star' is the brightest starlike object visible before the sun rises.' Frege insisted that the sense of a sentence is determined by the senses of the words that make it up, and that the sense of a word is its general capacity to determine the senses of sentences of which it is a part. Sense thus determines reference, but not vice versa. The sense of an expression is what we know when we know the meaning of an expression, or at least that part of the meaning of an expression that determines truth value.

Vygotsky gave the following example for his "meaning–reference" distinction.

Modern linguistics distinguishes between the meaning of a word, or an expression and its referent, i.e., the object it designates. There may be one meaning and different referents, or different meanings and one referent. Whether we say "the victor at Jena" or "the loser at Waterloo," we refer to the same person, yet the meaning of the two phrases differs. There is but one category of words – proper names – whose sole function is that of reference. Using this terminology, we might say that the child's and the adult's words coincide in their referents but not in their meanings. (1962, p. 73)

Vygotsky described the levels of generality and their relation to reference in terms of a geographical metaphor.

If we imagine the totality of concepts as distributed over the surface of a globe, the location of every concept may be defined by means of a system of co-ordinates, corresponding to longitude and latitude in geography. One of these co-ordinates will indicate the location of a concept between the extremes of maximally generalized abstract conceptualization and the immediate sensory grasp of an object – i.e., its degree of concreteness and abstraction. The second co-ordinate will represent the objective reference of the concept, the locus within reality to which it applies. Two concepts applying to different areas of reality but comparable in degree of abstractness – e.g., plants and animals – could be conceived of as varying in latitude but having the same longitude. (Vygotsky, 1962, p. 112)

The first coordinate is the degree of generality presented by a given "mode of presentation" of a word. The second coordinate is the objective referent, the object to which the term applies. The mode of presentation can vary from concrete, perceptual properties to the abstract relationships analogous to those that define Fregean senses. As in Frege, the key problem is to relate equivalence and generalization.

The higher levels in the development of word meanings are governed by the law of equivalence of concepts, according to which any concept can be formulated in terms of other concepts in a countless number of ways. . . . The manifold mutual relations of concepts on which the law of equivalence is based are determined by their respective measures of generality. (Vygotsky, 1962, pp. 112–113)

Vygotsky's developmental problem was to show how words embodied multiple levels of generality that gradually become differentiated as equivalences among items at the same level of generality. His example of how these levels can vary is the child's concept of number whose earliest forms have only a very simple level of generality, but whose later definition is in terms of interdefinable concepts (an example that Frege also uses).

Let us take two extreme examples; the child's early (presyncretic) words lacking any variation in degree of generality and the concepts of number developed through the study of arithmetic. In the first case, obviously, every concept can be expressed only through itself, never through other concepts. In the second case, any number may be expressed in countless ways, because of the infinity of number and because the concept of any number contains all of its relationships to all other numbers. "One," for instance, may be expressed as "1,000 minus 999" or, in general, as the difference between any two consecutive numbers, or as any number divided by itself, and in a myriad of other ways. This is a pure example of equivalence of concepts. In so far as equivalence depends on the relationships of generality between concepts and these are specific for every generalizational structure, the latter determines the equivalence of concepts possible within its sphere. (Vygotsky, 1962, p. 113)

The child's early concepts of number are not defined by "metasemantic" equivalences that define one concept in terms of another in a potentially infinite system of interchangeable concepts.

Frege was a logician, so he did not concern himself with "modes of presentation" other than those necessary for regimenting natural language into a form suitable for logical discourse. For Vygotsky, Frege's goal was the asymptotic limit of the development of thought, and he was concerned with the path the child had to travel to get to that point. Vygotsky's work on the development of word meanings was to show how different levels of generality associated with various modes of presentation determine the objective referents of words.

We compared the degree of generality of the child's real concepts with phases and stages reached by the child in experimental concept formation: syncretism, complex, preconcept, and concept. Our aim was to find out whether a definite relationship existed between the structure of generalization typified by these phases and the degree of generality of concepts. (Vygotsky, 1962, p. 111)

The clearest examples of Vygotsky's use of something like the sense–reference distinction is his contrast between complexes (especially what he calls "psuedoconcepts" and "spontaneous concepts") and true concepts. At the level of complexes, the words 'flower' and 'rose' are at the same level of generality. Their meaning is defined purely in terms of the objects they refer to (perhaps identified by certain perceptual features). Although the class of objects denoted by 'flower' includes that of a 'rose', both words are used to pick out objects defined solely by perceptual criteria. At a certain point the word 'flower' is seen by the child as naming a concept. A concept is not defined in terms of properties of its denotata, but by its relation to other concepts in a system of conceptual equivalences that then in turn determine a given denotational class.

A concept can become subject to consciousness and deliberate control only when it is part of a system. If consciousness means generalization, generalization in turn means the formation of a superordinate concept that includes the given concept as a particular case. A superordinate concept implies the existence of a series of subordinate concepts, and it also presupposes a hierarchy of concepts of different levels of generality. Thus the given concept is placed within a system of relationships of generality. (Vygotsky, 1962, p. 92)

Word meanings, however, are not only determined by the perceptual aspects of their denotata, but also by semantic properties defined in terms of the word's position in a system of sense relations. The clearest example of a system of such language internal relationships would be the concepts defined by a grammar. Concepts expressed by grammatical relations are not determined by perceptual qualities of the denotata of such concepts, but rather by their position in language internal "sense" systems defined by proportional differences and equivalences among signifiers and signifieds (in the Saussurean sense). Grammar is the way in which words are arranged to form sentences, with each morpheme or word containing a conceptual value determined by its ability to form sentences that express propositions. As the child differentiates the denotational level of word meaning, he simultaneously discovers the language internal equivalences in which words can participate and gradually begins to take certain concepts created by language internal grammatical relations as "objects" of cognition. The sense expressed by a word is now talked about or referred to.

An example of this dialectical interplay between sense and reference as mediated by grammar is Vygotsky's discussion of the relation between "spontaneous" and "scientific concepts." With everyday, spontaneous concepts (which are really "pseudoconcepts" in Vygotsky's other terminology), the child "has" a concept only in the sense that he knows to which objects the concept refers, but he is not conscious of his act of thought. The "sense" or mode of presentation of the concept is not the object of thought – what is referred to is language external reality, not language internal sense. Scientific concepts begin with verbal definition and are used in nonspontaneous operations. They are established by metasemantic definitional forms that talk about words as referring to concepts that are related to each other in a system of concepts. Each concept's relation to objects is mediated by some other concept. Spontaneous concepts are related to the world of denotation, to reference, and scientific concepts are related to the world of sense.

Though scientific and spontaneous concepts develop in reverse directions, the two processes are closely connected. The development of a spontaneous concept must have reached a certain level for the child to be able to absorb a related scientific concept. . . . In working its slow way upward, an everyday concept clears a path for a scientific concept and its downward development. It creates a series of structures necessary for the evolution of a concept's more primitive, elementary aspects which give it body and vitality. Scientific concepts in turn supply structures for the upward development of the child's spontaneous concepts toward consciousness and deliberate use. Scientific concepts grow down through spontaneous concepts; spontaneous concepts grow upward through scientific concepts. (Vygotsky, 1962, p. 109)

Grammar acts as the mediating device between the upward growth of spontaneous concepts and the downward growth of scientific concepts because the child's everyday uses of language follow certain grammatical regularities (they express them and are guided by them) without the concepts described by those regularities being talked about. On the other hand, scientific concepts are introduced by definitional equivalences established through the regimentation of sentences into full-fledged propositional or logical form. Such definitions require that sentences be treated as totally decontextualized. Because grammar is a system of language-internal, decontextualized equivalences, all scientific definitions presuppose a grammatical regimentation of language. The regimentation of speech by grammar allows grammar to be the link between discourse and logic.

Piaget demonstrated that the child uses subordinate clauses with "because," "although," etc., long before he grasps the structures of meaning corresponding to these syntactic forms. Grammar precedes logic. Here, too, as in our previous example, the discrepancy does not exclude union, but is, in fact, necessary for union. (Vygotsky, 1962, pp. 126–127)

The child's acquisition of scientific concepts provides a system of generality that changes the psychological structure of everyday concepts.

The differentiation of the representational function of egocentric speech and its subsequent application to the pragmatic aspects of language use begin the slow development of inner speech. Language can be used to represent the highly contextualized and interpersonal aspects of speech events. As spontaneous concepts move upward (become relatively more decontextualized), egocentric speech "goes underground," becoming inner speech. Inner speech obeys linguistic principles that are the inverse of grammar and logic. As Vygotsky repeatedly pointed out, psychological notions of topicality and given–new are structured along pragmatic discourse principles that are different from those that structure traditional notions of grammar. Whereas discourse using "scientific concepts" tends to have maximal elaboration of surface distinctions and explicit presuppositional structures (precisely because such discourse tends to be relatively decontextualized), inner speech obeys a principle of minimal surface elaboration and maximal presupposition and condensation. This reaches the point where all subjects are eliminated and thinking occurs only in predicates since the thinker already knows, and thus can presuppose, what the topics of his thoughts are. What is maximally presupposed in the context can be deleted in communication, and the efficiency of inner speech depends upon knowing what to omit as well as what to say.

These devices used by inner speech of condensation and ellipsis parallel the repertoire of mechanisms Freud postulated for the unconscious. This would not surprise Vygotsky, since inner speech is the asymptote of the process whereby egocentric speech "goes underground," and egocentric speech itself is the mediation of motivation by speech since it involves the use of language to represent and guide action. Inner speech is the means by which motivation and nonverbal thought can become regimented into external speech forms communicable to others. Although external and inner speech serve different functions (the former for communication with others, the latter self-regulation and communication for oneself), inner speech is still speech ("thought connected with words"). In external speech thoughts are expressed in words so that they can be communicated; in inner speech, words are merely routes to their meanings, "words die as they bring forth thought," and inner speech becomes "to a large extent thinking in pure meanings." This peculiar structure of inner speech allows it to be a mediator between nonlinguistic motivation and thought and external speech. As thought it is connected with nonverbal thought because all thought, according to Vygotsky, involves generalization; as *verbal* thought, it is still connected with external speech. Thus the psychological analysis of another's external speech is complete only when one understands its motivation.

We come now to the last step in our analysis of verbal thought. Thought itself is engendered by motivation, i.e., by our desires and needs, our interests and emotions. Behind every thought there is an affective–volitional tendency, which holds the answer to the last "why" in the analysis of thinking. A true and full understanding of another's thought is possible only when we understand its affective–volitional basis. (Vygotsky, 1962, p. 150)

Vygotsky's account of the development of scientific concepts and inner speech illustrates several of the more Marxist-inspired theses adumbrated earlier. First, the representational function is present in the means used in practical speech activity, but the child is unaware of this property of his speech. Yet it is precisely the fact that he uses speech forms that have the effect upon the adult of being interpreted as referring and predicating that the child is able to get adults to do things for him. When he differentiates out the representational function of speech during egocentric speech, he becomes aware of the possibility that was latent in his socially constituted "means of production." When this function is reapplied both to itself and the pragmatic aspects of language use, it creates new forms of consciousness by creating new interfunctional connections among psychological processes as well as giving them a new level of linguistically mediated generality. At the same time, this incorporation of language completely changes the child's psychological organization, and becomes the foundation for both abstract conceptual thought and more complicated motivational structures. In *Thought and Language* the development of abstract thought through the differentiation of the multiple levels of generality in words is presented in great detail; his analysis of the creation of higher forms of motivation is left to some rather cryptic remarks about inner speech. The connection between language and motivation becomes much clearer in his account of play.

Language, play, and motivation

Vygotsky's account of the development of scientific concepts and inner speech is a "microcosm" of how he interweaves Marxist themes and semiotic concerns. First, the representational function is present in the means used in practical speech activity, but the child is unaware of this property of speech. Yet is is precisely the fact that he uses speech forms that allow the adult to interpret him as referring and predicating that the child is able to get adults to do things for him. When this function is reapplied both to itself and other context-bound or pragmatic aspects of language use, it creates new forms of consciousness by creating new interfunctional connections among psychological processes as well as giving them a new level of linguistically mediated generality. At the same time, this incorporation of language completely changes the child's psychological organization and becomes the foundation for both abstract conceptual thought and more complicated motivational structures.

Thought and Language is a compilation of work written by Vygotsky almost at his deathbed. He never had a chance to complete his project for Marxist psychology; indeed, *Thought and Language* has been treated mainly as a psycholinguistic work, not as a general picture of the development of consciousness or as the application of a specific methodology that would integrate psychology with broader social institutional issues. However, at the same time that he was writing *Thought and Language,* he also completed an article on play that not only used the same approach, but dealth with how a child is socialized into a system of rules and norms, thus providing a development link between his Marxist framework and his empirical psychology.

Play is of critical importance in Vygotsky's theory because it is through play that the child develops the uniquely human forms of motivation.

These motivations have embedded within them a representation of rules as socially constituted and socially transmitted guides to behavior. The development of rule-guided behavior is, of course, linked to Marx's thesis about the uniqueness of human social activity as rule-governed. When looked at developmentally, play become the foundation for the child's development of second-order motivations necessary both for school and work. "At school age play does not die away but permeates the attitude to reality. It has its own inner continuation in school instruction and work (compulsory activity based on rules)" (Vygotsky, 1976, p. 554).

Play becomes the "leading edge" of the child's psychological development because it allows the child a "zone of proximal development" through which both these new motivations and a new kind of attitude toward reality are created. The critical point is that in play, the child creates an imaginary situation to guide his actions – a world of meaning is created that then has motivational force. These meanings, however, are not random, but have both a social and a linguistic origin.

Play creates a leading edge in the child's development because through it he begins to sever the direct connection between a thing, a situation, and an action. For the young child, a given situation dictates what he can do, given what he wants. A doorbell is to be rung, a rattle to be shaken. For the child, the meaning of an object is the interaction between the history of its effects upon his actions and his desires in the immediate moment. In play, the child sees one thing but acts differently in relation to what he sees. Both the situation and the action are imaginary; the child constructs a meaning to guide his action, and a symbolically mediated desire governs reality. A stick becomes a horse, a doll becomes a mother. Reality bends to the will of conception and action is dictated not by the object, but by the idea represented by it. However, a complete tie to reality is never severed in play – the arbitrariness of true symbolism is not present. In play, it is not the case that anything can stand for anything – a horse is a stick because it can be ridden on. In play, meaning is separated from the objects or sign vehicles that normally embody them, but in real life, this relation is unchanged.

Once meanings and ideas begin to determine action, rather than vice versa, a critical shift occurs in the child's relation to reality.

But all the same the basic structure determining the child's relationship to reality is radically changed at this crucial point, for his perceptual structure changes. The special feature of human perception – which arises at a very early age – is so-called reality perception. This is something for which there is no analogy in animal perception. Essentially it lies in the fact that I do not see the world simply in colour and shape, but also as a world with sense and meaning. I do not merely see something round and black with two hands; I see a clock and I can distinguish one thing from another. (Vygotsky, 1976, p. 546)

In play, a child treats an object as standing for something and as embodying a meaning. The meaning of the word 'horse' supplants the actual horse, the child foregrounds the meaning and backgrounds the object, thus experimenting with the link between object and meaning. In early play, this experimental foregrounding of the meaning over the object requires a "pivot" or mediational device. The stick severs the meaning of the word 'horse' from a real horse. The child transfers the meaning of the word from a real horse to a stick and then by treating the stick as if it were a horse he "acts out" a meaning.

The key to Vygotsky's analysis of symbolic play is that meaning and object separate, but that meanings of things are given by words. Play develops through the linguistic mediation of the meaning–object relation. Words stand for their objects, and when the child uses a stick to stand for a horse, he is really replacing the word 'horse' with another sign – a semiotic substitution of one sign vehicle for another. The stick does not stand for a real, existent horse, but rather for the meaning attached to the word 'horse'.

Separating words from things requires a pivot in the form of other things. But the moment the stick – i.e., the thing – becomes the pivot for severing the meaning of 'horse' from a real horse, the child makes one thing influence another in the semantic sphere. . . .Transfer of meanings is facilitated by the fact that the child accepts a word as the property of a thing, he does not see the word but the thing it designates. For a child the word 'horse' applied to the stick means, 'There is a horse'; i.e., mentally he sees the object standing behind the word. (Vygotsky, 1976, pp. 547–548)

Vygotsky linked play to the development of inner speech and the higher mental functions, all of which become mediated by meaning.

Play is converted to internal processes at school age, going over to internal speech, logical memory and abstract thought. In play, a child operates with meanings severed from objects, but not in real action with real things. A child first acts with meanings as with objects and later realizes them consciously and begins to think just as a child, before he has acquired grammatical and written speech, knows how to do things but does not know that he knows, i.e., he does not realize or master them voluntarily. (Vygotsky, 1976, p. 548)

It is the meanings given by words that become motivated rules that govern the child's play. In early play, the child constructs an imaginary situation in which there are guiding rules for behavior. The child plays at being a fireman or teacher, or he uses a stick to stand for a horse. In later play the rules set up an imaginary situation. Such play continuously demands that the child control his immediate impulses for the sake of the game, thereby creating a second-order desire, an affect that overcomes another affect not merely by supplanting it, but by incorporating it. In real life, obeying a rule and refraining from action often occur as renunciations, perhaps stirred by fear of punishment. In play, the reverse is true – voluntary subordination and restraint lead to pleasure. Play is "a rule which has become an affect" (Vygotsky, 1976, p. 549) and is the foundation for self-restraint, self-determination, and an "inner world" of adult fantasy.

Conclusion

Vygotsky's untimely death prevented him from expanding his ideas on the relation between Marxist social institutional level processes and the psychological functions that constitute human consciousness. His work on play, however, shows that his Marxist-inspired methodology not only was applicable to the relation between language and thought, but could be used to analyze the child's acquisition and understanding of social rules.

In both the development of play and inner speech, we have a dialectical opposition between an external, social form, and an internal, individual form, with each developing out of an originally undifferentiated social matrix through the differentiation of the representational function of signs. In each case, the external social form becomes more abstract and generalized while the inner forms move toward condensation and personal symbolism. External speech has as its asymptote scientific concepts, its internal counterpart being inner speech. Play's external forms develop into games with rules and ultimately the socially constituted forms of work, while "inner play" forms the foundation for the will and imagination. The "second-order" motivations that lie "behind" inner speech are the products of the history of the development of play; it is an effect of an earlier differentiation of speech functions that in the adult becomes a motivating cause for actions and allows a sociohistorical mode of meaning to touch human consciousness.

NOTES

1   Frege's influence on Vygotsky was indirect. Vygotsky's use of sense and meaning comes from Husserl's *Logical Investigations*, which was partially in direct response to Frege's work.

REFERENCES

Avineri, S. 1968. *The social and political thought of Karl Marx.* Cambridge: Cambridge University Press.
Husserl, E. 1970. *Logical investigations.* Translated by J. N. Findlay. New York: New York Humanities Press.

Marx, Karl. 1959. *Marx and Engels: Basic writings on politics and philosophy.* Edited by L. S. Feuer. Garden City, N.Y.: Doubleday.

Marx, Karl. 1973. *Grundrisse.* Translated by Martin Nicolaus. New York: Random House.

Sapir, Edward. 1949. *Language.* New York: Harcourt, Brace and World.

Vandenberg, B. Play: Dormant issues and new perspectives. *Human Development,* 24(6):357–65.

Vygotsky, L. S. 1956. *Izbrannie psikhologicheskie issledovaniya.* [Selected psychological research.] Moscow: Izdatel'stvo Akademii Pedagogicheskikh Nauk.

Vygotsky, L. S. 1960. *Razvitie vysshykh psikhicheskikh funktsii.* [The development of higher mental functions.] Moscow: Izdatel'stvo Akademii Pedagogicheskikh Nauk.

Vygotsky, L. S. 1962. *Thought and language.* Cambridge: MIT Press.

Vygotsky, L. S. 1972. The problem of stage periodization of child development. Translated by James V. Wertsch. Typescript.

Vygotsky, L. S. 1976. Play and its role in the mental development of the child. In: J. S. Bruner, A. Jolly, and K. Sylva (Eds.), *Play.* New York: Penguin.

Vygotsky. L. S. 1978. *Mind in society.* Edited by M. Cole, V. John-Steiner, S. Scribner, and E. Souberman. Cambridge: Harvard University Press.

Vygotsky, L. S. 1979. Consciousness as a problem in the psychology of behavior. *Soviet Psychology, 17*(4), 3–35.

Vygotsky, L. S. 1981. The genesis of higher mental functions. In J. Wertsch (Ed.), *The concept of activity in Soviet psychology,* Armonk, N.Y.: Sharpe.

4

Vygotsky's ideas about units
for the analysis of mind

V. P. ZINCHENKO

> It is impossible for the human intellect to grasp the idea of absolute con-
> tinuity of motion. Laws of motion of any kind only become comprehens-
> ible to man when he can examine arbitrarily selected units of that motion.
> But at the same time it is this arbitrary division of continuous motion into
> discontinuous units which gives rise to a large proportion of human error.
> Tolstoy (1957, p. 974)

In my view, an important theme of this volume is the analysis of the fate of
Vygotsky's ideas in contemporary science. This theme is reflected in the
book's subtitle, "Vygotskian Perspectives." Vygotsky did not leave any
well-developed account of his ideas about the units to be used in the
analysis of mind. Nonetheless, he discussed this problem at various points
in his scientific activity. This was the case in his critical analyses of others as
well as in his positive contributions. He always discussed this problem in
the context of major theoretical and methodological[1] issues, issues such as
the nature of an explanatory principle in psychology, the contradictory
and noncontradictory aspects of theory, and determinism and causality in
psychology. The problem of the units appropriate for analyzing mind had
an ontological as well as a methodological significance for him.

   For Vygotsky, the examination of the analytic units that lie at the basis of
a theory facilitated the reconstruction of the theory as a whole. This included the reconstruction of existing theories as well as the examination of
their premises and prospects. Following Vygotsky, we will attempt to
analyze and in particular to reconstruct the units for the analysis of mind
that lay at the basis of his theory, and we will trace their fate in the subsequent development of psychology.

The history of units used in the analysis of mind

The history of the search for units to analyze mind merits specific methodological and theoretical research inasmuch as it has had an enormous
role in the development of contemporary psychology. In this chapter,

94

however, we will limit ourselves to some general observations and illustrations. As is known, the problem of units for psychological research has confronted every school of scientific psychology. In the past, a variety of phenomena have been singled out in this capacity. For example, sensations (in associationism), figure–ground (in Gestalt psychology), the reaction or reflex (in reactology and reflexology respectively), set (in set psychology), and the behavioral act (in behaviorism) have served as units. In neobehaviorism in particular Tolman treated the problem of analytic units as central. Subsequently, Tolman's work has had a substantial influence on contemporary cognitive psychology. Tolman supplemented the stimulus–response scheme with a system of intervening, variable, cognitive maps organized in quasispatial form. In Western European psychology, Piaget discussed the problem in particular detail. He singled out reversible operations in this connection. These operations were part of a wider operative structure. According to Piaget, action is the source of these internalized operative structures. In contrast to reversible operative structures, other investigators have viewed mnemonic and motor schemes as the units of analysis. This is characteristic of Bartlett (1935) and several of his followers in contemporary Anglo-American psychology.

We have listed examples of relatively clear-cut, so to say "sterile," units of psychological analysis. In the history of psychology some investigators have also used integral, undifferentiated units of analysis. Only at higher stages of development do these begin to be differentiated into separate, more or less independent, and well-defined genera, species, and classes of mental processes. Representatives of the Leipzig school such as Krüger and Folkeldt introduced the concept of "emotionlike sensations" and spoke of the continuity of sensations and feelings in early stages of development. There is an analogous conception in Gestalt psychology. Koffka, for example, wrote that in the early stages of development the object is so dreadful (even black) for consciousness that the first emotionlike perceptions must be considered the point of departure for all subsequent development.

The approach within the Freudian tradition was quite different. In accordance with the concept of complex, stratified mental structure, we find a rejection of the notion of a universal unit for psychological research. It is suggested that a specific taxonomy of such units be constructed so that each level would have its own type of unit.

It is interesting that in the history of psychology, one can observe quite complex relationships between the analytic unit and the theoretical structure as a whole. Contradictions emerge more sharply at the level of units than they do at the level of overall theoretical structures. This frequently testifies to the fact that the founders of schools of psychology have given more content to the units of analysis than their opponents, or even their followers, understand. Nonetheless, in discussions of units for the analysis of mind, requirements for units, as well as for theory in general are typically formulated. Today, one can hardly doubt that it is impossible to build an image of an object on the basis of separate sensations. In precisely the same way, after Piaget's critique of Gestalt psychology one cannot doubt that it is impossible to derive operative structures or conceptual structures from perceptual structures.

Nonetheless, contemporary psychology, which is characterized by an unprecedented accumulation of new facts, has shown insufficient interest (and occasionally an astonishing carelessness) in isolating and defining units of mental analysis. This is particularly characteristic of cognitive psychology, which operates on the basis of the concepts of the functional block and operation and often relies on homunculi to solve the problem of how these blocks are coordinated into structures [see Velichkovskii and Zinchenko (1979) for more details].

The decreased interest in units for the analysis of mind is apparently linked with the excessive disillusionment resulting from the unjustified reliance on units such as sensations, reactions, and reflexes. It is also possible that the poor methodological standards of contemporary psychology are the cause of this collapse in interest. Indeed, one cannot find a strict definition of a unit for the analysis of mind in the psychological literature. The unit is instead characterized either as a universal constituent of mind, as its determinant, or, finally, as the genetically primary basis of mental development. In the first case it may be treated as either an elementary or structural universal. In the second, it emerges not so much in the role of a unit of analysis as in the role of an explanatory principle. Various schools of psychology deal with the interrelationships among these different treatments in a variety of ways. But common to them all is, first, insufficient consideration of the units of mental analysis. This weakness is expressed in carelessness in defining the methodological and ontological status of the units and also in carelessness in defining their functions. Secondly, and more critically, psychologists have failed to formulate normative requirements for the analytic units from the perspective of their role in a non-reductionistic psychological reality (on the onotological plane). An examination of this relationship often results in the redefinition of analytic units. Psychologists have also failed to formulate normative requirements for the units of analysis from the perspective of the logic of a particular philosophical tradition. Frequently, therefore, the motivation and basis for selecting units of analysis have remained beyond the boundaries of research, research that has often given a remarkable impression of a complete analysis.

But in reality, the identification of units is the beginning, not the conclusion of an analysis.

Vygotsky was a brilliant expert in the history of psychology and philosophy. In his analysis of the various periods and trends of psychology, he constantly formulated normative requirements for the units of mental analysis.

Requirements for the units of the analysis of mind

Vygotsky frequently argued that the outward relations among elements must not be mistaken for the internal relations of a unit.

By unit we mean a product of analysis which, in distinction from elements, possesses all the basic properties of a whole. Further, these properties must be a living portion of the unified whole which cannot be broken down further. . . .A psychology that wishes to study complex units must understand this. Psychology must replace methods of analysis that decompose the whole into elements with a method that is based on units. It must discover the indissoluble units that preserve the properties inherent in the unified whole. It must find the units in which contradictory properties appear. It must use this kind of analysis to settle the questions that face us. (Vygotsky, 1934, p. 9)

On the basis of this and other quotations from Vygotsky's work we will try to systematize his requirements for the units (and methods) of psychological analysis.

1. A unit must not be a diffuse, syncretic whole constructed of elements (i.e., by means of combining everything with everything else). Rather, it must be an integrated psychological structure. For example, Vygotsky agreed completely with Claperede that the weakest point of the James–Lange theory of emotions is that emotion is viewed as a completely unstructured formation, as an aggregate of sensations that are not interconnected in the mind, being comprised instead in accordance with physiological laws.

2. The unit must maintain the characteristics of the unified whole, though internal contradictions and oppositions may exist. The necessity of having different and even contradictory characteristics (or origins) might be called the requirement for the initial heterogeneity of the unit of analysis (see Zinchenko, 1978). With the acceptance of this requirement, it is much easier to understand the problem of the separation and subsequent "combination" of elements, their coordination of widely separate origins.

3. These units, though preserving the structural characteristics of the whole, must be capable of development, including self-development. They must possess the appropriate inherent properties and potential for being transformed into something that differs from their initial form. The

inclusion of units in the processes of real-life activity and, consequently, in the processes of active contact with the surrounding environment, is a necessary condition for development. Vygotsky always objected to viewing mental activity as completely autonomous from reality. He objected to the tendency to consider it as lying outside of nature and outside of life. He took exception to those who perceived it as a separate domain that, in Spinoza's words, is not a natural thing following the laws of nature, but a thing that lies beyond the boundaries of nature as though it were a state within a state.

4. The structural integrity of the analytic unit, its heterogeneity (i.e., the presence of contradictory origins), and its emerging properties, inevitably lead to yet one more characteristic of the unit on which Vygotsky insisted. The unit must be a *living* part of the whole. It must also be a unified system that cannot be further decomposed. A further decomposition of the whole into elements is possible, but this results in its destruction as a living and unified entity. From this, in particular, it follows that new units (in the ontological sense) do not arise gradually, but in a sudden leap.

5. For Vygotsky, a basic principle of research in psychology was that it must involve the study of the development, functioning, and structure (in general, the transition) of specific units. As a result, we can assume that he began with a taxonomic approach to the units of psychological analysis. This has been expressed somewhat later in a more distinct form in the works of Leont'ev (1972, 1975), which were devoted to the psychological analysis of activity. We would point out that any scheme for analyzing units from a taxonomic point of view must be made clear as is the case with the problem of psychological taxonomies in general.

6. An analysis that divides a complex whole into units has the advantage of allowing one to combine its results with the synthetic of the properties of any complex unity. It was precisely on this basis that Vygotsky considered analysis into units to be an effective way to study complex, dynamic systems of sense. For example, Vygotsky wrote that this kind of an analysis shows that

there exists a dynamic system of sense which is a unit of affective and intellectual processes. It shows that any idea contains, in a highly developed form, an affective relationship between humans and the reality represented in that idea. This kind of analysis permits one to reveal the direct movement from a human's needs and motivation to the direction of his/her thinking. It also permits the reverse movement, that is, from the dynamics of thought to the dynamics of behavior and the concrete activity of the individual. (1934, p. 14)

7. The units of analysis that are selected must not only reflect the internal unity of mental processes. They must also permit the investigation of the relationship between a specific psychological function (or process) and

the entire life of consciousness and to the various critical functions of consciousness. Consciousness was always the major object in Vygotsky's research. He evaluated the productivity of a particular psychological theory in terms of its actual or potential contribution to the study of consciousness. Vygotsky's opinion of Lange's theory is characteristic. He agreed with Lange that a mother who has lost a child will be resentful, perhaps even indignant, if she is told that what she is experiencing is weakness and sluggishness of the muscles and cold skin. In this connection Vygotsky wrote:

> The mother's resentment is justified; her indignation is appropriate. It is this resentment and indignation that they want to deprive of life and significance. In this process they remove the most powerful reality of emotional life simply because it steps beyond the limits of their psychology of elements, simply because it cannot be fit into its Procrustean bed. (Vygotsky, 1933, p. 362)

In this form, Vygotsky expressed one of the strongest protests in the history of psychology against reductionistic and epiphenomenal treatments of consciousness.

These requirements for the units of mental analysis were compiled on the basis of Vygotsky's critiques of others as well as on the basis of his own research. His strong reaction and concern with the methodological problems of science, and in particular with the units for the analysis of mind, is apparent. His approach to the analytic unit as a living, developing whole made it possible to overcome several difficulties encountered by psychology. In particular, it permitted psychology to overcome the difficulties inherent in combining what seemed to be incompatible requirements for the units of analysis (for example, homogeneity and heterogeneity).

At the same time, it is important to remember that Vygotsky the methodologist, who was concerned with the units of mental analysis, went beyond Vygotsky the psychologist. The issue was not only that Vygotsky failed to create a well-defined taxonomy of the units for the analysis of mind. Rather, the units he selected did not always correspond to the requirements that he had formulated. But how could it be otherwise? Vygotsky's efforts must be compared with the efforts in contemporary psychology where the problem of the units for mental analysis is rarely brought up at all, and then only in historical context. The problem of the levels in the organization of mind has frequently been substituted for this problem. Here the various levels function as units of analysis. But researchers, as a rule, have not concerned themselves with the units utilized in the characterization of the various levels. Too frequently we encounter the post hoc introduction of units into analytic schemas. In this connection one author has noted that gnostic neurons are included in the structure of psychological processes of recognition. These gnostic neurons may be involved in anything from the detectors of lines to detectors of corners, and thus. . .to detectors of my grandmother in a yellow Volkswagen. In other words, within each level the units can be heterogeneous, but the entire taxonomy of units must respond to the demand for homogeneity. Every unit must reflect characteristics of cognition, sensation, volition or purpose, intelligence, and activation. Otherwise it may be a unit of physiological or biomechanical analysis, but it is not a unit of psychological analysis.

Tool-mediated action as a unit for the analysis of mind

As we noted above, Vygotsky did not outline a well-developed taxonomy of units for psychological analysis. His clearest and most complete demonstration of the productivity of his approach can be found in his analysis of the processes of thinking and speech and the processes of generalization and social interaction. In this analysis, he utilized the category of meaning as a unit. Since Vygotsky's work on this topic is well known throughout the world, we do not need to expound on it here (see Vygotsky, 1934). Similarly, we will not attempt to construct our version of a taxonomy of units. We simply want to discuss the problem of the fundamental unit for the analysis of mind in light of Vygotsky's theory.

It seems to us that this problem involves the following considerations. First, meaning cannot be viewed as a universally or genetically primary unit for the analysis of mind. This was already demonstrated by P. I. Zinchenko (1939). Second, given the normative requirements established by Vygotsky, meaning cannot be accepted as a self-sufficient analytic unit since in meaning there is no "motive force" for its own transformation into consciousness. Much later, Leont'ev (1975) wrote that meaning is only one of the formators of consciousness. In the concluding chapter of his book *Thinking and Speech,*[2] Vygotsky himself recognized the insufficiency of meaning as a unit for the analysis of thinking (he was there no longer speaking of consciousness). In analyzing the internal plane of verbal thinking, Vygotsky wrote: "The thought is still not the last instantiation in this process. . . .Behind thought there is an affective and volitional tendency. Only it can provide an answer to the last 'why' in the analysis of thinking' (1934, p. 314). If one extends this idea of Vygotsky's, then one must say that only the cognitive aspect of thinking is fixed in meaning.

This statement indicates that even Vygotsky understood the inadequacy of the category of meaning as a unit for analyzing higher mental functions. In this connection it is interesting to trace what might be termed the reverse genesis of meaning, both in reference to its role as a primary unit for the analysis of mind and in reference to the units that constitute its immediate preconditions. We note immediately that the genetically primary units for analysis must meet one additional requirement that was not foreseen in Vygotsky's system of requirements. In proposing the genetically primary "cell" or "the undeveloped beginnings of the fully developed whole" as a unit of analysis, Davydov (1972) noted that such a "cell" must have an actual sensuous-contemplative form.

Some foundations for tracing the reverse genesis of units of analysis exist in Vygotsky's own work. Davydov and Radzikhovskii (Chapter 2, this volume) discuss in detail Vygotsky's treatment of object-oriented, practical activity (in the Marxist interpretation of this concept) as the aspect of reality that determines mind. They also present an interpretation of the category of activity as an explanatory principle in psychological theory. They reveal the significance of the concept of a "psychological tool" and its place in Vygotsky's version of the theory of internalization. We will not repeat their argument. But on the basis of the logic they use, we can infer several consequences for the problem of units of analysis.

The most important of these is that we see that tool-mediated action is a unit in the analysis of mind. We have not been able to find a direct indication in Vygotsky's work of the notion that tool-mediated action can function as a unit of analysis. But it does not seem to us that this proposal contradicts any of the requirements outlined above that units for the analysis of mind must satisfy. Moreover, Vygotsky himself treated meaning and the sign precisely as psychological tools.

Tool-mediated action appears in two forms, external and internal. The significance of the idea of internalization is that external tool-mediated action can be transformed into internal, mental action. Vygotsky and his followers studied in detail the conditions and circumstances under which this kind of transition takes place. Perhaps, however, they failed to note one subtlety, specifically, the fact that many tools do not have meaning. At one point, Bahktin (Voloshinov, 1929) correctly wrote that a tool has assigned purpose, but not meaning. That is, not every tool can function as a psychological tool, as a psychological means of activity. In other words, the question arises as to how internal psychological means (or tools), which have meaning, are formed on the basis of external tool-mediated action where the tool is devoid of meaning. The answer to this question was already partially developed during Vygotsky's lifetime. Bakhtin (1929) and Mandel'shtam (1922) introduced (apparently independently of one another) the concept of "object meaning." Much later, the Marxist psychologist Holzkamp (1973), while developing the psychological theory of activity of Vygotsky, Luria, and Leont'ev, once again introduced the concept of "object meaning." Holzkamp had in mind the subject's experience arising from individual practical activity. In principle, this experience is richer than the system of verbal categories that one masters. In Vygotsky's account of the development of concepts, the stage of generalization that he called "pseudoconcepts" corresponds most closely to the concept of "object meaning." It is possible to propose that object meaning is a bridge between external and internal tool-mediated action. It has its own kind of focus in which the processes of internalization and externalization are concentrated. In the process of joint activity, object meaning can be internalized, it can become a means of communication, and so forth. However, as Holzkamp has correctly pointed out, not all object meanings have this fate; that is, not all of them are transformed into meanings. This detail seems to us to be very important. By taking it into account, many puzzles about the internalization of tools are removed. Internalization is the activity–semiotic transformation not of tools, but of their meanings.

This possible mechanism for transforming object meaning into categorical meaning has an additional interesting property. The existence of the process that is the inverse of internalization, that is, externalization, is well known. It consists of the fact that having become the internal means of activity, meaning simultaneously becomes the prototype for new external modes of activity as well. And when these external modes are instantiated, they are already characterized not only (and in many cases even not so much) by object meaning, but by meaning in the real sense of the word. In other words, they are characterized not only by purpose, but by meaning.

In comparison with both the classical and nonclassical variants of the stimulus–response scheme, tool-mediated action (as actualized in either its external or internal form) provides a different ontology of mental reality. Vygotsky initially used the stimulus–means as a third link in the stimulus–response scheme. However, he soon rejected this terminology and began to utilize the concept of psychological means and the concept of tool-mediated activity.

We have given special attention to the characteristics of tool-mediated action as a unit for the analysis of mind since it was precisely this aspect of Vygotsky's research that was later developed most by his students and followers. Above all, it was utilized in the examination of perception, memory, and thinking as systems of perceptual, mnemonic, and cognitive actions. This approach was conceived in the 1930s and continues to be developed today. In his introduction to one of the first experimental investigations of memory understood as action, P. I. Zinchenko wrote:

Any mental process must be understood not as a metaphysical "function" or "capacity" of consciousness, not as the mechanical sum of the organism's reactions, but as a mental action. That is, it must be understood as a type of action that necessarily presupposes the reflection of reality in the form of some mental state. A mental state is necessarily mediated by action. Action itself is a real process in which the transition or "transmission" of objective reality into its ideal mental reflection, into the consciousness of the acting subject, occurs. (Zinchenko, 1939, p. 161)

In this examination of mnemonic action Zinchenko noted that its special feature is that the object of remembering no longer appears as a "stimulus," abstracted from the subject. Rather, it emerges as an essential feature of action, as an object with which the subject enters into a definite relationship. One should note that at that time the concept of "mental action" did not contain a distinct opposition between external material action and internal mental action. In our opinion, the concept of mental action is the equivalent of the concept of tool-mediated action, which, in accordance with the spirit of Vygotsky's ideas, is viewed as mental action independently of the form of its realization (external or internal).

In the 1930s, research began that was dedicated to the activity-oriented interpretation not only of the higher mental functions but also of motor skills and habits. This included the study of children's skill in the utilization of rudimentary tools. This research, which has continued up to the present time, led to the sharp differentiation of external and internal actions and refocused attention on the problem of the external and the internal. In the course of this research the initial treatment of tool-mediated action as mental action was long forgotten. The introduction of the opposition between external material action and internal mental action gave rise to a large number of problems. The most complex of these turned out to be the problem of obtaining evidence for the claim that external and internal activity have a common structure (see Leont'ev, 1975; Zinchenko, 1980). We will consider this problem only to the extent necessary for us to continue our line of reasoning concerning the units for the analysis of mind.

The problem of commonalities in the structure of external and internal activity

We have found that with the development of the Vygotsky–Luria–Leont'ev school, with the development of the activity-oriented treatment of higher mental functions, the category of action began to emerge alongside the category of meaning as a unit for the analysis of mind. As we have attempted to show, one can consider tool-mediated action as being very close to meaning as a unit of analysis. Of necessity, tool-mediated action gives rise both to object meaning and to categorical meaning. (For the moment, we will not address the question of whether action with tools is the sole source of object meaning.) In addition, in the course of these developments, the idea that tool-mediated action can function as a unit for the analysis of mind was not distinctly articulated by anyone. With reference to expanding the application of the category of action as a unit for the analysis of the higher mental functions, there were a number of important developments. First, the category of meaning was pushed into the background. Its restoration as a unit for the analysis of thinking and consciousness began only in the 1970s (see Leont'ev, 1975; Gordon, Komarova, and Puga, 1979). Second, the connection between tool-mediated action and action as such was gradually lost. In the characterization of the latter, its intentional aspects, rather than those aspects related to the use of tools, began to predominate. In other words, a generalization of the concept of action occurred. Concepts such as sensory, perceptual, mnemonic, and cognitive action came to be used in the capacity of genus–species distinctions. One could even say that a reverse "naturalization" of mind began to appear, something to which Vygotsky and Leont'ev had objected so sharply in the early 1930s. For example, instead of the tool, natural movements of the receptive apparati (i.e., movements of the hand, the eyes, the articulatory apparatus, etc.) became accepted as the means for carrying out perceptual action. This kind of generalization can, of course, be considered a departure from premises that are essential to Vygotsky's theory, but this does not seem to us to be the case. Rather, it seems to us that it is the next step in tracing the development of units of mental analysis back to their origins, that is, the elucidation of their preconditions. This problem has continued to be of interest in the Vygotsky–Luria–Leont'ev school to the present day and is of great significance for this chapter. Therefore, we will consider it in more detail.

Vygotsky was above all interested in the origin and the real-life functions of consciousness. Leont'ev, who had become the leader of the school after Vygotsky's death, was above all interested in the origin and real-life functions of the mind. Only after many years did Leont'ev return to the problem of the origin of consciousness. But it does not seem to me that this was a departure from Vygotsky's ideas. Rather, it was a rapprochement, although one equipped with a new arsenal of concepts and a new mode of research.

In a short chapter, it is not possible to review (or even summarize) the enormous amount of research on various cognitive actions that has been conducted by members of the Vygotsky–Luria–Leont'ev school. We will consider only one problem in connection with tool-mediated action. This problem is very similar to the one considered in the previous section. The question is how external, material action becomes internal mental action. In reality, even though the external tool is the result of the transformation of something (previously either external or internal) through subjective activity, the external tool itself does not contain so much as an ounce of mind.

In what manner does the combination of external, material (i.e., nonmental) tool-mediated action (also nonmental) give rise to mental action? In this regard, Vygotsky would probably have said that the maximum that we can obtain from this kind of combination is a mindless automaton. It is precisely with reference to this position that one can explain the tension and the ultimately unfulfilled character of Vygotsky's search for a way to "psychologize" tool-mediated action, the "psychologicalization" that he attempted to attain with the help of "pseudoconcepts" and "meaning." It is a paradox, similar to those often arising in science, that it is precisely this course that, it seems to us, extends Vygotsky's line of reasoning by following his own logic. It would seem that P. I. Zinchenko in the passage cited earlier on mental action provided the answer to this problem. But when the differentiation of external and internal was undertaken, this answer proved to be insufficient. More precisely, the concept of "mental action" was identified with internal action and forgotten. But the problem remained, and several dramatic attempts to solve it were made.

It is well known that the first investigations of the formation and development of perceptual, mnemonic, and cognitive actions were conducted with preschool and school-age children. In these instances, the problem of the separation of external and internal did not arise. External, material action, as it were, naturally entered into the fabric of what was a genuinely mental process. As investigations of the functional structure and microstructure of fully developed perceptual and mnemonic actions in adults began (especially studies of the microstructure of productive short-term processes), researchers began to encounter the following problem. It turned out that it became more and more difficult to identify specific, elaborated (i.e., accessible-to-registration) behavioral acts that correspond with specific forms of internal action (e.g., Zinchenko and Vergiles, 1969). These difficulties are further aggravated by the extensive lists of the cognitive actions, which have been isolated with the help of various techniques, and of the operations and functional blocks that make up these actions. Moreover, with the increased observations of internal actions it became difficult to imagine any direct analogue in external object activity (see Zinchenko, Velichkovskii, and Vychetich, 1980). Consequently, as short-term cognitive actions became the object of increasingly numerous and thorough experimental investigations, the activity-oriented approach encountered, with increasing frequency, situations in which actions occurred in forms that did not seem to involve external means. This is tied to the fact that the methods of cognitive psychology (including the principles for analyzing functional structure and microstructure) have provided a very detailed picture of the structure of the cognitive processes and have outstripped the methods of psychophysiological analysis of cognitive processes and the methods for registering the effector components in perception.

Of course, it would be premature to assert that all the possibilities have been exhausted in the search for the motor components of internal actions. The notion of internalizing external object-oriented activity in the form of internal activity remains in force.[3] But its future development requires serious theoretical and methodological work, as well as experimental substantiation.

At this point, we come to the extremely complex problem of defining action itself, that is, the problem of identifying the most essential and invariant properties that characterize all of its many forms. This definition must be sufficiently general to be suitable for both external and internal action (if this opposition is to be preserved). We are not the first to raise this problem, but it has not been satisfactorily resolved. Nonetheless, the school of Vygotsky–Luria–Leont'ev has a wealth of experience in the study and definition of various cognitive actions. That is, they have created the foundations for defining action as such. Meanwhile, action is a working theoretical concept in which many of the critical problems of psychology are concentrated. The problems of the relationship between the subjective and the objective, the psychological and physiological, and the external and internal are among these. The problem of the internalization and externalization of external mental functions is connected with this concept as well. Thus, the problem of action is the key problem of the psychological theory of activity. All of the theory's real achievements, as well as all of its errors and misunderstandings, are connected with the problem of action.

We will begin our discussion of this problem with the above-mentioned distinction between external, material, practical action and internal, ideal, mental action. This distinction has long been recognized in psychology, and a variety of perspectives on it have emerged. External and internal activity have been perceived as being absolutely distinct, as being identical, or, finally, as possessing structures that are – in principle – shared. As we noted above, the concept of internalization is a bridge between external and internal activity. The acceptance of the notion that external and internal activity are identical makes the concept of internalization meaningless and dismisses the problem of mental development. The acceptance of the notion that these forms of activity are absolutely distinct makes the problem irresolvable. It is impossible to present a logically consistent explanation of how the abbreviation and reduction of external activity can lead to the formation of the internal plane of activity (i.e., to an exclusively "mental" mode of its realization) if external material activity is not a mental formation or does not involve mind as an essential component.

The third perspective, which was expressed by Leont'ev (1975), is more constructive. Leont'ev saw an essential commonality of structure in the two forms of activity in the fact that both external and internal activity mediate the relationship between humans and the world in which their real life is carried out. The unity of various processes of activity that differ in form, as well as the transitions from one form of activity to another, underlay Leont'ev's line of reasoning, a line of reasoning that would permit the elimination or removal of the division of activity into two parts or aspects as if they belonged to two completely different domains. In this approach, Leont'ev directed attention not only to the internalization of external activity, but also to transitions in the reverse direction, from internal to external activity. The notion that external and internal activity share a common structure must not be understood as a position that they are identical. Leont'ev wrote that "the process of internalization is not the *transferal* of an external activity to a pre-existing, internal 'plane of consciousness': it is the process in which this internal plane is *formed*." (1975, p. 98).

In this manner, the theory of activity overcame the notion of an absolute distinction between external and internal activity. In order to solve this problem it was necessary to overcome the absolute opposition of the subjective and objective that is still so widespread. This includes the concretization and expansion of what is ideal and what is objective. The latter can include such things as the description of objects that contain the accumulation of the transformations of reality through subjective activity (see Zinchenko and Mamardashvili, 1977). In the same manner, an expansion of the concept of the subjective, or the mental, is also necessary. Subjectivity must be included in reality, and the primitive distinction between mind and body must be overcome. When subjectivity becomes included in the objective reality of a science, it plays an important role in defining it. It cannot be situated somewhere above the science as a phantom twin of physical events that has to be eliminated, and it cannot be outside of science in the form of a mysterious spirit. In this connection one cannot avoid recalling that Marx had very serious objections to contemplative materialism in which consciousness "was accepted in a completely naturalistic manner, simply as a given that *inherently contrasts* with being or nature" (Marx and Engels, n.d., p. 34; emphasis added).

As a result, we come to the thesis about the relativity of the opposition of subjective and objective and of internal and external. But the question remains as to what concrete significance this has for psychological research and theory and for empirical work and practice. To further complicate the picture, assume that we will not be able to find traces of external activity in internal activity in the foreseeable future. Does this mean that the activity-oriented interpretation of mind will come to ruin? We showed earlier that it is theoretically possible to limit the opposition between the external and internal. But can we restrict this opposition in practice? We think so. Moreover, this is based not only on methodological and theoretical foundations, but also on the basis of experimental methods. If the former were already clearly formulated in the preexperimental period of psychology,[4] the latter are the achievement of recent decades. It is difficult to deny that the overwhelming majority of research in psychology has been devoted to cognitive processes. Executive processes,[5] and above all the form of activity that has come to be referred to as external, material, and practical, were studied significantly less. But external, material, practical activity is also a form of activity. Whatever descriptive phrases we might use to describe it, it is still composed of actions, operations, and so forth. Having accepted our conditional assumption concerning the futility of searching further for the external in the internal, let us try to turn the problem on its head (while not rejecting it completely). Might it be advisable to attempt to find the internal in the external? In other words, perhaps it is necessary to attempt to "mentalize" external, material, practical action. This must be accomplished not with the help of a "spirit" that is foreign to external action, but through the identification of the mental components in external action itself. If this effort is successful, then many problems are either solved or no longer arise. The first of these is the problem of how internal ideal action is formed from external material action.

External material action, which has mental components within its biodynamic fabric, can actually serve as the source for the emergence and development of various transformed forms of action. This includes internal actions that have become isolated and autonomous and have been freed from an external form. But even when internal actions become autonomous, they retain a genetic connection with material, practical actions, they continue to be tied to their origins. Moreover, a functional connection is preserved. That is, the connection manifested in the transitions between external and internal actions (about which Leont'ev wrote) is preserved.

This line of reasoning is completely consonant with ontological claims of Marxist psychology. Such claims are always constructed on the basis of the primacy of the subject's practical activity. Lektorskii (1976) in particular has demonstrated how "the principle of object-oriented activity that has been formulated in Marxist philosophy permits the genetic reconstruction of the varied forms of human activation. It allows them to be genetically 'derived' from a single base. In the Marxist conception, this base is sensuous-object activity, that is, material practice" (1976, p. 60). The philosophical category of sensuous-object activity and the corresponding psychological concept of sensuous-object actions are fundamental to all of psychology, as well as to related applied fields.

The utilization of these concepts as a *genetically* primary foundation has made it possible to oppose methodological pluralism with a unified methodology that opens up the potential for penetrating into the actual nature of the human mind and consciousness. According to Leont'ev, the theory of activity is the concretization of Marxist-Leninist methodology in psychology. The theory of activity is the foundation of a unified, monolithic psychology that makes possible a consistent, coherent reconstruction of nonreductionistic psychological reality.

It is important to note that an integrated picture of mental phenomena can be found in sensuous-object action. For precisely this reason sensuous-object action can emerge as a genetically primary unit for the analysis of the human mind. It emerges as a "cell" of this genus, as the "origin of the developed whole" that has the same actual sensuous–contemplative form. Sensuous-object action contains the most important components of mental action: cognitive, executive, and emotional–evaluative components. Only if we take these components as given from the very beginning can we single out objective processes (i.e., those that operate independently of observation and self-observation). That is, we can select those aspects of the object of psychological research that are subject to objective description where the use of terms such as "consciousness," "will," "subject," "personality," and so forth is inevitable and, moreover, necessary. If we begin with these terms, it is already too late to unite consciousness with natural phenomena and the terms with which they are described. In a similar manner, if we do not accept as given from the very beginning the connections among these components of sensuous-object action, it is then already too late to unify movement and sensation, or image and action. In light of this, consciousness and intentional and emotional mental processes are brought into the analysis *from the very outset* not in their relationship to reality, but in their relationship *in* reality (Zinchenko and Mamardashvili, 1977).

This gives still more significance to the search for the internal in the external. This search must seek support from the analysis of the primary forms of action, or even "living movement" [to use the terms of Bernshtein (1966)]. This is also in accord with the spirit of the activity-oriented interpretation of mind. The notion of action, the basic component of which is actual movement, lies at the basis of this theory. This idea arose as a product of the study of sensory and perceptual action (Zaporozhets, 1967; Zinchenko, 1961, 1967; Zinchenko and Vergiles, 1969; Leont'ev, 1959), the study of the development of voluntary movements (Zaporozhets, 1959), and the study of the formation of intellectual actions and concepts (Gal'perin, 1959; Davydov, 1972).

These investigations, which were carried out within the limits of the theory of activity, assume that ideal, intellectual action incorporates some form of real movement. Therefore, the path of the study of the structure of actions must proceed through a description of various forms of actual movement. But the entire problem consists of the question of how movement should be represented, that is, whether biomechanical, physiological, or psychological characteristics should be used.

The problem of living movement and liberated action

In developing our argument so far, we have arrived at concepts and terms that seem foreign to Vygotsky's theory. They appear to be much closer to Bernshtein's (1966) theory of the structure of movement. Currently, one finds more and more points of contact between these two traditions in Soviet science. It seems to me, however, that this is in accordance with the spirit of both theories. I would remind the reader that Vygotsky took the following statement of Spinoza as an epigraph to his book *The Psychology of Art* (1968):

No one has hitherto laid down the limits to the powers of the body. . . .But, it will be urged, it is impossible that solely from the laws of nature considered as extended substance, we should be able to deduce the causes of buildings, pictures, and things of that kind which are produced only by human art; nor would the human body, unless it were determined and led by the mind, be capable of building a single temple. However, I have just pointed out that the objectors cannot fix the limits of the body's power, or say what can be concluded from a consideration of its sole nature. (*Ethics*, Part III, Postulate 2, Scholion)

In these remarkable words, Spinoza provided support for the construction of the materialistic psychology that Vygotsky accepted. It is a separate matter that Vygotsky constantly sought to explain consciousness as his basic goal. As we attempted to show above, his efforts – and above all his genetic research method for the study of the mind – steadily led him not only to the analysis of activity, but also to the analysis of action. One can even propose that, in a certain period of his work, he considered the treatment of mind as action to be self-evident. Already in 1926 (that is, two years before Janet) Vygotsky defined memory as activity in the strict sense of the word (1926, p. 153).

If Vygotsky was interested in the structure, potential, and actual functions of human consciousness, then Bernshtein (1966) was interested in the structure, potential, and actual functions of human movement. Vygotsky was interested in the morphology of consciousness, whereas Bernshtein was interested in the morphology of movement. Vygotsky viewed consciousness as an organ of individuality. Bernshtein considered living movement in precisely the same manner. These two schools of thought intersected at a point which can be designated "human action." Vygotsky came to it from above; Bernshtein from below.

In this chapter we cannot provide a systematic review of the characteristics of living movement. We will highlight only the most essential features. These are the features that provide a basis for its acceptance as a genetically primary unit in the analysis of mind, a unit that lies at the basis of sensuous-object action. In their research, Bernshtein (1966) and Zaporozhets (1959) convincingly demonstrated the possibility of providing a psychological characterization of living movement. Factors such as the movement task, the program of movement, the image of the situation and of the actions that must be carried out, the image of the intended result of the action, sensory corrections, set, and so on enter into the characterization of living movement. Moreover, in the description of movement, one is dealing with its internal picture. Accordingly, the methods developed by Bernshtein and Zaporozhets for investigating movements presuppose not only an external picture of voluntary movement, but also a characterization of the internal structure of the process that controls it. It includes a consideration of the internal, not yet realized motorics. In other words, both in the Bernshtein school and in the Zaporozhets school, movements have been understood and studied as actions that have definite biological and personal sense. Movements were understood and studied as actions directed toward the resolution of a particular problem, as actions that carry the stamp of the individual's needs.

The results of these investigations made it possible to consider living movement as a morphological object, as an organ of individuality with its own complex structure: "Movement is not a chain of details but a structure which is differentiated into details; it is an integral structure with the simultaneous presence of highly differentiated elements and several options for their interrelationships. This justifies my earlier figurative characterization of living movement as a biodynamic fabric" (Bernshtein, 1966, p. 179). This kind of approach to movement also made it possible to find the internal in the external and to identify the common feature in the structure of external and internal activity. The application of the principles of microstructural analysis to research on executive activity (e.g., Gordeeva, Zinchenko, and Devishvili 1975) is a development of the methods and ideas of Bernshtein and Zaporozhets. This analysis was aimed at elucidating the internal structure of the motor act. The formation and functioning of each of the functional blocks singled out in the motor act (i.e., the block for the formation of programs, the block for execution or realization, and the block for control and corrections) were subjected to extensive study. Results showed that the complexity of the motor act is completely commensurate with the complexity of the cognitive act. The results also showed that there is actually a place for the elements of memory and foresight in the motor act. All this is evidence for the fact that the structures of external and internal activity share not only a common genesis, but a common functional nature as well. As we noted above, the common nature of this structure does not mean certain features and characteristics are not unique to each of these forms of activity. On the contrary, these characteristics must become the object of intensive research.

It seems to us that many of the parameters of living movement that have recently been identified correspond completely with Vygotsky's requirements for units for the analysis of mind. Beginning with living movement and continuing with sensuous-object action and liberated action, an interesting path is revealed for the analysis of consciousness as an organ of individuality. Bernshtein viewed living movement in exactly the same way. The two approaches intersect at the point that could be labeled human action.

Finally, both of these investigators used a dialectical materialistic approach. This is particularly in evidence in their rejection of atomism, in their insistence on the nonreducibility of the whole to its parts or elementary processes, and in their understanding of the fact that it is possible to reveal the structural and functional unity of the whole only when we examine phenomena in their active state.

We will clarify this discussion with the use of one example. According to specialists in the prevention of aviation catastrophes, in complex flying conditions humans and machines turn out to be, as it were, outside of time (we have in mind here the "time" of consciously controlled decisions and actions). It is precisely this fact that provides the potential for avoiding catastrophes. But where does this potential originate? Or must we assume in such cases, as a minimum, a double reading of time – that is, actual situational time and a suprasituational time that flows in the space of the activity itself? And must we also assume their coordination? But by whom are they coordinated? Is there a subject who is responsible for this act of coordination?

The obvious precondition here is the subject's loss of self-control (i.e., the separation of the personal "I" from the situation and, consequently, its separation not only from the time of objects but from the time of the subject as well). This means that the "I" is "outside of time."[6] This kind of "switching off" may not affect the possibility of self-reflection on the actions being performed. But the subject does not plan or control their realization. It is the subject's observing beyond himself or herself that may give him or her the possibility of fixing actions in memory. A split in the personality emerges in which the observing "I" has a very restricted potential for interfering in the conduct of the acting "I." In this kind of situation, it is difficult to say which "I" is primary and which is secondary. This would lead us to ask whether the psychological origins of epiphenomenalism might not lie in this dual personality and the passivity of the observing "I." However, one can argue that such self-observation and occasional surprise at what the subject can do in critical situations is actually an important element in the formation of a conscious personality, including the mastery of professional activities. With respect to such situations, Vygotsky wrote:

In a period of strong excitation a sensation of colossal power frequently appears. The feeling appears suddenly and raises the individual to a new and higher level of activity. In these strong emotions the excitement and sensation of strength merge. This liberates reserve energy (which had been unknown up to that time), and brings to consciousness the unforgettable sensation of possible victory. (1933)

It is useful to compare this with Spinoza's statement that "no one has hitherto established the limits of the body's power."

In fact, we find that in such situations we are faced with liberated or unloosed action. And as the ancients said, a liberated person does not make mistakes. At the same time, it is only here that we find ourselves in the midst of quite special phenomena. These are psychological phenomena proper, phenomena that are acts but not facts (in this sense the concept of fact itself must be reviewed in psychology).

The origins of such liberated actions must be sought in the characterization of living movement. But living movement, in turn, must be considered not as the displacement of a body in space, but as the surmounting of space. It is sufficient to consider the task of structuring movement in a specific object situation (Bernshtein). In order to carry it out, mind and body must comprehend, through some sort of nonrational, nonreasoned means, the most complex physics of the concrete object situation (i.e., statics, dynamics, kinematics, etc.) and coordinate this with bodily biomechanics (which possess an enormous range of degrees of freedom that must be overcome in every motor act). It did not occur to anyone to describe these acts in terms of an act that is controlled and structured through the conscious presence of the individual subject and his or her volition. From here come the terms "blocks," "operations," "functional organs," "organs of individuality," "montage of blocs" (and as the ultimate notion, "spiritual organism") and the categories "space," "time," "the whole," and "life." What does all this mean?

This means one simple thing, but a thing that is nonetheless extraordinarily difficult to master. Just as we accommodated ourselves to the idea of relativity in physics with great difficulty, our patterns of thinking in our psychologized culture make it difficult for us to master the thought that dual phenomena operate, and can be distinguished, in consciousness. These are (1) phenomena that are controlled and developed by consciousness and volition (and that are in this sense "ideal–constructive"), and (2) phenomena and connections that though acting in the same consciousness, are not obvious to it and are controlled by it (in this sense they are uncontrolled by the subject and, in general, are subjectless.) We emphasize that we are referring to a distinction of the contents of consciousness itself, not one relating to the objects of the outside world that influence consciousness. It is important to remember that something in consciousness has "vital" characteristics that defy objective analysis in relation to consciousness in the sense of an individual psychological reality. Human action is the source of these vital characteristics of consciousness. This is the real content of the principle of the unity of consciousness and activity (see Zinchenko and Mamardashvili, 1979).

In his analysis of Feuerbach's views in "The Historical Significance of the Crisis in Psychology" Vygotsky (1982) argued that we can identify two layers of thinking and consciousness. One of these is consciousness of consciousness. The second is objective reality in consciousness. In our view, various forms of action are the source of objective reality in consciousness. A result of this is the mysterious structure of consciousness, a structure characterized both as a sense structure (reality for oneself according to Leont'ev) and in terms of reality in the strict sense that appears in images, representations, meanings, programs of action, and so on.

The degree and extent of the manifestation (or action) of reality in consciousness is inversely proportional to the degree and extent of the reflection by it. It is inversely proportional to the stamp of the "I" in the act, of its objects in the world. In this context, it is clear that the concepts of "physical action," the "objective" (i.e., independent of consciousness), the "external," the "spatial," and so forth must be reviewed and broadened. It is also apparent that the temporary states of dissolution in object-oriented activity that are revealed in the phenomenon of liberated action must be related to consciousness, not to the unconscious as it is understood in the traditional sense. The timelessness of liberated action in situations that are critical for the subject is like the timelessness of acts of creation, acts of brutality, and acts of discovery. In all of these the necessary condition is the liberation or unfettering of the subject, the repudiation of strict subjectivity. The analysis of liberated human action is a serious challenge to psychology.

Conclusion

It would be naïve to expect a chapter of this kind to resolve the numerous problems that arise in connection with a taxonomy of the units for the analysis of mind. We have only attempted to reconstruct Vygotsky's ideas on units of analysis and to show that the requirements he formulated for these units are requirements for current and future efforts in psychology. We considered the units of analysis that, in my view, possess inherent characteristics and that can emerge as genetically primary relative to many formations that subsequently arise in the course of mental development. We include here units such as living movement, sensuous-object action, liberated action, and tool-mediated action. These are able to create object meaning and categorical meaning. A special problem that has not been considered at all in this chapter is connected with that which gives rise to new formations. According to Marx, this occurs through the organs of individuality (it could be said "individuation"), themselves acquiring inherent characteristics, including even the influence on its own origin. In other words, we stand before a dynamic and complex organizational system of phenomena, for which Vygotsky's lessons on description and explanation are very useful.

In concluding this chapter, I would like to say a few words about Lev Semenovich Vygotsky himself. In the opinion of my teachers, he was a very kind man. From his work it is apparent that he was a very fervent man who was relentless in his scientific efforts. He was demanding of others as well as of himself. Knowledge, feeling, and will were harmoniously combined in him. This made him a true psychologist whose life and works served as the example for training many generations of Soviet psychologists. We close with his words, which reveal the Consciousness, Personality, and Activity[7] of this great scholar:

The very attempt to approach the mind *scientifically*, the strength of free thought to master the mind. . .contains within itself the entire past and future paths of psychology. This is so because science is the path to the truth, though it may be a path which leads through delusion. But this is precisely the way it is with us and our path in science: in our struggle, in overcoming mistakes, in the incredible difficulties, and in our superhuman skirmishes with thousand-year-old prejudices. We do not want to be Ivans who have forgotten their heritage; we do not suffer from a delusion of grandeur, thinking that history begins with us; we do not want to obtain from history a clean but trivial name; we want a name on which the dust of centuries will settle [he is alluding here to the discussions concerning the renaming of psychology]. In this we see our historical right, our historical role, our goal of realizing psychology as a science (Vygotsky, 1982, p. 428).

NOTES

1 Here, as in Soviet psychology in general, the terms "methodology" and "methodological" are not used in connection with the problems of designing and conducting empirical research. Rather, they are used to refer to the study of general theoretical and metatheoretical issues that underlie any investigation of psychological phenomena. [J.V.W.]
2 The title of the abridged English translation of this volume is *Thought and Language* (1962). We have used the more accurate translation of the volume's title here since it reflects the orientation toward action and activity that dominates Zinchenko's discussion. [J.V.W.]

3 Incidentally, Vygotsky made some interesting observations about the early reaching movements of the infant. He argued that these movements become indicatory (i.e., acquire a semiotic function) before, or at least at the same time as, they are comprehended and used intentionally. (For more details on this, see Chapter 7 in this volume by Wertsch and Stone.) The remarkable property of such "natural" movements is that they are equally directed at an object and at an adult in the context in which they occur. In such cases we are not only dealing with the type of socialization of the child's behavior noted by Shtern. The mastery of movements with a semiotic function is the condition for its preservation and repetition; it is a condition for the construction of an image and standard of activity. It also creates the prerequisite for the subsequent acquisition of external, artificial semiotic means.

4 Let us illustrate this idea with a quotation from St. Augustine about the connection between memory and action. "Expectation is related to things in the future, memory – to things in the past. In contrast, the tension found in an action is related to the present; through it the future passes into the past, inasmuch as expectations about the end of an action in progress are impossible without memory. . . . Consequently, there must be something in action that related to what does not yet exist" (St. Augustine, *Collected works*, Part 2, pp. 302–303, Kiev, 1901–1915). Thus action is not only a mode that unites the past with the future; it also contains elements of memory and foresight (about which Sherrington wrote at a much later point in history). It is because of this that action is a unique mode for overcoming time and space and hence for mastering them.

5 Zinchenko is using the term "executive" processes here to refer to processes that represent the *execution* of a plan. In his theoretical approach, executive processes follow a latent planning stage and precede a stage of control and correction (See Kochurova et al., 1981). [J.V.W.]

6 In this connection, the following quotation by Faulkner (1943) is quite interesting: "It was as if he had swung outward at the end of grape vine, over a ravine, and at the top of the swing had been caught in a prolonged instant of mesmerized gravity, weightless in time" (p. 5).

7 *Activity, Consciousness, Personality* is the title of A.N. Leont'ev's last book (Leont'ev, 1975). [J.V.W.]

REFERENCES

Bakhtin, M. M. 1929. *Problemy tvorchestva Dostoevskogo*. Moscow–Leningrad. [Translated as M. M. Bakhtin, *Problems of Dostoevsky's poetics*, Ann Arbor, Mich.: Ardis, 1973.]

Bartlett, F. C. 1935: *Remembering: A study of experimental and social psychology*. Cambridge: Cambridge University Press.

Bernshtein, N. A. 1966. *Orcherki po fiziologii dvizhenii i fiziologii aktivnosti*. [Essays on the physiology of movements and the physiology of activation.] Moscow: Meditsina.

Davydov, V. V. 1972. *Vidy obobshcheniya v obuchenii*. [Forms of generalization in instruction.] Moscow: Pedagogika.

Faulkner, W. 1943. Barn burning. In *Collected stories of William Faulkner*. New York: Random House.

Gal'perin, P. Ya. 1959. [The development of research in the formation of cognitive actions.] In *Psikhologicheskaya nauka v SSSR* (T. 1). [Psychological science in the USSR (Vol. 1).] Moscow: Izdatel'stvo APN, RSFSR.

Gordeeva, N. D., Zinchenko, V. P., and Devishvili, V. M. 1975. *Mikrostrukturnyi analiz ispolnitel'noi deyatel'nosti*. [The microstructural analysis of executive activity.] Moscow.

Gordon, V. M., Komarova, N. N., and Puga, N. B. 1979. [The investigation of some subjective and objective determinants of the process of problem solving.] *Ergonomika: Trudy VNIITE*. [Ergonomics: Works of the VNIITE.] Moscow: Vsesoyuznyi Nauchno-Issledovatel'skii Institut Tekhnicheskoi Estetiki, Issue 18.

Holzkamp, K. 1973. *Sinnliche Erkenntnishistorischer Ursprang and gesellschaftliche Function der Wahrnehmung*. Frankfurt: Athenaeum.

Kochurova, E. I., Visyagina, A. I., Gordeeva, N. D., and Zinchenko, V. P. 1981. Criteria for evaluating executive activity. In J. V. Wertsch (Ed.), *The concept of activity in Soviet psychology*. Armonk, N.Y.: Sharpe.

Lektorskii, V. A. 1976. [Principles of object-oriented activity and the Marxist theory of knowledge.] *Ergonomika: Trudy VNIITE*. [Ergonomics: Works of the VNIITE.] Moscow: Vsesoyuznyi Nauchno-Issledovatel'skii Institut Tekhnicheskoi Estetiki, Issue 10, 60-67. [Translated as V. A. Lektorskii, Activity with objects and the Marxist theory of knowledge, *Soviet Psychology*, 16 (4), 1978, 47–55.]

Leont'ev, A. N. 1959. [Mechanisms of sensory reflection.] *Voprosy Psikhologii*. [Problems in psychology,] No. 1, 19–41.

Leont'ev, A. N. 1972. *Problemy razvitiya psikhiki*. [Problems in the development of mind.] Moscow: Izdatel'stvo Moskovskogo Gosudarstvennogo Universiteta. (Translated as A. N. Leont'ev, *Problems in the development of mind*, Moscow: Progress, 1981.)

Leont'ev, A. N. 1975. *Deyatel'nost', soznanie, lichnost'*. [Activity, Consciousness, Personality.] Moscow: Izdatel'stvo Politicheskoi Literatury. (Translated as A. N. Leont'ev, *Activity, consciousness, and personality*, Englewood Cliffs, N.J.: Prentice-Hall, 1978.)

Mandel'shtam, O. E. 1922. *O prirode slova*. [On the nature of the word.] Khar'kov: Istoki.

Marx, K., and Engels, F. (n. d.) *Collected works,* vol. 20.

Tolstoy, L. N. 1957. *War and peace*. Translated Edmonds. Harmondsworth, England: Penguin Books.

Velichkovskii, B. M., and Zinchenko, V. P. 1979. [Methodological problems of contemporary cognitive psychology.] *Voprosy Filosofii*. [Problems in philosophy], No. 7, 67–79.

Voloshinov, V. N. 1929. *Marksizm i filosofiya yazyka*. Leningrad: Gosizdat. (Translated as V. N. Voloshinov, *Marxism and the philosphy of language*, New York: Seminar Press, 1973.) [*This volume was published under the name of Voloshinov, but the basic text belongs to M. M. Bakhtin. – V.P.Z.*]

Vygotsky, L. S. 1926. *Pedagogicheskaya psikhologiya*. [Pedagogical psychology.] Moscow: Rabotnik Prosveshcheniya.

Vygotsky, L. S. 1933. Uchenie Spinozy o strastyakh v svete sovremennoi psikhonevrologii. [Spinoza's doctrine on the passions in light of modern psychoneurology.] Manuscript. Moscow: (Translated as Spinoza's theory of the emotions in light of contemporary psychoneurology, *Soviet Studies in Philosophy,* Spring, 1972, 362–382.)

Vygotsky, L. S. 1934. *Myshlenie i rech'*. [Thinking and speech.] Moscow–Leningrad: Sozekgiz. (Translated as L. S. Vygotsky, *Thought and language.* Cambridge: MIT Press, 1962.)

Vygotsky, L. S. 1968. *Psikhologiya iskusstva.* [The psychology of art.] Moscow: Iskusstvo. (Translated as L. S. Vygotsky, *The psychology of art.* Cambridge: MIT Press, 1971.)

Vygotsky, L. S. 1982. Istoricheskii smysl psikhologicheskogo krizisa. [The historical significance of the crisis in psychology.] In L. S. Vygotsky, *Sobranie sochinenii.* [Collected essays (Vol. 1).] Moscow: Pedagogika.

Zaporozhets, A. V. 1959. *Razvitie proizvol'nykh dvizhenii.* [The development of voluntary movements.] Moscow: Izdatel'stvo Akademii Pedagogicheskikh Nauk RSFSR.

Zaporozhets, A. V. 1967. (Ed.) *Vospriyatie i deistvie.* [Perception and action.] Moscow: Proveshchenie.

Zinchenko, P. I. 1939. [The problem of involuntary memory.] *Nauchnye zapiski Khar'kovskogo Gosudarstvennogo Pedagogicheskogo Instituta Inostrannykh Yazykov.* [Scientific record of the Khar'kov State Pedagogical Institute of Foreign Languages]1, 146–187. (Translated as The problem of involuntary memory, *Soviet Psychology,* Fall 1983.)

Zinchenko, V. P. 1961. [Perception and action.] *Doklady APN RSFSR* [Papers of the RSFSR Academy of Pedagogical Sciences], Nos. 2, 5.

Zinchenko, V. P. 1967. [Perception and action.] *Voprosy Psikhologii* [Problems in psychology], No. 1.

Zinchenko, V. P. 1978. [Set and activity: The need for a paradigm.] *Bessoznatel'noe,* T. 1. [The unconscious, Vol. 1] Tbilisi: Metsniereba.

Zinchenko, V. P. 1980. [The problem of the commonality of structure of external and internal activity.] *Ergonomika: Trudy VNIITE.* [Ergonomics: Works of the VNIITE.] Moscow: Vsesoyuznyi Naucho-Issledovatel'skii Institut Tekhnicheskoi Estetiki, Issue 19.

Zinchenko, V. P., and Mamardashvili, M. K. 1977. [The problem of an objective method in psychology.] *Voprosy Filosofii* [Problems in philosophy], No. 7, 109–125.

Zinchenko, V. P., and Mamardashvili, M. K. 1979. [The study of higher mental functions and the evolution of the category of the unconscious.] In *Razvitie ergonomiki v sisteme dizaina.* [The development of ergonomics in a system of design.] Borozhomi.

Zinchenko, V. P., Velichkovskii, B. M., and Vychetich, G. G. 1980. *Funktsional'naya struktura zritel'noi pamyati.* [The functional structure of visual memory.] Moscow: Izdatel'stvo Moskovskogo Gosudarstvennogo Universiteta.

Zinchenko, V. P., and Vergiles, N. Yu. 1969. *Formirovanie obraza.* [Formation of the visual image.] Moscow: Izdatel'stvo Moskovskogo Gosudarstvennogo Universiteta. (Translated as: V. P. Zinchenko and N. Yu. Vergiles, *Formation of the visual image.* New York: Plenum, 1972.)

5

Vygotsky's uses of history

SYLVIA SCRIBNER

"History" is not a distinctive subject-matter to be inquired into. It is rather at once a trait of all subject-matters, something to be discovered and understood about each of them; and a distinctive way of inquiring into any subject-matter.

Randall, Jr. (1962, p. 28)

This chapter is a beginning exploration of the question "What is history?" in the psychological theory of L. S. Vygotsky.

Although the uses psychologists make of history is a topic worthy of analysis in its own right (White, 1976), the present inquiry addresses a special concern. Since the early 1970s social scientists have shown heightened interest in the relationship between culture and cognition. In spite of many advances in research methods and findings, however, conceptual difficulties continue to limit the enterprise. Principal among these difficulties is the problem of determining for any given domain of intellectual functioning (e.g., conservation, memory, logical reasoning) which aspects are universal in nature and which are specific to particular social environments. Theories of psychological development are of propaedeutic value here, and among them, Vygotsky's theory would seem to hold special promise for construction of an integrative account of cultural variations in thought. Some of us have attempted to develop this promise and use Vygotsky's framework as a guide to our work (Cole and Scribner, 1977; Scribner and Cole, 1981) but the implications of his theory for comparative studies of cognition have proved ambiguous. One source of ambiguity is that Vygotsky, like other developmental theorists, applies his concepts of development to the careers of both the child and the "primitive." These actors walk hand-in-hand through his pages in a relationship we find difficult to define yet impossible to ignore. Are we to infer from these passages that Vygotsky believed that in some cultures characterized as "primitive" adults are "childlike"? If not, are we forced to dismiss Vygotsky's child–primitive comparisons as an unfortunate aberration in an otherwise bril-

119

liant and useful approach to the social foundations of thought? More is at stake in these vexing questions than the accomplishment of a balanced appraisal of Vygotsky. Child–primitive comparisons continue to dominate many studies of cultural influences on thought [Hallpike (1979) is a recent anthropological effort using this framework] and continue to arouse controversy and debate (Cole and Scribner, 1977; Lave, 1981). In this context, clarification of Vygotsky's views seems essential; without it, his writings are subject to misuse; with it, we can hope for further constructive development of a sociohistorical theory of mind.

Clarifying Vygotsky's views of primitive thought, however, turns out to be no simple matter. If we want to go beyond a mere restatement of what Vygotsky said, we need to determine the function child–primitive comparisons played in his system as a whole. To conduct this analysis we are forced to shift our starting point. We need to begin, not with "child" or "primitive" but with more inclusive and fundamental categories in Vygotsky's theory. And this brings us to "history," the topic of this chapter. Vygotsky declares that historical analysis is the key to his system. The essence of a dialectical approach, he states, is to study something historically, to study "phenomena in movement"; "the historical research of behavior is not an additional or auxiliary aspect of theoretical study but forms the very basis of the latter" (DHF, p. 105; for sources and their designation, see note 1).

Accepting this view, we can examine how Vygotsky worked out his historical research of behavior, anticipating that this analysis might help us understand the significance of his methodology involving child and primitive thought. A complete analysis of Vygotsky's historical approach is, of course, a large undertaking and beyond the scope of this chapter. Here I will offer a series of preliminary observations, concentrating on the "sequences of moving phenomena" to which Vygotsky applied the term "history" and their functional role in his theory. Although certain of Vygotsky's concepts have been superceded or substantially modified by Soviet psychologists (see, for example, Leont'ev and Luria, 1968) I have chosen to conduct this analysis in Vygotsky's own terms. I am interested in following the logic of his method of theory construction rather than in evaluating the status of the theory.

Historical approach: Vygotsky's leading contribution

Of Vygotsky's many contributions to psychological theory, he has perhaps been most widely acclaimed for introducing the historical approach to the development of higher mental processes. Graham (1972) tells us that Soviet historians of science, who hold different assessments of Vygotsky's work, agree in honoring him as the first to explicate the historical forma-tion of the mind. This approach is so central to evaluations of Vygotsky that it has been elevated over other constructs to serve, in various compound forms, as the *name* for the theory as a whole. Soviet psychologists refer to Vygotsky's theory as "cultural *historical* theory" (Davydov, and Radzikhovskii, Chapter 2, this volume) or "social *historical* theory" (Leont'ev and Luria, 1968); and U.S. psychologists often seem to have Vygotsky's position in mind when they speak of the "Soviet *sociohistorical* approach" to mental development (as for example, Wagner and Paris, 1981).

In using the compound term "*sociohistorical*" rather than the simple term "*historical*," commentators appear to be singling out for emphasis one of Vygotsky's uses of history – history as the chronology of events involving humanity as a whole. Vygotsky refers to this series of events as general his-tory and we will follow his usage as we begin our analysis.

General history: the first level of history

Singling out general history as the foundation for the entire theoretical edifice seems consistent with Vygotsky's own view of his enterprise. He begins, "The Development of Higher Mental Functions" with a quotation from Engels: "The eternal laws of nature to an ever greater extent are changing into laws of history." Vygotsky invites us to read this work as the unravelling of the mechanisms by which this transformation from the natural to the historical takes place in the phenomena of mental life.

To follow his course, we need to begin with the central questions about mental phenomena that Vygotsky sought to address. As we know, he was absorbed with the problem of the higher forms of behavior or higher psy-chological functions (we will not concern ourselves with the distinction here). To understand the development of the child, he said, psychology must be able to account for such complex phenomena as acquisition of speech and development of planning and self-control, the outstanding accomplishments of early childhood. But such an account was exactly what the various schools of psychology were unable to construct. Vygotsky devotes more than a fourth of his manuscript to an intricate analysis of the limitations in psychological theory and method responsible for this failure. This critique is not easily epitomized, but it pivoted around two seemingly irreconcilable approaches within psychology to the study of higher be-havior. Briefly stated as a reminder of Vygotsky's view of the state of psy-chology in his day: Empirical psychologists conceived of higher forms of behavior as simply more complicated varieties of elementary processes and, like them, products of biological evolution; accordingly, they tried to explain both classes of phenomena by the same laws (the naturalist or natural science camp). Speculative philosopher–psychologists contended that higher functions are *sui generis;* they are not regulated by biological laws or deterministic laws of any kind; as expressions of "human nature," they are, by nature, inexplicable (the idealist or cultural psychology camp).

Vygotsky's diagnosis of the difficulty was a brilliant penetration beneath the surface of the argument. The limitations of both camps arose from a *common* source: Neither understood the true origin of higher mental processes. These are discontinuous with elementary processes because they do not originate in biological evolution and cannot be explained by "natural" laws (i.e., laws of nature). But they are not lawless. Rather, their roots are to be found on another level of explanation – the regularities of the laws of history. Vygotsky put it this way: "Neither the eternal laws of nature nor the eternal laws of the spirit" but "historical laws" are the key to discovering the development of higher forms of behavior (DHF, p. 20).

What are these historical laws? In his discussion of the current state of psychology, Vygotsky presents and dismisses historical approaches offered by several schools, most notably psychoanalysis and "understanding psychology" (represented by the works of E. Spranger). Vygotsky called these metaphysical, unscientific positions: "It is not enough to formally bring psychology and history closer to one another; it is necessary to ask: what psychology and what history are we dealing with?" (DHF, p. 32).

As we know from his many citations, Vygotsky was, in the first place, dealing with the materialist history of Marx and Engels. One of their kernel ideas was that the human species differs from all others because, through its manipulation of nature, it frees itself from biological determinism and begins to fashion its own nature. Productive activities (generically "labor") change in the course of history as new resources and new forms of society come into being. This history is material because it establishes the material activities of people and their intercourse with one another as the source of ideas and mental life (Marx and Engels, 1846).

In adopting this outlook, Vygotsky committed himself to two propositions that it entails: (1) Because socially organized activities change in history, the human nature they produce is not a fixed category that can be described once and for all; it is a changing category. Questions about what human nature is, or more appropriately to Vygotsky's enterprise, what human mental life (the "psyche") is, cannot be separated from questions about how human mental life becomes what it is. Questions of genesis thus move to the forefront of the scientific enterprise; psychological study of human nature (thought and behavior) must concern itself with the processes of formation of human nature. (2) Changes in social activities that occur in history have a directionality: hand-powered tools precede machines; number systems come into use before algebra. This movement is expressed in the concept of historic *development* in contrast to the generic concept of historic *change,* and its reflection in human mental life is expressed as mental *development.*

Here is a passage in the opening chapter of *"The Development of Higher Mental Functions"* in which Vygotsky introduces some of these concepts. He has been laying out the deficiencies in the two camps of psychology and he summarizes them in this manner:

The higher forms of behaviour originated by mankind's *higher development,* are either placed alongside the physiological, organic processes. . .or are totally set apart from all that is material and begin a new and this time eternal life in the realm of ideas. . .Either one or the other. Physiology or mathematics of the spirit, but under no circumstances the *history of human behavior* as a part of *mankind's general history.* (DHF, p. 20; emphasis added)

Vygotsky expresses his main conclusion – the need to search for specifically human behavior in history rather than biology – in this way:

Human behavior differs from animal behavior in the same qualitative manner as the entire type of adaptability and historical development of man differs from the adaptability and development of animals, because the process of man's *mental development* is part of the *general historic development of mankind.* (DHF, pp. 95, 96; emphasis added)

Many years later, Leont'ev and Luria (1968), in a retrospective assessment, credited Vygotsky's theory of "the sociohistorical formation of higher mental processes" as the key to his solution of the crisis in psychology (p. 341). One might say that Vygotsky used the category of "general history" to achieve a synthesis in psychology between "nature" and "culture" (see Toulmin, 1978).

All aspects of the historical progress of humankind were not of equal importance to Vygotsky. He was concerned with those forms of social life that have the most profound consequences for mental life. As we know, he thought these to lie primarily in the symbolic–communicative spheres of activity in which humans collectively produce new means for regulating their behavior. Vygotsky called these means "cultural" and the new forms of behavior "specifically cultural forms" (DHF, p. 46). Historical laws of development, as they apply to human mental life, are therefore laws of development of cultural forms of behavior, and the other way around: Cultural forms appear slowly, each new stage building on a preceding one, so that everything cultural is "in its very nature, an historic phenomenon" (DHF, p. 21). Thus, we find Vygotsky introducing the term "cultural development" in his discussion of the origins of higher psychological functions and in some contexts using it interchangeably with "historical development."[2]

By situating the origin and motor force of the higher mental processes in human cultural history, Vygotsky at the same time redefined the nature of psychological explanation. Insofar as its object of inquiry is regulated by historical rather than biological processes, psychology's search for laws of development (formation of human nature) must be conducted on the sociocultural level of reality, and it must devise a methodology appropriate to this enterprise.

For Vygotsky, then, the transformation of phylogeny (biological evolution) into general history (historical development) is more than a backdrop for a Marxist psychology; it is a first building block in the construction of this science, setting before it the task of explaining the genesis and development of cultural forms of behavior and developing a method for this purpose.

Ontogeny: the second level of history

The second level of history that enters into Vygotsky's system is the "subject's individual history" (T&S, p. 27) or the "history of the child" (T&S, p. 63). Although Vygotsky's concern with the course of human history distinguishes him from other developmental psychologists, his attention to individual growth and change seems to require no theoretical prolegomenon. Individual history appears to many U.S. psychologists to be the natural subject of Vygotsky's psychology or, more conservatively, the domain in which Vygotsky's psychology coincides with the field of developmental psychology as it is customarily defined.

Vygotsky's analysis of child history centers on the same topic as his analysis of general history: the characterization of "uniquely human aspects of behavior" (Vygotsky, 1978; p. 19). Just as Vygotsky rejected the notion that biological laws can explain the emergence of higher forms of behavior in general history, he rejected their explanatory value for these behaviors in child history as well. He claimed that on the individual level of organization, as well as on the species level, two lines of development must be distinguished – the biological (sometimes referred to as natural; see note 2) and the cultural. Natural processes regulate the growth of elementary psychological functions in the child – forms of memory, perception, and practical tool-using intelligence, for example, that are continuous with the mental life of apes and other species. Social and cultural processes regulate the child's acquisition of speech and other sign systems, and the development of "special higher psychological functions" such as voluntary attention and logical memory (DHF, p. 35). These acquisition processes constitute the cultural development of the child, or what Vygotsky claims is the same statement (we will return to this equivalency later), the cultural development of behavior (DHF, p. 17). The cultural line of development is closely linked to the child's "social history," the particular societal and cultural medium in which he or she grows up (T&S, p. 27). It proceeds by the child's mastery of the means and forms of behavior "elaborated in the course of the historical development of human society" (El'konin, 1967, p. 35).

Although most of Vygotsky's work is a sustained argument for psychology's recognition of a separate cultural line of development in the child, he tends to retain the biologically derived term "ontogeny" as a generic term to refer to *all* processes of child development (see note 2). Vygotsky makes a crucial distinction between ontogeny and phylogeny, however. In contrast to phylogenesis, in which the line of historical–cultural development *displaces* the biological, in ontogenesis both lines of development co-occur and are fused. As children grow in size and gain control over locomotion (biological development), they are also acquiring use of tools and speech (cultural development).

We now have two series of changes, each of which involves a line of cultural development, one taking place on the level of general world history and the other on the level of individual history. On both levels specifically human aspects of human nature are in the process of formation.

How do these two series of cultural development relate to each other? Before we try to work out the answer to this question, it seems necessary to justify why it should be raised in the first place. We might take Vygotsky's discussion of the historical development of human nature as an independent topic in its own right. It clearly served the theoretical function of carrying the critique against dualist positions in psychology and establishing the main directions for a new science of behavior. Having served these functions, the concept of general history might silently leave the scene. Adoption of this position would imply that the sociohistorical aspect of Vygotsky's theory plays no significant functional role in his systematic study of higher mental processes in child development.

Vygotsky's writings, however, do not readily lend themselves to such an interpretation. He not only engages in general theoretical discussion on cultural development, but he laces his texts with detailed descriptive material on human behavior in early history and primitive cultures – material culled from the writings of ethnologists, the French sociological school and the field of "ethnic psychology." (Levy Brühl and Wundt are two well-quoted sources in the latter fields.) This material always involves "primitive man," a term variously referring to the prehistoric species at the threshold of humanity, to *Homo sapiens* in the earliest historical epochs, or to "the most primitive man of the now living tribes" (Vygotsky, 1966, p. 18). Vygotsky insists that the data of ethnic psychology need to be taken into account in child psychology if effective approaches are to be worked out for the study of higher processes. And to emphasize the point, as it were, he follows a practice of interweaving material from both these fields in discussions of substantive topics and he does so within an avowedly comparative framework. Thus, Vygotsky seems to be saying that it is not merely history in the abstract but some actual stuff of history that is critically important to theory and research on child development. Let us consider the kind of information he uses from history and anthropology and the contexts in which he considers such material relevant.

Child and primitive

I have selected illustrative material dealing with the two classes of phenomena Vygotsky defined as branches of the development of higher functions – organization of functional systems and acquisition of sign systems. (Unless otherwise indicated, all emphasis in quotations is mine.)

Example 1: Memory. In the essays in "Tool and Symbol," Vygotsky undertakes an analysis of sign operations in the child, focusing on their role in integrating elementary processes into higher systems. He elects to begin with the "history of child memory" since memory is an "exceptionally advantageous subject" for a "comparison of elementary and higher functions" (p. 83). But he immediately introduces material from general history. "The phylogenetic investigation of human memory shows that, even at the most primitive stages of psychological development, we can clearly see two, principally different types of memory functions" (p. 85). When he completes the description of stages of memory in early history, Vygotsky presents a series of studies he and his colleagues conducted on the development of memory operations in children.

Example 2: Counting. In "Development of Higher Mental Functions," Vygotsky includes an important theoretical section analyzing the first forms of sign-mediated activities. He describes as one such activity finger-counting systems among the Papuans of New Guinea: "Counting fingers was once an important cultural triumph of mankind. It served as a bridge over which man passed from natural arithmetic to cultural. . . . Finger counting underlies many scales of notation. It is widely represented to this very day among primitive tribes" (p. 28). "Studying these primitive counting systems, we may observe in developed and active form the same process that is present in rudimentary form during the *development of a child's arithmetic reasoning,* and, in certain cases in the behavior of grown-ups" (p. 129).

Example 3: Prehistory of writing. This discussion (Vygotsky, 1978) presents a clear revelation of the movement of Vygotsky's thought from child to human history to the history of writing to the writing of a traditional people and back to the child. (The passage is continuous but several sentences are omitted for condensation purposes.)

The gesture is the initial visual sign which contains the *child's* future *writing* as an acorn contains a future oak.

. . . Wurth pointed out the link between pictorial or pictographic writing and gesture in discussing the *development of writing in human history.* He showed that figurative gestures often simply denote the reproduction of a graphic sign; on the other hand, signs are often the fixation of gestures. For example, the *pictorial writing of Indians* represents a line connecting points by one that indicates motion of the hand or index finger.

. . . Now we will point out two other domains in which gestures are linked to the *origin of written signs.* The first concerns *children's scribbles.*" [And the second, Vygotsky goes on to say, concerns children's play]. (Vygotsky, 1978, p. 107).

Does ontogeny recapitulate general history?

Reading these passages, we hear echoes of many other comparisons between primitive and child mentality in the history of psychology. Developmental psychology, in particular, has rarely escaped such comparisons. Implicitly or explicitly they are present in the major theories and were certainly a prominent feature of the genetic psychology movement of Vygotsky's day. Most of these comparisons take the form of parallelism, a framework developed in biology that proposes that stages of ontogeny correspond to sequences of life forms in phylogeny. The most conspicuous version of parallelism attempted to account for these correspondences through a biological law of repetition (the biogenetic law) whose workings are inscribed in memory in the famous aphorism that "ontogeny recapitulates phylogeny."

One particular feature of recapitulation theory is of special interest to our present inquiry. Whereas all species have always consisted of both immature and mature members, evolutionary history has been conventionally depicted as a sequence of successive adult stages; and whereas ontogeny is, properly speaking, the entire life history of an individual, conventionally it has been studied with respect to stages of development up to the point of maturity or adulthood (Gould, 1977, p. 484). Accordingly, most ontogeny–phylogeny comparisons take the form of finding resemblances between immature members of higher species and mature members of lower species. When Hall and other genetic psychologists at the turn of the century extended recapitulation theory from anatomy to behavior, they left this form of comparison intact; they proposed that the biogenetic law reproduces forms of thought and behavior in ontogeny that correspond to various stages of cultural evolution. According to the theory, the white Western child passes through all earlier and lower stages to arrive at "civilization"; individuals in traditional societies, however, retrace only part of this ancestral cultural history and remain arrested at one of the lower levels. In this scheme, the term "primitive" applied to early humans of all ages, adults in contemporary traditional societies, and children in industrial societies. [See Grinder (1967) for readings of genetic psychology and Hallowell (1967) and Gould (1977) for critiques.]

As Gould (1977) documents, recapitulation theory supported racist ideology and practices and persisted in psychology long after its repudiation in biology as scientifically worthless.

With this historical background, it is understandable that questions have arisen on the meaning of child–primitive comparisons in Vygotsky's work. Vygotsky's view of higher mental functions as having social–historical, rather than biological, origins sets his theory apart from others and certainly distinguishes it from the thinking of the genetic psychology movement. Still, without diminishing the significance of his theoretical break with biologically oriented psychologies, we need to consider the following possibility: In displacing the biological concept of phylogeny with the social concept of history, did Vygotsky nonetheless leave the structure of the older theories intact? Does ontogeny recapitulate history? Or, in the weaker version, does the child parallel stages of culture on its way to mature intellectual functioning?

These questions are not idle: A biological orientation to intellectual development is not logically necessary to a recapitulationist or parallelist view. And several surface features of Vygotsky's comparative remarks resemble those of classic parallelist theories. For one thing, Vygotsky frequently compares characteristics of the modern child to those of the primitive adult; or, to put it the other way around – for it is in this version that the "shoe pinches" – he compares the primitive adult to the modern child. A second resemblance, as we have pointed out, is that Vygotsky adopts the tradition of using the term "primitive" to refer not only to ancient forebears but to living men and women in contemporary societies whose technological means are primitive.

As an example of the interpretive problems Vygotsky's comparisons pose, consider Luria's (1976) cross-cultural research and the controversy it aroused. In the early 1930s, Luria undertook to test the sociohistorical aspects of Vygotsky's theory in a remote area of the Soviet Union that was undergoing rapid changes in modes of production and social life. In a series of studies among adults, he found conceptual and reasoning differences between nonliterate peasants and others who had participated in agricultural collectives or in literacy and training experiences. These differences were similar to age-related changes psychologists had identified in ontogeny, and Luria tended to interpret them within a development perspective. For example, he considered the grouping of objects by perceptual–functional attributes (common among his nonliterate respondents and young children in other studies) developmentally lower than grouping by taxonomic class membership (the preferred mode of literate, schooled respondents and other children). Luria presented these findings as confirmation of Vygotsky's thesis that the higher psychological processes change as a function of sociohistorical changes. But did this work and its interpretation imply that the "unchanged" Uzbekistanian peasants were childlike? Some critics apparently thought so. Cole (1976, p. xiv) points out that Luria's research received a mixed reception when it was first reported; some believed it insulting to ethnic minorities in the Soviet Union; other commentators faulted not merely this piece of research, but the general theory for its imputation that certain classes and sections of the population who were carrying out Soviet policy were not capable of abstract thought (cited in Cole and Griffin, 1980).[3]

Disagreements as to the implications of Vygotsky's sociohistorical views are not confined to the Soviet Union or the past (see Cole and Griffin, 1980). As I hope my presentation has shown, Vygotsky's writings in the context of the history of developmental psychology provide grist for controversy.

If ambiguities are present in Vygotsky's work; it is not the function of interpretation to "get rid" of them. What I want to show is that some, if not all, of the sources of controversy disappear when we go beneath the surface and examine the functional role of ontogeny–history comparisons in Vygotsky's theory. Before doing that, however, I think it useful to draw attention briefly to material that refutes a recapitulationist position and cautions against an assimilation of Vygotsky's views to classical parallelist positions as well [for descriptions of these theories, see Gould (1977)].

I will confine my remarks to four points.

1. First, Vygotsky vigorously denies that his is either a recapitulationist or a parallelist position. He was quite aware of the possibility that his citation of ethnopsychological material might be interpreted as supporting such

positions and he was concerned to set the record right. One passage (others might be cited, viz. T&S, p. 129) illustrates the tone of his argument:

In the child's development, we find represented (but not repeated) both types of psychological development which we find in phylogenesis in isolated form: the biological and the historic. In ontogenesis both processes have their analogies (not parallels). This is a fundamental and central fact. . . .By this we certainly do not wish to say that ontogenesis in any form or degree repeats or reproduces phylogenesis or runs parallel to it. (DHF, p. 47)

2. A recapitulationist position requires that the same processes operate on both the individual and species level; in biological theories this requirement was met by postulating a biogenetic law of repetition. Vygotsky, however, repeatedly points out that the child's acquisition of tool and sign use does not follow that of primitive man (e.g., DHF, p. 49). He judged Spranger's cultural psychology deficient, in part, because it tried to equate "such different life processes as the historical development of mankind and the child's psychological development" (DHF, p. 32). Equation of these life processes is precluded by the distinctive characteristics of child and general history: The child is an assimilator of sign systems and develops higher functions through processes of internalization. Adults in the course of history are the inventors and elaborators of sign systems, as well as users. Assimilative and creative processes are not psychologically the same. The contrast is well illustrated in Vygotsky's discussion of the development of cultural forms of memory. Children of a certain age learn to use external aids for remembering. In the history of society we also find a stage in which adults rely on external memory aids (notched sticks, knotted ropes). Vygotsky recalls an anecdote related by Levy-Brühl: A missionary observed a man in a preliterate culture carving figures in a piece of wood to help him remember a sermon that impressed him. Vygotsky says that Levy-Bruhl saw this as an example of the way primitive man relies on memory instead of thought,but "we are prone to see the contrary in this example, how man's intellect leads to the formation of new forms of memory. . .how much thought must have been necessary to inscribe a speech by carving figures on a piece of wood" (DHF, p. 125). What is memory to a child (use of an aid to remember) is thought for the adult (preparation of an aid to remember).

3. Turning to parallelism: Classical positions set up correspondences in the *content* of child behavior and the *content* of adult behavior in earlier epochs. In the genetic psychology movement, fears, ideas, and beliefs about the world were the material proof of the affinity of child and cultural developments. [See Gould (1977) for some startling examples. Grinder (167) reports that Hall, a founder of genetic psychology in the United

States, launched his work with a volume on *The Content of Children's Minds.*]
Vygotsky makes no claim for phenotypic similarities and severely criticizes
psychologists who do. "It goes without saying," he points out, that "to base
oneself on ethnopsychological data does not mean to transpose them
directly to the doctrine of ontogenesis" (DHF, p. 38) nor does it mean there
is a correspondence between actual phenomena of cultural development
in the child and in history. Vygotsky's refusal to assume likenesses in
mental content across time and place is consistent with his view of sociohistorical shaping of mind: Ontogentic development is influenced by its particular sociocultural milieu; not only are modern children unlike primitive
adults in "real life" but they are unlike children in other times and places.
In an obvious reference to Piaget's early work, Vygotsky protests that, in
certain psychological research

the world outlook and causal concept of the contemporary European child of
intellectual background and the same outlook and concept of a child coming from
some primitive tribe, the outlook of a child from the Stone Age, that of the Middle
Ages, and that of the XX century – these are all conceived as being basically identical; one and the same in principle, always equal one to the other. (DHF,
p. 22, 23)

4. Finally Vygotsky's position lacks a principal feature of classical
parallelist theories – a "stage theory" of culture that can be brought into
correspondence with stages in ontogeny. I find no evidence that Vygotsky
incorporated a Spencerian (1888) or other doctrine of cultural stages in his
theory. According to Spencer, societies develop over history, becoming increasingly complex and more highly organized, each marked by more advanced forms of thought. According to Vygotsky, the decisive moment in
history is marked by the *advent* of culture – more exactly, the invention of
cultural means for regulating behavior. The transition from nature to culture is the lever for movement from lower to higher forms of thought. In a
generic sense, all cultures exhibit some higher forms of behavior and
thought; indeed these define the human species. For what makes an individual a primitive human rather than an animal is the fact that he or she
uses tools and signs to mediate interactions with nature and with others. All
humans participate in the most powerful, most basic of all sign systems,
speech. Because every language incorporates a system of socially created
significances, all human adults who have mastered this system will have a
human, that is, semantic, consciousness. And because all human societies
known to us engage in processes of dialogue and communication, we must
make the assumption that in childhood, speech has gone inward and has
reorganized some forms of psychological functioning in at least some
domains. Vygotsky says just that "should it be exposed enthnologically, we
would witness an all-encompassing stage of culture which has been

reached during different epochs and in differing forms by all nations" (DHF, p. 108). Such a framework – holding that adults in all cultures have higher sign-mediated systems of some kind – imposes a substantial constraint on developmental interpretations of cognitive differences among adult populations. Over and beyond the "all-encompassing stage of culture," differences will be located in the particular characteristics of higher systems and the functions they serve, not in the absence or presence of "higher thought." Because cultural means have developed over history, and will continue to develop, we expect to find continual changes in the structure and form of higher systems.

It would be possible, of course, to order higher systems in a progression according to their different characteristics, assigning one level to a certain historical period and another more advanced level to a nearer point in time. But just as Vygotsky does not offer a "progression of cultural stages," he does not offer a stagelike progression of higher forms of behavior. One reason, I believe, is that he does not represent higher systems as general modes of thought or as general structures of intelligence in a Piagetian sense. Vygotsky addressed the question of general processes of formation of particular functional systems, a project quite at variance from one aimed at delineating a particular sequence of general functional systems. In the passages quoted above, we note that Vygotsky's comparisons are always made with respect to some particular system of sign-mediated behavior – memory, counting, writing. As we will see, each of these systems has its own course of development; all of them ("higher" or "cultural" by definition) advance from rudimentary to more advanced forms. But there is no *necessity* in theory for all functional systems characterizing the behavior of an individual, or behaviors in a given social group, to be at the same level. Vygotsky's theory allows for the possibility, for example, that highly developed forms of memory or planned behavior will coincide with the use of primitive counting systems, or the other way around. Various combinations are theoretically conceivable. In actuality, because cultural means have a single line of historical development according to Vygotsky, all combinations are not likely to be realized: looking backward at early human societies, we find no examples of highly advanced mathematical systems in the absence of written notational systems. Thus Vygotsky sometimes refers globally to the "psychology of primitive man" (DHF, p. 41) and contrasts it, in dichotomous fashion, to the "higher psychology of modern man." His theoretical scheme, however, does not itself impose such global comparisons. Since his child–primitive comparisons are made with respect to particular functional systems, it is in Vygotsky's studies of the formation of these systems that we expect to locate their functional significance.

Higher psychological functions: a third line of history

Higher psychological functions have their own genesis and stages of development, – in the broadest sense, a history. This history, is, of course, embedded in the history of real people and is therefore realized on the two planes of phenomena we have already examined – general history and child history: "These functions, which from the point of view of phylogenesis arc [products of] the historical development of the human personality possess also from the point of view of ontogenesis, their own particular history of development" (T&S, p. 64).

As compared to the history of humanity or child history, the history of the development of the higher psychological functions (this is Vygotsky's terminology) is "an absolutely unexplored field of psychology" (DHF, p. 1). Yet, Vygotsky argues, to understand the cultural development of the child, we need to know the specific features of structure and function that characterize higher systems, their origin and development to "full maturity and death" (DHF, p. 6), and the laws to which they are subject. The title of Vygotsky's "Development of Higher Mental Functions" now becomes clear. He proposes to accomplish psychology's mission – achieving an understanding of the formation of human nature (see the discussion under the heading "General history. . .") through studies of the origin and development of higher psychological functions *as such*. This is a radical enterprise for it amounts to nothing less than constructing a new object of scientific investigation. In the essays collected in "Tool and Symbol," Vygotsky set his exposition in the framework of approaches to child psychology and made it clear that his topic was human ontogeny. But in the later work, he equally clearly distinguishes his inquiry from the study of the child as a whole (DHF, p. 3). For purposes of theory construction, he takes as his conceptual object "higher psychological systems" and separates it from the natural object, the "child." [Glick (1983) makes this distinction between conceptual and natural objects in a penetrating analysis of Piaget's theory of development.]

Since Vygotsky took a new object for investigation, he needed a new method for this task: "The study of any new field must always begin by a search for and elaboration of method. . .the object and the method of study emerge as closely linked to each other" (DHF, p. 68).

How to begin? The psychologies of Vygotsky's day offered few leads. Cultural psychology was concerned with the products, not the processes, of cultural development. Traditional approaches in child psychology, including experimental psychology, did not recognize the separate status of cultural forms of behavior and offered neither concepts for thinking about them nor techniques for their investigation. It seemed necessary to begin at the beginning, with information about actual forms of cultural behavior. Where could one turn to find such material? Because the history of higher functions appears twice, once in child history and once in general history, it might appear that information derived from either of these two sources would serve as a suitable point of departure. Not so, says Vygotsky. We cannot follow the obvious path of sifting through the thousands of accumulated facts on child behavior, because this behavior is the product of two lines of development, the natural and the cultural, fused into a "common although complex process" (DHF, pp. 37). The two can be disentangled through a process of abstraction, but such a process empties child development of the concrete content the theory builder needs. The way out of the difficulty is to turn to facts of behavior that are the product of the cultural line of development exclusively; these are to be found in the data of ethnic psychology, where higher psychological functions appear before our eyes in clear outline (DHF, p. 44). In phylogenesis,

both these processes – that of the biological and cultural development of behavior – are represented as independent and self-sufficient lines of development.
    . . .Therefore we must turn to phylogenesis which shows no such unification and fusing of both lines so as to untie the complicated knot inherent in child psychology (DHF, p. 36, 37).

As this passage reveals, it was not only to demonstrate the validity of a historical materialist approach that Vygotsky ventured into folk psychology. His excursion was obligatory for methodological reasons: "For the clarification of the basic concepts. . .must by necessity, considering the present level of our knowledge of this issue, base itself on an analysis of how man's psyche developed during consecutive stages of historical development" (DHF, pp. 37, 38).

We now have an additional answer to the question that motivated this exploration of Vygotsky's approach: Why does Vygotsky place such emphasis on the facts of primitive life as the ethnopsychology of his day revealed them? They were the only available source of evidence about changing human behavior that could be used for a psychological analysis of the cultural development of behavior, or, what to Vygotsky was the same thing, the development of cultural forms of behavior. Ethnopsychological material was the only available source because Vygotsky's ideas about two lines of development in ontogeny precluded his use of facts of child behavior for this purpose until they were refracted through the evidence of general history.

This is a broad answer. But we can be more precise in Vygotsky's uses of historical data. He turned to ethnopsychology for discovery purposes and, if we follow his account, we can determine what discovery he made there.

What follows is my logical reconstruction of Vygotsky's steps in building a method for the study of formation of cultural behavior. (We have no way of knowing, of course, whether or not the logical order coincided with the chronological order in which he actually carried out the work and developed his ideas.)

Constructing a model: general history as the middle link

Beginning with Vygotsky's stated goal of achieving a complete dynamic analysis of higher psychological systems, encompassing their genesis, structure, and function, we can identify four moments in his theory-building procedure. The first concerns the discovery of the structure of higher psychological systems. Although Vygotsky tells us he must turn to ethnic psychology to untie the knot in child psychology, in fact he begins to untie the knot with observations about the behavior of *contemporary*, not primitive, adults! As Vygotsky presents it, his starting points were little noticed, but everyday cultural forms of behavior. Certain phenomena, trivial in themselves, are significant to the psychologist for revealing in pure form the defining properties of all higher systems of behavior. Vygotsky called these phenomena "rudimentary forms" – vestiges of behavior developed early in cultural history, now functioning as "living fossils" removed from the contexts that gave them social meaning but valuable as prototypes or blueprints for study. Vygotsky singled out three such rudimentary cultural forms for analysis: casting lots, tying knots, and counting fingers. Each reveals the tripartite structure of cultural forms of behavior consisting of environmental stimulus and response and a human-created symbolic stimulus mediating between the two. Casting lots represents a situation in which a person creates an artificial stimulus to determine her choices in a situation in which a response is blocked by two equipotent and opposing stimuli; tying knots exemplifies the invention of a stimulus to ensure retrieval of information when it is needed; finger counting is the adaptation of always-available objects to support intellectual procedures with a high potential for inaccuracy. Each form reveals the "key to higher behavior" (DHF, p. 129) – the transition point in which the species became human by creating symbolic means to master its own activity.

These rudimentary forms, however, have been superceded in modern societies by different forms of symbolic mediation. Although they are useful in helping the psychologist identify the structural components of higher systems and the primary instrumental function of signs, they cannot reveal their own future. To determine how rudimentary forms change to new forms requires a shift away from observations of everyday contemporary behavior to another domain of behavior. It is at this point, the second moment of theory building concerned with the transformation of structures, that the stuff of general history plays a critical role. At least with respect to some psychological functions, sufficient information is on hand to permit reconstruction of the phases of transformation through which rudimentary forms pass on the way to becoming higher systems. Examining the evidence from ethnopsychology, Vygotsky found that the history of transformation appears similar for various systems of higher behavior. External means of regulation of behavior (e.g., knots) "go inward," passing through a series of stages until symbolic regulation has an entirely intrapsychological form. In this sequence of interiorization, Vygotsky believed he had found a model of the formation of higher psychological functions that might apply to the cultural line of development in ontogeny as well as history. Such a model, of course, was hypothetical, since it was derived by the interpretative mode from documentary evidence. To be established as a scientific scheme, it required testing and elaboration. Observation of child behavior was not the optimal method of test for the reasons that limited the usefulness of facts of child behavior as a method of discovery in the first place: The fusion of two lines of development in child behavior conceals the pure form of cultural development.

Vygotsky's genius now takes hold – the historical sequence can serve as a model for an aritificially evoked process of change in children, a process evoked through experimental means. If children of different ages are used as subjects and the experiment is appropriately set up [see chapter 5 in Vygotsky (1978)], the investigator will be able to follow the way in which children make the transition from rudimentary to higher psychological forms. The experiement will reveal in "pure and abstract form" (DHF, p. 130) how cultural development proceeds in ontogeny.[4] In the terms in which we have been laying out the logic of Vygotsky's procedure, the experimental–genetic method constitutes the third moment of theory building and the source, Vygotsky claimed, of the richest and most vital evidence. The experiment reveals the very essence of the genetic process. By its means, we can witness the drama of the formation of human nature unfolding according to its own laws of development.

Leont'ev's (1964) research on memory development is an especially clear example of the movement from ethnopsychological to experimental data that we have just described. His introduction to that research begins with a review of the phylogenetic history of human memory that traces the creation and elaboration of external signs as memory aids in history and their replacement by self-generated signs or behaviors that are solely internal. He presents this progression as conjectural. It serves only as a "hypothesis" for experimental investigations, whose task is to reproduce artificially under laboratory conditions the process of development of memory (Leont'ev, 1964).

At this juncture, material on the behavior of primitive humans does not represent as great a leap from descriptions of child behavior as the passages quoted so far first suggested. From a systematic point of view, primitive history comes into play to supplement knowledge of certain forms of behavior among contemporary adults with information about adults in earlier times. Ethnopsychology is thus related to child psychology only indirectly through the scheme it presents of how rudimentary cultural forms develop into higher forms.

The rudimentary functions. . .furnish us with a fulcrum for the historical approach to the higher psychological functions and for establishing a link between the psychology of primitive man and that of man's higher psychology. At the same time they furnish the scale by which we may transpose the data of ethnic psychology to experimental psychological research. (DHF, p. 104)

In the present interpretation, the stuff of general history prepares the way for experimental modeling of higher psychological systems. What about the stuff of child history? Observations about the actual developmental progress of contemporary children constitute the fourth moment of theory building. Vygotsky believed that models emerging from experimental studies are, of necessity, schematic and simplified (DHF, p. 221). The experiment fails to inform us about how higher systems are actually realized by the child; an experimentally induced process never mirrors genetic development as it occurs in life (Vygotsky, 1962, p. 69). Nor do experiments capture the rich variety of child behavior in the many settings in which children grow up and acquire culturally elaborated means made available to them in their particular social milieus. Although the experiment models the process, concrete research is required to bring the observations made there into harmony with observations of naturally occurring behavior. Child history provides the material to corroborate or correct the model and reveal how higher processes are formed in everyday activities (DHF, p. 222). Thus Vygotsky begins with and returns to observations of behavior in daily life to devise and test models of the history of higher systems. Starting from behavioral observations of contemporary adults, he moves to observations of primitive adults documented in ethnopsychological records and then, by way of experiment, to behavioral observations of children in modern times.

Vygotsky's sociohistorical approach turns out on analysis to be not only the foundation of his theory of development but a crucial element in his methodology as well. With this in mind, we can understand his somewhat scornful comment that only "sloth" (DHF, p. 48) would assimilate his theory to recapitulationist or parallelist positions. A final verdict is not yet in. But whatever ambiguities his works present, it is clear that he used ethnopsychological material principally for heuristic purposes. Vygotsky was advancing a complicated proposition for psychologists to consider: Look to cultural history for hypotheses about the origin and transformation of higher functional systems. His work may be read as an attempt to weave three strands of history – general history, child history, and the history of mental functions – into one explanatory account of the formation of specifically human human aspects of human nature.

Conclusions: extending the historical approach

Our analysis of Vygotsky's historical approach was motivated by current concerns in research on cultural variations in thought. Sociocultural changes are not a matter of past history but constitute a major condition of life in our times. Whereas investigators of cultural influences on thought have tended to concentrate their studies in traditional societies, new cultural means are being elaborated at an accelerating rate in industrialized nations as well. Hardly have we approached the problem of understanding the intellectual impact of the printing press (Eisenstein, 1979) than we are urged to confront the psychological implications of computerization (Tikhomirov, 1981). Technological and social changes occurring in all societies create a need for comprehensive theories of learning and development; at the same time they provide the context for fundamental research that can contribute to those theories and to more effective programs of education.

For these reasons, it would seem shortsighted to look upon Vygotsky's sociohistorical approach as past achievement rather than as guide to the present. In what ways might we enhance the usefulness of this framework for contemporary cognitive science? One step is to arrive at a more balanced interpretation of Vygotsky's views on cultural differences in thought and a better appreciation of his methodology. Most of this chapter has been directed to that end. However, our analysis also points to certain inadequacies in Vygotsky's historical approach that may limit its current application. We might more accurately describe these as "incompletenesses." Some of the theoretical ambiguities we have noted seem paradoxically to result from Vygotsky's failure to use the historical approach to the fullest: He did not encompass the full range of "phenomena in movement" on the level of either general history or individual history.

Consider general history. In Vygotsky's theory, this history appears as a single unidirectional course of sociocultural change. It is a world process that informs us of the genesis of specifically human forms of behavior and their changing structures and functions in the past. For Vygotsky's model-building purposes, it might have been sufficient to look back at history and view it in this way as one stream of development. But for purposes of concrete research, and for theory development in the present, such a view seems inadequate. Societies and cultural groups participate in world history at different tempos and in different ways. Each has its own past history influencing the nature of current change. Particular societies, for example, may adopt the "same" cultural means (e.g., writing system) but, as a result of their individual histories, its cognitive implications may differ widely from one society to the other. Saxe (1982) provides a dramatic example in his studies of the Oksapmin people of Papua New Guinea. Until recently, this aboriginal group relied exclusively on a rudimentary number system based on body parts to carry out simple quantitative operations needed in daily life. Saxe documents how the organization of the system is changing as a result of new occupational and trading activities. At the same time that this ancient system is undergoing modifications, indications are that the Oksapmin will soon be learning to use hand-held calculators to keep accounts in the number of trade stores in the country (Edwards, 1981). Americans are also learning to use hand-held calculators that are displacing highly routinized paper-and-pencil calculations that have long dominated arithmetic practice in school and personal life. In world history, written arithmetic precedes electronic arithmetic, and there is only this one course of cultural development. This sequence, however, is realized in United States history but not in Oksapmin history. Would we expect psychological implications of computer use to be equivalent in the two societies? Could this question be appropriately addressed in empirical research based on the world history model alone?

Many such discontinuties come to mind, but the import of this single comparison is clear. Individual societal histories are not independent of the world process, but neither are they reducible to it. To take account of this plurality, the Vygotskyian framework needs to be expanded to incorporate a "fourth-level" of history – the history of individual societies. [For a discussion on issues in integrating the history of human society in general with the history of individual societies, see Semenov (1980).]

This expansion of the scheme would have the added advantage of firmly anchoring all studies of social and psychological change in the present. "The most primitive of now living tribes" is a member of a live culture and not a past one. This means that hypotheses about psychological change need to be informed by knowledge of conditions in cultures here and now, and not derived solely from historical reconstructions.

Now let us turn to the level of individual history. In Vygotsky, as in other classic developmental theories, ontogeny stops with the attainment of adolescence. Biological theories of parallelism, as we have pointed out, also work with this truncated ontogenetic sequence; perhaps there is some justification for this practice in biology inasmuch as maturational processes are most marked in early life stages. But what is the justification for a restricted individual biography in a psychological theory emphasizing the "cultural line of development"? Vygotsky himself said that it is not until adolescence that the "problems of cultural psychology" clearly emerge (DHF, p. 26). Whatever one's views about the nature of maturational processes in childhood, it is certain that in youth and adulthood normal psychological change is not attributable to these processes. Flavell (1970) described adulthood as a pure experiment in nature of the effect of experience, and Vygotsky acted on that concept when he resorted to observations of adult behavior to develop his experimental schemes. It is fascinating to consider why Vygotsky's group did not follow through on the logic of the method – why, with the exception of Luria's cross-cultural studies, adults dropped out of the research program. Whatever the reasons, opportunities are now present to fill in the missing link of adult cognitive change.

Basic theoretical questions are at issue. Do adults acquire new sign-systems and new sign-mediated functions in the same way as children? For example, is the learning-to-read process the same for adults with fully developed language competencies as for children? (Weber, 1977). Will Oksapmin adults and children assimilate calculators into their problem-solving routines differently? Does cognitive change in adults proceed in all cases, as with children, from the social interpsychological to the intrapsychological plane? Opportunities to investigate such questions are multiplying and, compatibly, so are the interests of developmental psychologists and educators in extending research to encompass the entire life span. It seems desirable, therefore, to enlarge Vygotsky's framework by replacing "child history" with "life history."

When we incorporate these revisions into Vygotsky's scheme, we have a historical framework consisting of four levels of "culture development" (depicted in Figure 1) in which to locate particular theoretical and research questions. It is customary for investigators concerned with culture and thought to single out for emphasis one or another level of change as seems suitable for the inquiry at hand. Psychologists, for example, tend to conceive of the individual as a dynamic system while assuming in their research designs that history on the societal level is static; anthropologists often make the reverse assumption. When Vygotsky turned his attention to specific topics of child development [e.g., play (Vygotsky, 1978)], he also followed the practice of assuming that only child history was in movement

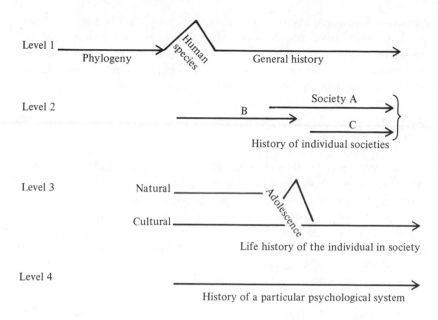

Figure 1. Vygotsky's levels of history – a modified scheme. (As explained in the text, we have modified the scheme to include level 2 and to extend level 3 to encompass adulthood.)

and other lines of cultural development remained constant. Extracting one process of change for study in this manner is a useful and often necessary technique. But Vygotsky's work in its totality makes clear the levels of cultural development are interrelated, that they are proceeding concurrently and mutually influencing each other. His framework is thus a useful guide for researchers who, increasingly today, confront the need to deal simultaneously with more than one level of change. Life-span developmental psychologists, for example, are challenging the dominant view that individual change can be studied independently of sociocultural change. Over a long period of time, the assumption of social stasis is untenable; an eighth-grade education may have been the national norm of half-century ago, but a high school education is the norm today. In this new field, investigators are devising and testing new techniques for studying concurrent changes in individual and social histories (see Schaie, Labouvie, and Buech, 1973).

Cross-cultural researchers are also discovering that presuppositions about the independence of individual and cultural change may need scrutiny. The typical paradigm for studying cognitive development cross-culturally assumes that in each society some stock of cultural means – language, number systems, and the like – is in place and has been mastered by adults who then, informally or formally, help children achieve competency in these systems. As our earlier discussion of Oksapmin society indicated, such assumptions may be unwarranted. We reported that in this aboriginal culture, three arithmetic systems may be competing with one another in the near future – the indigenous body-parts number system (itself undergoing change), paper-and-pencil school arithmetic, and calculator arithmetic. Parents may be shifting over from one or another system or devising inventive combinations of several systems at the very time their children are acquiring their first number concepts. A simple transmission model with arrows running from adult to child seems insufficient here. Novel questions arise. One might ask how adult–child dyadic learning relationships are affected when both members of the dyad are novices and are acquiring new number facts and computationl skills together. Or we might want to inquire into the development of "binumeracy" (drawing an analogy with biliteracy) among adults and children and investigate how uses of one or another number system are influenced by the characteristics of the particular arithmetic tasks that Oksapmin now encounter in their communities. We might be concerned to document whether social pressures are being generated for conversion to a modern number system at a faster rate than some adults are prepared to accept and what consequences such a situation might have for their children's learning progress.

These are among the intriguing questions posed by a consideration of Vygotsky's uses of history. Vygotsky presents us with a mode of theory-building that calls for the integration of all levels of history into one explanatory account of the sociohistorical formation of mind. Few may be ready to concern themselves with such a grand design, but whatever our disciplinary backgrounds, many of us will find it profitable to follow Vygotsky's invitation and explore new ways of bringing an historical perspective to the study of human nature.

NOTES

1 My major sources were English translations of unpublished manuscripts by Vygotsky. One is a collection of essays under the title "Tool and Symbol in the Development of the Child" (referred to as T&S), and the second is the book-length manuscript "The Development of Higher Mental Functions" (referred to as DHF). Most of "Tool and Symbol" and some sections of "The Development of Higher Mental Functions" are available in published form in Vygotsky (1978). An abridged version of "The Development of Higher Mental Functions" is included in Leont'ev, Luria, and Smirnov (1966); Wertsch (1981) has a complete text of Vygotsky's chapter 5. The views I have credited to Vygotsky

are all expressed in these published works, but I have followed the practice of citing the manuscripts because these contained his fullest discussion of methodological choices.

In preparing this chapter I found that Vygotsky's essays in *Thought and Language* [published in English as Vygotsky (1962)] could not easily be integrated with material in the other manuscripts. *Thought and Language* contains Vygotsky's writings on generalization and the semantic structure of consciousness; in these essays, he presents *word meaning* as a critical unit of analysis for the psychology of thought. In "Tool and Symbol" and "The Development of Higher Mental Functions," on the other hand, Vygotsky deals with the role of speech and other sign systems in intellectual operations and treats higher psychological systems as a unit of analysis for developmental psychology. Piaget's distinction between figurative and operative aspects of thought comes to mind, though I do not mean to imply that this classification is appropriate for Vygotsky's work. As additional writings become available, Vygotsky scholars may achieve a better integration of these approaches. For my purposes, I thought it best to confine my account to the two works on higher mental systems because it is in these that Vygotsky engages in the most extensive discussion of methodology.

Because of these limitations in source material, the interpretation I present here has to be considered incomplete.

2 Vygotsky's terminology presents a number of problems, some of which I have flagged in the text. He uses the terms "historical development" and "cultural development" interchangeably. On some occasions he uses the term "phylogeny" to refer to the biological evolution of species and distinguishes this sequence of development from general history. But, on other occasions, he uses "phylogeny" in a superordinate sense to encompass both biological and historical development. In discussing child development, Vygotsky sometimes contrasts the *biological* and cultural lines of change, and at other times draws the contrast between *natural* and cultural lines. Wertsch (pers. commu.) believes that Vygotsky was not consistent in his use of the term "natural": "Sometimes he equated it with biological phenomena, but sometimes it also seems to have included elements of what Piaget would later call sensorimotor intelligence."

3 Luria's studies appear to have been inspired principally by Vygotsky's work on concept formation and generalization, as reported in *Thought and Language*, rather than by the work on higher mental functions [see account in Luria (1971)]. Vygotsky's treatment of concept formation seems to imply a stronger developmental approach to sociohistorical changes in thought than do his other writings, but further analysis is needed.

4 The account given here of the methodological significance of Vygotsky's experimental–genetic studies is substantially the same as that presented by El'-konin (1967). He asserts that the aim of Vygotsky's research was modeling, rather than empirically studying, developmental processes. But he also observes that this interpretation has not been widely recognized.

REFERENCES

Cole, M. 1976. Introduction. In A. R. Luria, *Cognitive development: Its cultural and social foundations*. Cambridge: Harvard University Press.

Cole, M., and Griffin, P. 1980. Cultural amplifiers reconsidered. In D. R. Olson (Ed.), *The social foundations of language and thought*. New York: Norton.

Cole, M., and Scribner, S. 1977. Developmental theories applied to cross-cultural cognitive research. *Annals of the New York Academy of Sciences, 285*, 366–373.

Cole, M., and Scribner, S. 1978. Introduction. In L. S. Vygotsky, *Mind in society*. Cambridge: Harvard University Press.

Edwards, A. 1981. Papua New Guinea: Calculating the way to numeracy. *Bulletin 12*. Reading, England: University of Reading Agricultural Extension and Rural Development Center. May, pp. 20–21.

Eisenstein, E. L. 1979. *The printing press as an agent of change*. New York: Cambridge University Press.

El'konin, D. B. 1967. The problem of instruction and development in the works of L. S. Vygotsky. *Soviet Psychology, 5*(3), 34–41.

Flavell, J. H. 1970. Cognitive changes in adulthood. In P. Baltes and L. R. Goulet (Eds.), *Life-span developmental psychology*. New York: Academic Press, pp. 247–253.

Glick, J. 1983. Piaget, Vygotsky and Werner. In S. Wapner and B. Kaplan (Eds.), *Towards a holistic developmental psychology*. Hillsdale, N.J.: Erlbaum.

Gould, S. J. 1977. *Ontogeny and phylogeny*. Cambridge: Harvard University Press.

Graham, L. R. 1972. *Science and philosophy in the Soviet Union*. New York: Knopf.

Grinder, R. E. 1967. *A history of genetic psychology, the first science of human development*. New York: Wiley.

Hallowell, A. I. 1967. The recapitulation theory and culture. In A. I. Hallowell, *Culture and experience*. New York: Schocken.

Hallpike, C. R. 1979. *The foundations of primitive thought*. New York: Oxford University Press.

Lave, J. 1981. Review of *The foundations of primitive thought* by C. R. Hallpike. *Contemporary Psychology, 26*, 788–790.

Leont'ev, A. N., and Luria, A. R. 1968. The psychological ideas of L. S. Vygotsky. In B. B. Wolman (Ed.), *Historical roots of contemporary psychology*. New York: Harper & Row.

Leont'ev, A. N., Luria, A., and Smirnov, A. (Eds.) 1966. *Psychological research in the U.S.S.R.* (Vol. 1). Moscow: Progress Publishers.

Leontiev, A. N. 1964. *Problems of mental development*. Washington, D.C.: U.S. Joint Publications Research Service.

Luria, A. R. 1971. Towards the problem of the historical nature of psychological processes. *International Journal of Psychology, 6*, 259–272.

Luria, A. R., 1976. *Cognitive development: Its cultural and social foundations*. Cambridge: Harvard University Press.

Marx, K., and Engels, F. 1846. *The German ideology* (reprint. ed.). New York: International Publishers, 1970.

Randall, Jr., J. H. 1962. *Nature and historical experience: Essays in naturalism and in the theory of history*. New York: Columbia University Press.

Saxe, G. B. 1982. Developing forms of arithmetic thought among the Oksapmin of Papua New Guinea. *Developmental Psychology 18*, 583–594.

Schaie, K. W., Labouvie, G. V., and Buech, B. U. 1973. Generational and cohort-specific differences in adult cognitive functioning. *Developmental Psychology, 9*, 151–166.

Scribner, S., and Cole, M. 1981. *The psychology of literacy*. Cambridge: Harvard University Press.

Semenov, Y. I. 1980. The theory of socioeconomic formations and world history. In E. Gellner (Ed.), *Soviet and Western anthropology*. New York: Columbia University Press.

Spencer, H. 1888. *The principles of sociology* (Vol. 1) (3rd ed.). New York: Appleton.

Tikhomirov, O. K. 1981. The psychological consequences of computerization. In J. V. Wertsch (Ed.), *The concept of activity in Soviet psychology*. Armonk, N.Y.: Sharpe.

Toulmin, S. 1978. The Mozart of psychology. *New York Review of Books*, Sept. 28.

Vygotsky, L. S. 1962. *Thought and language*. Cambridge: MIT Press.

Vygotsky, L. S. 1966. Development of the higher mental functions (abridged). In *Psychological research in the U.S.S.R.* (Vol. 1). Moscow: Progress Publishers.

Vygotsky, L. S. 1978. *Mind in society: The development of higher mental processes*. Cambridge: Harvard University Press.

Vygotsky, L. S. 1981. The genesis of higher mental functions. In J. V. Wertsch (Ed.), *The concept of activity in Soviet psychology*. Armonk, N.Y.: Sharpe.

Wagner, D. A., and Paris, S. G., 1981. Problems and prospects in comparative studies of memory. *Human Development*, *24*: 412–424.

Weber, R. 1977. Learning to read: The linguistic dimension for adults. In T. P. Gorman (Ed.), *Language and literacy: Current issues and research*. Teheran: International Institute for Adult Literacy Methods.

Wertsch, J. V. (Ed.) 1981. *The concept of activity in Soviet psychology*. Armonk, N.Y.: Sharpe.

White, S. H. 1976. Developmental psychology and Vico's concept of universal history. *Social Research*, *43*, 659–671.

6

The zone of proximal development: where culture and cognition create each other

MICHAEL COLE

I have chosen the rather unwieldy title of this chapter to highlight an aspect of current psychology that has bothered me for some time – the intellectual separation of its subfields that should, according to its own principles, be closely related. Recently published work by Soviet psychologists following in traditions established by L. S. Vygotsky hold great promise, in my estimation, for promoting reintegration of psychology and its sister science of anthropology.

In the present instance the subfields I have in mind are typically referred to as developmental, cognitive, and cross-cultural psychology and the anthropological efforts known as social, cultural, and cognitive anthropology. With a few exceptions, textbooks on cognitive and developmental psychology are written as if data on cognition and cognitive development were separable from an understanding of the cultural circumstances in which people grow up. Psychological processes are just as routinely downplayed in anthropological texts.

There are both historical precedents and contemporary intellectual justifications to support the separation of these approaches to the study of human nature. Early in the history of psychology as a discipline, Wilhelm Wundt promoted the separation of cultural factors in cognition by invoking a distinction between elementary and higher psychological functions according to individual and social levels of analysis. Elementary functions were the object of controlled, laboratory-based analysis of the introspective accounts of individual human subjects. Evidence concerning higher psychological functions had to be gleaned from data provided by ethnologists, folklorists, and philologists because they represent "mental products which are created by a community of human life and are, therefore, inexpliable in terms merely of individual consciousness, since they presuppose the reciprocal action of many" (Wundt, 1916, p. 3).

After several decades of research applying models and methods of cognitive and developmental psychology in widely different cultures, great uncertainty remains about the utility of the information obtained.

Table 1. *Psychology and anthropology: conceptual polarities*

Anthropology	Psychology
Culture	Cognition
Higher functions	Elementary functions
Products	Process
Content	Process
Group	Individual
Independent variable	Dependent variable
Observation	Experimentation
Field	Laboratory
Holistic	Analytic
Description	Explanation

Whether from the viewpoint of psychology (Jahoda, 1980) or anthropology (Edgerton, 1974) thoughtful observers have noted the severe interpretive difficulties that accompany cross-cultural comparisons. In Table 1, I have compiled two lists of terms that summarize the set of methodological/ conceptual contrasts that have dominated these discussions.

Although a simplification, Table 1 faithfully represents the division of labor that has created what can fairly be called a dualistic approach to mind and society in which psychology is assigned the task of relating individual cognitive processes to group cultural products, which presumably have been described and catalogued by anthropology. In the standard formulation provided by texts on cross-cultural psychology, culture is an important source of independent variables for the study of psychological dependent variables (e.g., Brislin, Lonner, and Thorndike, 1973).

We have discussed the strengths and weaknesss of this approach to the study of culture and psychological processes at length elsewhere (Cole, 1981; Laboratory of Comparative Human Cognition, 1979; Scribner and Cole, 1981). It is not my intent to repeat such a discussion here. Rather, I would like to concentrate my attention on one of the problems posed by the division of labor schematized in Table 1: Nowhere in the table are we provided with a specification of how cultural independent variables become transformed into psychological, individual cognitive processes. How are different cultural contents transformed into cultural differences in cognitive processes? So long as the interlocking set of antinomies contained in Table 1 controls our research, this question will be difficult if not impossible to answer. We are restricted to a relatively crude black-box formulation which can correlate (anthropological) input and (psychological) output. But a direct analysis of the process of change is precluded. And without a systematic method for demonstrating the intimate mechanisms transforming culture into cognition, there is unlikely to be any serious integration of cognitive, developmental and cross-cultural psychology with each other or with their parallel concerns in anthropology; each is trapped in its own set of phenomena, sealed off methodologically from the other.

Searching for common ground

The sociocultural approach

With these remarks as background, I can outline reasons why Vygotsky's work provides a rich source of ideas about ways to reconcile the study of culturally organized experience with the study of cognition and cognitive development.

As described by Luria (1979), Vygotsky set out in the middle 1920s to reconstruct psychology in a manner that would overcome the dualisms emanating from Wundtian psychology and its successors. Central to this effort was an approach that denied the strict separation of the individual and its social environment. Instead, the individual and the social were conceived of as mutually constitutive elements of a single, interacting system; cognitive development was treated as a process of acquiring culture. The normal adult cognitive processes, Wundt's higher psychological functions, were treated as internalized transformations of socially prevalent patterns of interpersonal interaction.

Vygotsky and his students called their approach a "sociocultural" or "sociohistorical" theory of psychological processes. The basic idea was expressed in the "general law of cultural development," where Vygotsky proposed that any higher psychological function appears "twice, or on two planes. First it appears on the social plane and then on the psychological plane. First it appears between people as an interpsychological category and then within the individual child as an intrapsychological category." (Vygotsky, 1978, p. 57).

The tight connection between the social organization of behavior and the individual organization of thinking is further emphasized in Vygotsky's claim that "the levels of generalization in a child correspond strictly to the levels in the development of social interaction. Any new level in the child's generalization signifies a new level in the possibility for social interaction" (Vygotsky, 1956, p. 432, cited in Wertsch, 1983, p. 26).

In the main, these ideas were tested in experiments with children, the work for which Vygotsky is best known. However, even in their early writings, Vygotsky and his students also pointed to a variety of data from the ethnological literature to substantiate the notion of cultural development as a historical process. So, for example, Vygotsky (1978) cited the Inca *quipu,* a record-keeping device, as a historically elaborated logical memory function, and Luria (1932) pointed to the use of drumming during collective work among primitive agriculturalists as a culturally mediated form of will.

In the early 1930s, Luria led two expeditions to remote parts of Central Asia to investigate the hypothetical links between socially organized modes of interaction and cognition. He sought to take advantage of the massive and rapid changes in basic modes of production that followed upon the program of mechanization and collectivization undertaken all over the Soviet Union in the late 1920s. Within a period of two to three years millions of peasants had been organized into collective farms, introduced to modern farming methods, and provided the rudiments of education built around literacy. In the Soviet republics of Central Asia, these changes meant a drastic shift in modes of social control, abandonment of a pastoral existence for sedentary farming, learning a new language, and exposure to a foreign ideology.

Although Luria and his colleagues made many interesting observations, Soviet cross-cultural research carried out within the sociohistorical tradition must be considered of very limited success. Research on perception of Gestalt figures demonstrated cultural variation where universal, biologically coded modes of perception had been hypothesized (leading the enthusiastic Luria to wire Vygotsky with the news that "Uzbekis have no illusions!"). Luria also demonstrated, in a series of clinical interviews, that Uzbekis who had changed their way of living to conform with literate, collectivized modes of production changed the way they responded to classification and reasoning tasks. Uzbekis who retained the traditional patterns of their culture responded to such problems using concrete examples based on their own experience. Uzbekis who had become collectivized (some of whom had learned to read and write) responded to syllogisms as logical puzzles; they also based their classifications of verbally presented items on taxonomic relations rather than the common functions that the objects named could fulfill (Luria, 1976).

Other parts of the research program failed to provide evidence of hypothesized shifts in the organization of mental processes. For example, a key element in analyses of the consequences of literacy was the notion that there would be a shift in the structure of remembering from direct, unmediated recall to mediated, logical remembering. This idea was tested in one study using techniques that mixed free recall and cued recall procedures that had proved useful in developmental studies of recall with children (Vygotsky, 1978). Another large study employed "pictograms" wherein people were asked to use pencil and paper to draw some graphic representation of a to-be-remembered word or phrase. This work, too, had shown interesting age-related changes in children's memory as the graphic representation became integrated into the process of recall.

In neither case did Luria obtain clearly interpretable data when he contrasted collectivized and traditional Uzbekis. The free recall studies produced a marked shift in remembering performance only at relatively high levels of education, and people in all groups displayed mediated patterns of recall for some items. The pictogram data were not sufficiently orderly to permit any generalizations (Luria, pers. comm.).

The resulting mixture of results posed some serious problems of interpretation. At a global level, there were performance differences on some tasks to support the hypothesis of basic shifts in cognition corresponding to differential exposure to collectivized activities. There was, as Luria put it, a shift from "functional" to "abstract" responses for some tasks. However, according to the theory, distinctive modes of thought would be associated with distinctive modes of interaction. In fact, only the contents of Uzbeki culture, in the narrow sense of Uzbeki objects and vocabulary, were represented in the clinical interview. Specifically Uzbeki modes of interaction were never studied, so that only the barest outline of the factors responsible for the differences observed in the clinical interview could be speculated upon.

If these initial observations had been followed up, the cultural–historical aspect of the theory might have undergone proper development. But history itself intervened. The initial reports of this research evoked angry criticism in Moscow where the historical–developmental parallels were taken as evidence that Luria was denigrating the peoples among whom he had worked (see Cole, 1976). His shortcuts and simplifications had made this critique plausible, and it was not until many years later that part of the research was published and new studies undertaken (Tulviste, 1979).

It is a striking fact that the tasks upon which the experimental evidence for the theory rested, tasks conducted for the most part using children as subjects, were absent from Luria's account of research conducted in Uzbekistan. His cross-cultural studies of color and object perception, classification, and logical reasoning were chosen not for their role in the cultural theory, but for the role they had played in Western European studies aimed at specifying general principles of mental function and cognitive development, just the approach he had set out to criticize! Gone were the clever studies of mediated remembering and problem solving, experiments that studied cognition as process in change.

Lacking a detailed theory of Uzbeki adult activities, Luria had fallen back upon general psychological indices of cognitive development. Having substituted indices of mental development and the clinical interview for experimental models of real activity, he compromised the essential principles upon which his theory is based.

The concept of activity

The shortcomings of the cross-cultural research and the need to provide a framework that would allow one to observe the actual processes by which culture shapes cognitive development were well known to Luria, Vygotsky, and their students. But for reasons sketched earlier, they found it more productive to attempt a solution in contexts other than the cross cultural arena.

The seminal formulation in a Vygotskian approach of a unit of analysis that could serve as the basis for a cultural theory of cognition was provided by A. N. Leont'ev, the third founder, with Vygotsky and Luria, of the sociohistorical school. Leont'ev's ideas are beautifully summarized in a relatively recent article (Leont'ev, 1972, reprinted in Wertsch, 1981).

Leont'ev begins by reviewing the shortcomings of research carried out in a "two-part scheme" (by which he meant all manner of stimulus–response theories), because such approaches exclude "the process that active subjects use to form real connections with the world of objects." This exclusion, he says, leads to unconstrained theorizing about internal processes or denies the possibility of principled psychological analysis altogether. As I have characterized it, this criticism applies to virtually all cross-cultural psychological research, including Luria's.

Leont'ev insists on the need for a three-part scheme in which the third part, encompassing the other two, is the subject's *activity (deyatel'nost')*, including the goals, means, and constraints operating on the subject.

The centrality of *activity* to a cultural theory of cognition is reflected in Leont'ev's assertion that

> human psychology is concerned with the activity of concrete individuals, which takes place either in a collective – i.e., jointly with other people – or in a situation in which the subject deals directly with the surrounding world of objects – e.g., at the potter's wheel or the writer's desk. . . . if we removed human activity from the system of social relationships and social life, it would not exist. . . .*the human individual's activity is a system in the system of social relations. It does not exist without these relations.* (Leont'ev, 1981, pp. 46–47; emphasis added)

Following Marx, Leont'ev (as suggested by his reference to the potter's wheel and writer's desk) emphasizes that "intellectual activity is not isolated from practical activity," which he understood to include "ordinary material production" as well as activities that we count as intellectual.

Leont'ev conceived of activity as a nested system of coordinations bounded by general human motives. In contemporary ethnographic terminology, an activity is coextensive with the broadest context relevant to ongoing behavior. Activities are composed of actions, which are systems of coordination in the service of goals, which represent intermediate steps in satisfying the motive. As he puts it, "an activity is usually carried out by some aggregate of actions subordinated to *partial goals,* which can be distinguished from the *overall goal.*" (Leont'ev, 1981, p. 61; emphasis in original). Actions, in turn, are composed of operations, the means whereby an action is carried out under specified constraints.

Leont'ev's concept of activity provides the basic unit of analysis that Vygotsky and his colleagues had been using in a partially articulated way in their research. It also pinpoints the weakness of Luria's cross-cultural research (and, by extension, the work of most cross-cultural psychologists). Working in his own culture, Luria could present a psychological task (defined by Leont'ev as "the goal under certain conditions") and be relatively certain that the goal and conditions were a part of adult activities; hence it made sense to inquire into the way that children come to be guided by those goals and constraints. Knowing the structure of external activity, Luria had an empirical framework within which to interpret their internal concomitants. But he had no such knowledge of Uzbeki activities and their associated congeries of goals and means. Hence, he was on shaky grounds when he attempted to draw inference about thought (e.g., internal activity).

Contributions from Western European and American social sciences

If my account is correct, extension of the precepts of the sociocultural school to actual cognitive activities in other cultures was weakened by the failure properly to deal with real contexts of activity found in the host culture, substituting European-derived tasks for indigenous ones. Psychological research originating with Western European and American researchers can be submitted to the same criticism (e.g., Laboratory of Comparative Human Cognition, 1978). However, there has been research carried out by cultural anthropologists that strongly supports the basic proposals put forth by sociocultural theorists and that illustrates the usefulness of their conceptual framework. This research fits surprisingly well with modern ideas growing up in cognitive psychology.

Contributions from cultural anthropology

Cultural anthropology is not a highly elaborated enterprise in the USSR, but it is in Western Europe and the United States, where it has been a major source of ideas concerning basic units of analysis for the systematic study of traditional cultures. My reading of this literature has impressed me strongly with the correspondence between the Soviet concept of activity and the anthropological notion of an event or context (e.g., Frake, 1977). Two classic formulations will illustrate my point.

In his monograph on *Foundations of Social Anthropology*, S. F. Nadel directly addresses the problem of units of analysis, arriving at a formulation quite similar to Leont'ev's notion of activity.

First, he explicitly acknowledges that it is necessary to determine if "the units we seek to isolate satisfy the condition of the whole, that is, if each bears the characteristics pertaining to that total entity, culture or society" (Nadel, 1951, p. 75). He goes on to define a basic unit that contains both culture and the individual.

Society and culture are broken down, not to, say, individuals, nor to the "works of man" (Kroeber), but to *man-acting.* In this sense no legitimate isolate can be discovered other than that of a standardized pattern of behavior *rendered unitary and relatively self-contained by its task-like nature* and its direction upon a single aim. (Nadel, 1951, p. 75 emphasis added)

At about the same time that Luria was conducting his research in Central Asia, Meyer Fortes was engaged in a field study of the Tallensi of northern Ghana. The object of his study was, as he phrases it, "the entire society and its culture." Like Nadel, Fortes chose a unit of analysis that included both individuals and society. He called it a "social space." Relationships between children and adults were, he says, determined by the child's social space. More generally,

An individual's social space is a product of that segment of the social structure and that segment of the habitat with which he or she is in effective contact. To put it in another way, the social space is the society in its ecological setting seen from the individual's point of view. The individual creates his social space and is in turn formed by it. On the one hand, his range of experiences and behavior are controlled by his social space, and on the other, everything he learns causes it to expand and become more differentiated. In the lifetime of the individual it changes *pari passu* with his psycho-physical and social development. . . .In the evolution of an individual's social space we have a measure of his educational development. (Fortes, 1970, pp. 27–28)

Nadel provides a basic unit of activity that is both individual *and* social. To this Fortes adds the notions that (1) the nature of activity changes over time and (2) activities are mutually constructed by participants.

I will return presently to provide examples of anthropological analyses of people acting in mutually constructed activities that are also important contexts of development. First, however, I want to show how these anthropological concepts parallel important formulations in cognitive and developmental psychology.

Scripts, schemata, and events

Since the early 1970s it has become fashionable to characterize cognitive processes in terms of units variously labeled scripts (Schank and Abelson, 1977) frames (Minsky, 1975), and schemata (Rumelhart and Norman, 1980).

Consider the recent characterization of schemata by Rumelhart (1978). Condensing his discussion slightly, we can say that such theories attempt to account for the representation and application of human knowledge in terms of basic units called schemata.

When we look to the hypothetical content of schemata, the relationship to anthropological units such as "person-acting" become immediately apparent. Rumelhart tells us that there are schemata representing our knowledge of objects, situations, events, sequences of events, actions, and sequences of action. "A schema contains, as part of its specification, the network of inter-relations that is believed normally to hold among constituents of the concept in question" (Rumelhart, 1978, p. 3).

Since schemata are closely identified with the meaning of concepts, word meanings are assumed to represent the typical or normal situations and events that are instances of the schema.

Katherine Nelson (1981) discusses the mechanisms of schema acquisition in a manner that brings us directly back to Vygotsky. Schemata, she tells us, are built up from recurrent events occurring in social contexts. She terms the basic representations of event knowledge "scripts." She then points out that

young children's scripts are initially acquired within contexts that are highly structured for them by adults. . . . one of the salient facts about the social events that they participate in is that they are most often directed by adults *and that the goals involved are the goals of others.* Thus the children's parts in the interactions are determined for them. . . . Adults provide directions for the activities, and often even supply the lines. (Nelson, 1981, p. 106; [emphasis added]).

Here several ideas come together. Nelson is reporting in script terminology on the way that children are incorporated into *adult* activities. These activities are described in terms that fit neatly Nadel's notion of man-acting and Fortes's characterization of a social space as the basic education/culture acquisition unit. Nelson adds the essential idea that children are frequently operating in someone else's scripts, subordinate to the control of others. This brings us to the final Vygotskian concept I want to consider.

The zone of proximal development

Given the strong lines of convergence toward a culturally based conception of cognition that exists in modern cognitive psychology and anthropology, as well as the sociocultural school, we can now turn to the concept that provides the title of this chapter.

When Vygotsky and his students observed the actual processes by which children came to adopt the role of adults in culturally organized activities, they emphasized, like Fortes, and Nelson, the interactional nature of the changes we call development. They found it useful to characterize the behavioral changes they observed in terms of shifts in control or responsibility. In 1934 (translated in 1978) Vygotsky coined the term "zone of proximal development" to describe this shifting control within activities. He first applied the idea in the context of instruction and testing. He said that the zone of proximal development is the difference between a child's *"actual development as determined by independent problem solving"* and the higher level of *"potential development as determined through problem solving under adult guidance or in collaboration with more capable peers"* (p. 86).

Educational applications of this concept have become well known in recent years (Brown and French, 1979; Bruner, Chapter 1, this volume; Cazden, 1981; Wertsch, 1978). This diagnostic and experimental work demonstrates the ways in which more capable participants structure interactions so that novices (children) can participate in activities that they are not themselves capable of; with repeated practice, children gradually increase their relative responsibility until they can manage the adult role.

Here, I would like to treat the idea of a zone of proximal development in terms of its general conception as the structure of joint activity in any context where there are participants who exercise differential responsibility by virtue of differential expertise. I find it significant that Vygotsky's notion of a zone of proximal development provides an excellent summary of Fortes's description of the basic mechanism of education in African Tale society. For example, Fortes tells us that

as between adults and children in Tale society, the social sphere is differentiated only in terms of relative capacity. All participate in the same culture, the same round of life, but in varying degrees, corresponding to the stage of physical and mental development. Nothing in the universe of adult behavior is hidden from children or barred to them. They are actively and responsibly part of the social structure, of the economic system, the ritual and ideological system.

. . .Education, it is clear, is regarded as a joint enterprise in which parents are as eager to lead as children to follow. . . .A child is never forced beyond its capacity. (Fortes, 1970, pp. 19, 23)

Fortes goes on to describe how, within a social sphere that strikes him as remarkable for its unity, responsibility is regulated in a process that provides for the transfer of control to children, to succeeding next generations, as its overall function.

More recent psychoanthropological research describes zones of proximal development within culturally organized activities in some detail.

Alfred Kulah (1973) analyzed an unusual kind of zone of proximal development in his study of the use of proverbs in the formal and informal rhetorical discussions of the Kpelle elders of Liberia. He was interested in the way that young Kpelle children come to learn the meaning of the proverbs. His investigation showed that in a very important sense, proverb content and interpretation are not taught, they are "arranged for." The arranging starts long before any child is expected to know or use proverbs. All Kpelle children engage in a variety of verbal games, including riddling and storytelling. One genre of this game requires teams of children to pose riddles to each other. The riddles consist of two parts roughly akin to a "question" or an "answer". Both questions and answers are part of the traditional lore of the group. They must be learned as pairs. The children line up in two rows ordered by the age of the participants from youngest to oldest. They sequentially challenge each other with riddles. The team that answers the most riddles correctly is the winner.

The teams of children are age-graded. Children of a wide span of ages (say, from 5 to 12) may play, with the oldest on each team taking the first turn, then the next oldest, down to the youngest. In this way, even the youngest member of a team is important, and even the youngest is around to learn many new riddles.

This activity is related to adult proverb use in the following way. The question and answer halves of the riddles that the children learn are key phrases that appear in adult proverbs. It is as if the riddle learning serves to teach children the "alphabet" along the way to learning to "read words." For example, a "question" might be something like "rolling stone" and the answer, "gathers no moss."

Kulah's research shows that the potential meaning in combining "rolling stone" and "gathers no moss" is not well understood by young children, even if they know a lot of riddle question–answer pairs. In a task designed to see if the children would group different riddles by the common meaning that the adult interpretation specifies, young children did not respond as if one riddle was related in any way to another. But as the children grew older, they came more and more to approximate adult groupings of riddles according to their "message." By the time they are old enough to participate in the adult discussions where these proverbs are a rhetorical resource, they show the adult pattern of proverb interpretation. They are ready to learn how to use their now-organized "alphabet" in a new context, as a component in new, adult tasks.

An even closer parallel to the context that Fortes and Vygotsky had in mind is provided by Childs and Greenfield's (1982) description of learning to weave among Zinacantecan weavers of south-central Mexico. Zinacantecan women weave using backstrap looms on which they fashion a variety of basic garments. The role of social guidance in this process is very clear.

The process of weaving can be divided into six basic steps, beginning with setting up the loom to finishing off the woven product. The first time a novice reaches any step the adult or adults in attendance can be found to intervene heavily; after practice they intervene seldom or not at all. On the child's first garment, the adults observed by Childs and Greenfield spent 93% of the time weaving with the child. If a girl had completed one garment, adult participation was reduced to about 50%. After as many as four garments, adults were still involved directly in weaving about 40% of the time.

Childs and Greenfield showed that adult talk is also tied to the level of the child's skill and the specific task at issue. Early in learning, their talk is dominated by commands of the sort "Do x." In later stages of learning, when novice weavers' actions are more skillful, adult talk shifts to comments on salient aspects of the work in progress.

A second important feature of Zinacantecan weaving as an instructional zone of proximal development is that the successive steps toward mastery are experienced by the novice as part of the overall adult activity. From an early age, long before they might notice that they are learning to weave, girls are witness to the whole process. Before they actually take responsibility for any of the six steps described by Childs and Greenfield, they have been witness to the entire process countless times. In an important sense, at the point where Childs and Greenfield begin their analysis, girls are beginning to "practice what they already know."

This manner of arranging instruction provides powerful facilatory constraints on the physical process of learning. In the parlance of contemporary cognitive psychology, the girls are provided powerful "top-down" constraints on learning.

These same points are reinforced in Lave's (1978) study of tailoring in Liberia. Lave carefully analyzed the organization of tailoring practice in shops where several masters and their apprentices produced a variety of men's garments. Like Childs and Greenfield, Lave found that tailors had evolved a systematic ordering of instruction. From time to time, she observed explicit instruction; for example, a master might demonstrate how to sew a button or mend a zipper, or a young apprentice would be asked to practice sewing on a discarded scrap of material. Far more important was the way in which apprentices were kept busy in productive activities while getting exposure to – and practice in – subsequent steps in the tailoring process.

Lave emphasizes the economic importance of the tailor's methods, where instruction of apprentices was a part of the larger system of adult activities aimed at wresting a living under competitive, economically marginal conditions. Virtually *never* is a novice permitted to engage in a task where costly failure is likely. At the same time, apprentices are eager to take over as much of the production process as possible both as a measure of their manhood and a necessary step toward economic independence.

Summary of common ground achieved

From my remarks so far I hope I have established the following points:

1. There is a basic unit common to the analysis of both cultures' and individuals' psychological processes.

2. This unit consists of an individual engaged in goal-directed activity under conventionalized constraints. This unit is variously designated an "activity," a "task," an "event."

3. In the main, particularly where children are concerned, these activities are peopled by others, adults in particular.

4. The acquisition of culturally appropriate behavior is a process of *interaction* between children and adults, in which adults guide children's behavior as an essential element in concept acquisition/acculturation/education.

From this common starting point, different analysts move in different directions according to their special interests. Anthropologists, in general, eschew the implications of activities as the basis for internal activity (e.g., cognition), looking instead to the social structure of which it is the basic unit. Psychologists, in general, eschew analysis of links between activities (e.g., social structure) in their attempts to discern laws of internal (mental) organization and the emergence of more abstract categories of knowledge.

These separate lines of analysis are, of course, but a recapitulation of the division of labor that I described at the opening of this chapter. What I hope has been added is the realization that in circumstances where we do *not* want to take the cultural content of activity as given, we now have common ground that can serve as the basis for a culturally grounded theory of cognition.

Culture and cognition as the object of study

In circumstances where we do *not* want to take the cultural context as given, but seek rather to study the role of culture in organizing systematic differences between people, the sociocultural approach in combination with concepts developed in Anglo-American cultural anthropology and cognitive psychology offers a very fruitful framework because of its militant insistence on linking individual and social activity. "Man-acting" and "schema" may be the "inside" and "outside" versions of the same sphere of activity, as I have suggested. But the mutual indifference of psychologists and anthropologists to the phenomena that they study quickly induces mutual indifference and robs the social sciences of the benefits that might result from the interactions that a common unit of analysis might provide.

A sociocultural approach militates against this separation because of the two-sided nature of *activity* as a basic concept. As Leont'ev states,

In activity the object is transformed into its subjective form or image. At the same time, activity is converted into objective results and products. Viewed from this perspective, activity emerges as a process of reciprocal transformations between the subject and object poles. (Leont'ev, 1981, p. 46)

When we add to this Leont'ev's insistence that activities are systems in the system of social relations it is clear that the study of culture and cognition must incorporate the study of *both the systems of social relations and of internal (cognitive) activity.*

In my opinion, American scholars are in a particularly advantageous position to exploit the insights of the sociocultural theorists. In recent years there has been a great deal of interest among scholars of many disciplines in the "real activities of real people," the necessary starting point of analysis. There has also been an increasingly heavy emphasis on human activity as mutually constituted in interaction.

For reasons that go beyond the confines of this chapter, our Soviet colleagues have not pursued the techniques necessary to fulfill their own theoretical prescriptions [however, see Wertsch (1981) for some interesting beginnings]. Using insights gathered in disparate areas of the social sciences within a sociocultural framework, I foresee the opportunity to solve some of those fundamental problems in the analysis of human nature that Vygotsky confronted a half-century ago and we continue to confront today.

NOTE

Preparation of this chapter was supported by a grant from the Carnegie Corporation. I would like to thank Professor V. V. Davydov, Director of the Institute of Psychology, Academy of Pedagogical Sciences, Moscow, and his colleagues for making possible the discussion of the ideas contained here.

REFERENCES

Brislin, R. W., Lonner, W. J., and Thorndike, R. M. 1973. *Cross-cultural research methods.* New York: Wiley.

Brown, A. L., and French, L. A. 1979. The zone of potential development: Implications for intelligence testing in the year 2000. *Intelligence, 3,* 255–277.

Cazden, C. 1981. Performance before competence: Assistance to child discourse in the zone of proximal development. *Quarterly Newsletter of the Laboratory of Comparative Human Cognition, 3,* 5–8.

Childs, C. P., and Greenfield, P. M. 1982. Informal modes of learning and teaching: The case of Zinacenteco Weaving. In N. Warren (Ed.), *Advances in cross-cultural psychology* (Vol. 2). London: Academic Press.

Cole, M. 1976. Foreword to Luria, A. R. *Cognitive development.* Cambridge: Harvard University Press.

Cole, M. 1981. *Society, Mind, and Development.* Paper prepared for the Houston Symposium IV on Psychology and Society: The child and other cultural inventions. April 30–May 2.

Edgerton, R. 1974. Cross-cultural psychology and psychological anthropology: One paradigm or two? *Reviews in Anthropology, 1,* 52–65.

Fortes, M. 1970. Social and psychological aspects of education in Taleland. In J. Middleton (Ed.), *From child to adult: Studies in the anthropology of education.* New York: Natural History Press.

Frake, C. 1977. Plying frames can be dangerous: Some reflections on methodology in cognitive anthropology. *Quarterly Newsletter of the Laboratory of Comparative Human Cognition, 1,* 1–7.

Jahoda, G. 1980. Theoretical and systematic approaches in cross-cultural psychology. In H. C. Triandis and W. W. Lambert (Eds.), *Handbook of cross-cultural psychology* (Vol. 1). Boston: Allyn and Bacon.

Kulah, A. A. 1973. The organization and learning of proverbs among the Kpelle of Liberia. Doctoral dissertation, University of California, Irvine.

Laboratory of Comparative Human Cognition. 1978. Cognition as a residual category in anthropology. *Annual Review of Anthropology, 7,* 51–69.

Laboratory of Comparative Human Cognition. 1979. What's cultural about cross-cultural cognitive psychology? *Annual Review of Psychology, 30,* 145–172.

Lave, J. 1978. Tailored learning: Education and cognitive skills among tribal craftsmen in West Africa. Manuscript, University of California, Irvine.

Leont'ev, A. N. 1972. Problema deyatel'nosti v psikhologii [The problem of activity in psychology], *Voprosy Filosofii* [Problems of philosophy]. No. 9, 95–108.

Leont'ev, A. N. 1981. The problem of activity in psychology. In J. V. Wertsch (Ed.), *The concept of activity in Soviet psychology.* Armonk, N.Y.: Sharpe.

Luria, A. R. 1932. *The nature of human conflicts.* New York: Liveright.

Luria, A. R. 1976. *Cognitive development.* Cambridge: Harvard University Press.

Luria, A. R. 1979. *The making of mind. A personal account of Soviet psychology.* Edited by M. Cole and S. Cole. Cambridge: Harvard University Press.

Minsky, M. 1975. A framework for representing knowledge. In P. H. Winston (Ed.), *The psychology of computer vision.* New York: McGraw-Hill.

Nadel, S. F. 1951. *Foundations of social anthropology.* London: Cohen and West.

Nelson, K. 1981. Social cognition in a script framework. In J. H. Flavell and L. Ross (Eds.), *Social cognitive development.* Cambridge: Cambridge University Press.

Nelson, K. 1982. The syntagmatics and paradigmatics of conceptual development. In S. Kuczaj (Ed.), *Language, thought, and culture,* vol. 2, *Language development.* Hillsdale, N.J.: Erlbaum.

Rumelhart, D. E. 1978. Schemata: The building blocks of cognition. In R. Spiro, B. Bruce, and W. Brewer (Eds.), *Theoretical issues in reading comprehension.* Hillsdale, N.J.: Erlbaum.

Rumelhart, D. E., and Norman, D. A. 1980. *Analogical processes in learning*. CHIP No. 97. Center for Human Information Processing, University of California, San Diego.

Schank, R., and Abelson, R. 1977. *Scripts, plans, goals, and understanding: An inquiry into human knowledge structures*. Hillsdale, N.J.: Erlbaum.

Scribner, S., and Cole, M. 1981. *Psychology of literacy*. Cambridge: Harvard University Press.

Tulviste, P. 1979. On the origins of theoretic syllogistic reasoning in culture and the child. *Quarterly Newsletter of the Laboratory of Comparative Human Cognition*. *1*(4), 73–80.

Vygotsky, L. S. 1956. *Izbrannie psikhologicheskie issledovaniya*. [Selected psychological investigations]. Moscow: Izdatel'stvo Akademii Pedagogicheskikh Nauk.

Vygotsky, L. S. 1978. *Mind in society: The development of higher psychological processes*. Edited by M. Cole, V. John-Steiner, S. Scribner, and E. Souberman, Cambridge: Harvard University Press.

Wertsch, J. V. 1978. Adult–child interaction and the roots of metacognition. *Quarterly Newsletter of the Institute for Comparative Human Development*, 2, 15–18.

Wertsch, J. V. (Ed.) 1981. *The concept of activity in Soviet psychology*. Armonk, N.Y.: Sharpe.

Wertsch, J. V. 1983. The role of semiosis in L. S. Vygotsky's theory of human cognition. In B. Bain (Ed.), *The sociogenesis of language and human conduct*. New York: Plenum.

Wundt, W. 1916. *Elements of folk psychology*. London: Allen and Unwin.

7

The concept of internalization in Vygotsky's account of the genesis of higher mental functions

JAMES V. WERTSCH and C. ADDISON STONE

Introduction

One of psychology's most persistent problems is how to conceptualize the relationship between external and internal activity. As authors such as Leont'ev (1981), Luria (1981), and Toulmin (1972, 1979) have pointed out, the failure to deal with this problem has been the cause of many blind alleys in psychology and philosophy. The Cartesian assumption that the only true domain of psychological study is internal mental activity has encouraged investigators to focus on issues such as innate competence and to view the problem of how the social and physical context influences individuals' mental processes as unimportant or secondary. Conversely, the assumption of various behavioristic approaches that external behavior is the sole object of study in psychology has encouraged investigators to ignore the complexities of internal psychological processes. The tendency to focus solely on one or the other pole of this dichotomy has not been productive because it has consistently produced incompatible theories.

Leont'ev (1981) has argued that one of Soviet psychology's major accomplishments has been to recognize the integral relationship between external and internal activity and thus to develop a principled account of the relationship between these two domains of human activity. In his words, psychology has recognized that "internal activity, which has arisen out of external, practical activity, is not separate from it and does not rise above it; rather, it retains its fundamental and two-way connection with it" (1981, p. 58).

The connection Leont'ev sees between external and internal activity is sometimes investigated by using the approach suggested by Zinchenko (chapter 4, this volume). Zinchenko and his colleagues (e.g., Zinchenko and Gordon, 1981; Kochurova et al., 1981) have studied the process of externalization, or the transformation of internal activity into external activity. Our concern here will be with the complementary research problem, that of internalization, or the transformation of external activity into internal activity.

162

In the West the notion of internalization has been a part of many twentieth-century psychological theories. It has been studied by figures as diverse as Janet (1926–1927, 1928), Mead (1934), Piaget (1926), and Watson (1924). However, Western investigators have seldom singled it out for explicit definition or analysis. Claims about the internalization of behaviors, action patterns, or social and emotional attitudes have often been quite vague and have masked a wide range of unexplored and undefended assumptions. As a result, there have often been undetected but important differences among investigators in their ideas about internalization. The fact that the same terms are used has often proved to be a source of misinterpretation and confusion rather than an aid to mutual understanding.

In contrast, Soviet theorists have often focused explicitly on the relationship between external and internal activity in general and the problem of internalization in particular (see Gal'perin, 1969, 1976; Leont'ev, 1972, 1975, 1981; Luria, 1981; Rubinshtein, 1957; Vygotsky, 1960, 1962, 1978, 1981a). This is a reflection of the importance attached to these issues in the Marxist–Leninist philosophical foundations of Soviet psychology in which a central concern is the relationship between material reality and human consciousness. In this chapter we will explore one of the major Soviet accounts of internalization, that proposed by Vygotsky and his students.

As noted by Zinchenko (Chapter 4, this volume), the Vygotskian approach begins by rejecting both the assumption that the structures of external and internal activity are identical and the assumption that they are unrelated. He points out that the first position makes the very notion of internalization uninteresting and trivial, whereas the second makes it unresolvable. Vygotsky argued that there is an inherent relationship between external and internal activity, but that it is a *genetic* or *developmental* relationship in which the major issue is how external processes are *transformed* to *create* internal processes. In Leont'ev's words: "the process of internalization is not the *transferal* of an external activity to a preexisting, internal 'plane of consciousness': it is the process in which this plane is *formed*" (1981, p. 57).

At first glance it might seem that there is nothing new in this formulation for Western cognitive psychology. After all, Leont'ev's claim seems to be compatible with the Piagetian notion of internalization or "interiorization" via reflective abstraction (Furth, 1969) that has dominated recent developmental theory. We will argue, however, that the Vygotskian formulation involves two unique premises (premises that are implicit in the term "activity" as used by Leont'ev). First, for Vygotsky, internalization is primarily concerned with *social* processes. Second, Vygotsky's account is based largely on an analysis of the semiotic mechanisms, especially language, that mediate social and individual functioning. Thus, internalization is viewed as part of a larger picture concerned with how consciousness emerges out of human social life. The overall developmental scheme begins with external social activity and ends with internal individual activity. Vygotsky's account of semiotic mechanisms provide the bridge that connects the external with the internal and the social with the individual.

In order to understand the role of these two premises in Vygotsky's account of internalization, they must be explicated within the framework of his genetic analysis. In the words of Vygotsky (1978), we must use a "developmental analysis that returns to the source and reconstructs all the points in the development of a given structure"(p. 65). In the case of higher mental functions (e.g., voluntary memory, voluntary attention, thinking) this means beginning with social phenomena. Vygotsky viewed the failure to do this as one of the fundamental weaknesses of the psychology of his day.

To paraphrase a well-known position of Marx's, we could say that humans' psychological nature represents the aggregate of internalized social relations that have become functions for the individual and forms of his/her structure. . . .Formerly, psychologists tried to derive social behavior from individual behavior. They investigated individual responses observed in the laboratory and then studied them in the collective. . .Posing the problem in such a way is, of course, quite legitimate; but genetically speaking, it deals with the second level in behavioral development. The first problem is to show how the individual response emerges from the forms of collective life. (1981a, pp. 164–165)

Like Marx (1959) and Engels, Vygotsky saw this line of reasoning as applying to social history, but he also utilized it in the study of ontogenesis. In this connection he formulated the following "general genetic law of cultural development."

Any function in the child's cultural development appears twice, or on two planes. First it appears on the social plane, and then on the psychological plane. First it appears between people as an interpsychological category, and then within the child as an intrapsychological category. This is equally true with regard to voluntary attention, logical memory, the formation of concepts, and the development of volition. (1981a, p. 163)

The general genetic law of cultural development provided the groundwork for Vygotsky's approach to many of the ontogenetic issues he studied. For example, one of its instantiations is his notion of the "zone of proximal development" (*zona blizhaishego razvitiya*). He defined this zone as the difference between a child's "*actual developmental level as determined by independent problem solving*" and the higher level of "*potential development as determined through problem solving under adult guidance or in collaboration with more capable peers*" (1978, p. 86). Vygotsky introduced the notion of the zone of proximal development in an effort to deal with two practical issues in educational psychology: the assessment of children's cognitive abilities and the evaluation of instructional practices. In the case of psychological assessment his concern was that a single-minded focus on intrapsychological functioning had restricted psychological assessment (especially testing) to the measurement of a child's past accomplishments. He argued that in order to address the crucial issue of a child's growth potential, testing procedures must examine the realm of the activity where growth takes place. For him this meant examining interpsychological functioning. Thus his proposal was to assess both the child's level of individual performance (i.e., the actual development level) and the level of performance he or she is capable of attaining in interpsychological functioning (i.e., the level of potential development). For detailed explication of these issues, see Brown and Ferrara (Chapter 12, this volume).

Vygotsky's second use of the notion of the zone of proximal development, the evaluation of instruction, was similarly motivated by his claim that intrapsychological functioning grows out of interpsychological functioning. In this case his argument was that

instruction is good only when it proceeds ahead of development, when it *awakens and rouses to life those functions that are in the process of maturing or in the zone of proximal development*. It is in this way that instruction plays an extremely important role in development. (1956, p. 278)

Here again, the issue is how to evaluate interpsychological processes and relate them to their intrapsychological outcomes.

Up to this point we have purposely avoided introducing specific points about Vygotsky's semiotic analysis in order to provide an independent review of the "social origins" premise of his argument. However, one cannot proceed very far in this review without realizing that it is inextricably tied to his "semiotic mediation" premise. For example, when expanding on the general genetic law of cultural development he borrowed a central idea from the French psychiatrist Pierre Janet (1926–1927, 1928) to produce the following semiotic reinterpretation of the genetic law.

The history of signs. . .brings us to a much more general law governing the development of behavior. Janet calls it the fundamental law of psychology. The essence of this law is that in the process of development, children begin to use the same forms of behavior in relation to themselves that others initially used in relation to them. . . .With regard to our area of interest, we could say that the validity of this law is nowhere more obvious than in the use of the sign. A sign is always originally a means used for social purposes, a means of influencing others, and only later becomes a means of influencing oneself.

. . .the mental function of the word, as Janet demonstrated, cannot be explained except through a system extending beyond individual humans. The word's first function is its social function; and if we want to trace how it functions in the behavior of an individual, we must consider how it is used to function in social behavior (1981a, pp. 157, 158)

Vygotsky's semiotic mechanisms served to bind his ideas concerning genetic analysis and the social origins of behavior into an integrated approach. Namely, he argued that it is by mastering semiotically mediated processes and categories in social interaction that human consciousness is formed in the individual. It is within a theoretical framework based on these points that internalization was considered by Vygotsky. The general line of his reasoning can be seen in the following passage:

For the first time in psychology, we are facing the extremely important problem the relationship of external and internal mental functions. . . .everything internal in higher forms was external, i.e., for others it was what it now is for oneself. Any higher mental function necessarily goes through an external stage in its development because it is initially a social function. This is the center of the whole problem of internal and external behavior. . . .When we speak of a process, "external" means "social." Any higher mental function was external because it was social at some point before becoming an internal, truly mental function. (1981a, p. 162)

Among other things this passage reinforces our claim that, for Vygotsky, internalization is viewed as part of the more general picture of how human consciousness emerges out of social life. For him, the reason behind a process's external form is its social nature.

In the rest of this chapter we will examine some of the implications of Vygotsky's account of internalization in light of its role in this general theoretical approach. We will utilize genetic analysis to examine the formation of an internal plane of functioning that derives from social life. In doing so, we will place particular emphasis on the semiotic processes involved in both interpsychological and intrapsychological functioning. Much of our discussion will revolve around a seeming contradiction that arises in Vygotsky's approach. On the one hand Vygotsky argued that internal psychological processes retain certain properties that reflect their social origins, that, in fact

all higher mental functions are internalized social relationships. . . .Their composition, genetic structure, and means of action – in a word, their whole nature – is social. Even when we turn to mental processes, their nature remains quasi-social. In their own private sphere, human beings retain the functions of social interaction. (1981a, p. 164)

Thus Vygotsky envisioned a functional and structural relationship between external social processes and internal psychological processes. On the other hand, however, he made it quite clear that he did not see a simple isomorphism between the two. Indeed, he explicitly rejected this idea as is evident, for example, in his critique of Watson's (1924) account of inner speech (an account in which inner speech is identical with external speech in all respects except its vocalization). In contrast to assuming that external and internal processes are copies of one another, Vygotsky stated that "it goes without saying that internalization transforms the process itself and changes its structure and functions" (1981a, p. 163).

How is it possible to reconcile this apparent contradiction? We will argue that the answer lies in Vygotsky's genetic analysis of semiotic functioning. In order to make this point, we will analyze two examples of the general semiotic mechanism that plays a major role in his account of the formation of an internal plane of functioning.

We will call this semiotic mechanism "the emergence of control over external sign forms." As we will argue below this mechanism serves a crucial function in Vygotsky's account of higher mental processes. It is an example of the following general claim by Leont'ev (1981) about the necessity of transmitting human experience in an external form.

Humans' activity *assimilates the experience of humankind*. This means that humans' mental processes (their "higher psychological functions") acquire a structure necessarily tied to the sociohistorically formed means and methods transmitted to them by others in the process of cooperative labor and social interaction. But it is impossible to transmit the means and methods needed to carry out a process in any way other than in external form – in the form of action or external speech. (p. 56)

One of the correlates of the fact that interpsychological semiotic processes require the use of external sign forms is that it is possible to produce such forms without recognizing the full significance that is normally attached to them by others. As a result, it is possible for a child to produce seemingly appropriate communication behavior before recognizing all aspects of its significance as understood by more experienced members of the culture. One of the mechanisms that makes possible the cognitive development and general acculturation of the child is the process of coming to recognize the significance of the external sign forms that he or she has already been using in social interaction. In more informal terms our claim is that children can say more than they realize and that it is through coming to understand what is meant by what is said that their cognitive skills develop.

The two phenomena that we will analyze are the development of word meaning and the evolution of egocentric and inner speech. In both cases we will see by examining the ontogenesis of sign-mediated activity, we can understand how Vygotsky's claims form part of an internally consistent approach.

The development of word meaning

One of Vygotsky's major concerns when considering the influence of speech on human activity was how the use of words leads to a categorized reflection of reality. For him categorization is an inherent aspect of semiotic functioning both in the social and in individual activity, and it provides an important key to understanding the nature of human consciousness. As in the case of all his claims, he based this argument on the results of genetic analysis. For example, he argued that ontogenesis leads ultimately to the appearance of abstract, generalized categories and systems of categories:

We have attempted to investigate the relationship of the word to reality. We have tried to study experimentally the dialectical transition from sensation to thinking and to show that reality is reflected differently in thinking than in sensation, that the basic distinguishing characteristic of the word is the generalized reflection of reality, (1956, p. 383).

Vygotsky's genetic analysis of this issue begins with the axiom that categorization or generalized word meaning is inextricably tied to human social interaction. Borrowing from Sapir (1921), he wrote:

In order to transmit some experience or content of consciousness to another person, there is no other path than to ascribe the content to a known class, to a known group of phenomena, and as we know this necessarily requires *generalization*. Thus it turns out that *social interaction necessarily presupposes generalization and the development of word meaning*, i.e., generalization becomes possible with the development of social interaction. Thus higher, uniquely human forms of psychological social interaction are possible only because human thinking reflects reality in a generalized way. (1956, p. 51)

In accordance with the requirements of genetic analysis Vygotsky went on to examine how the development of categorization is tied to the development of social interaction in childhood. In this connection he argued that: "the levels of generalization in a child correspond strictly to the levels of development in social interaction. Any new level in the child's generalization signifies a new level in the possibility of social interaction" (1956, p. 423).

Vygotsky's analysis of the interrelated development of word meaning and social interaction is based on the semiotic distinction between meaning (*znachenie*) and reference (*predmetnaya otnesennost'*). Borrowing from Husserl, he pointed out that

it is necessary to distinguish. . .the meaning of a word or expression from its referent, i.e., the objects designated by the word or expression. There may be one meaning and different objects or conversely, different meanings and one object. Whether we say "the victor at Jena" or "the loser at Waterloo," we refer to the same person (Napoleon). The meaning of the two expressions, however, is different. (1956, p. 191)

For Vygotsky, the distinction between meaning and reference had great significance for understanding the ontogenesis of human consciousness; it "provides the key to the correct analysis of the development of early stages of children's thinking" (1956, p. 192). The importance of the distinction derives from the fact that it allowed Vygotsky to deal with the function of referring, or picking out particular objects, independently of the function of categorizing these objects in terms of generalized meanings. This was essential for his account of ontogenesis since he saw agreement on reference as the key to understanding the initial stages of adult–child interaction. It was in this connection that he introduced the notion of the "indicatory function of speech."

Our initial words have indicatory meaning for the child. In this, it seems to us that we have identified the *original function of speech*, which has not been appreciated by other researchers. The original function of speech is not that the word has meaning for the child; it is not that a corresponding new connection is created with the help of the word. Rather, *the word is initially an indicator*. The word as an indicator is the primary function in the development of speech, from which all others may be derived. (1981b, p. 219)

Thus Vygotsky's genetic analysis of word meaning begins outside the realm of meaning itself. His argument was that agreement on reference provides an "entry point" for children to participate in social interaction with more experienced members of a culture. He cautioned that this agreement on reference can easily be mistaken for agreement on meaning. He argued that although it is tempting to attribute an understanding of meaning to children when they begin to use word forms in what appear to be appropriate ways, the appearance of new words marks the beginning rather than the end point in the development of concepts. He considered this to be an essential point that is often not appreciated by investigators of the ontogenesis of human cognition.

The outward similarity between the thinking of the 3-year-old and the adult, the practical coincidence in the child's and adult's word meaning that makes verbal social interaction possible, the mutual understanding of adult and child, the functional equivalence of the complex and the concept – all these things have led investigators to the false conclusion that the 3-year-old's thinking is already present. True, they assumed that this thinking is undeveloped, but they nonetheless assume that it has the full set of forms found in adult intellectual activity. Consequently, it is assumed that during this transitional period there is no fundamental change, no essential new step in the mastery of concepts. The origins of this mistake are very easy to understand. At a very early age the child acquires many words whose meanings for him/her coincide with those in adults. Because of the possibility of understanding, the impression has been created that *the end point of development in word meaning coincides with the beginning point*, that a ready-made concept is given from the very beginning, and consequently that there is no room for development. Those investigators (e.g., Ach) who equate the concept with the initial meaning of the word thereby inevitably arrive at false conclusions, based on illusion. (1956, pp. 179–180)

In making his counterproposal, Vygotsky outlined an ontogenetic progression from "unorganized heaps" to "complexes" and then to "concepts" on the basis of his well-known block sorting and classification tasks. The transition between complexes and concepts is possible because of the existence of "pseudoconcepts" or "concept complexes." In many ways these appear to be genuine concepts, but certain aspects of their properties reveal that they are in fact still complexes. According to Vygotsky, one of the most important functions of pseudoconcepts is that they make possible a more advanced form of an adult–child interaction. However, even at this new level genuine agreement about meaning does not exist between child and adult.

Although the child agrees with the concept in its outward form, he/she in no way agrees with the adult in the mode of thinking or in the type of intellectual operations that he/she brings to the pseudoconcept. It is precisely because of this that the meaning of the pseudoconcept takes on great functional significance as a *special, two-sided, internally contradictory form of childhood thinking*. (1956, p. 181)

Vygotsky argued that this "two-sided" nature of adult–child interaction provided the motivating force behind the transition from pseudoconcepts (as well as other types of complexes) to concepts. He argued that until the child has reached an advanced stage in the mastery of word meanings, adult–child interaction is asymmetrical in an essential way. Whereas children's understanding of words may be based on relatively simple, context-bound sign–object relationships, adults understand them in terms of a complex semiotic system that involves sign–sign relationships. As Silverstein (chapter 9, this volume) points out, Vygotsky's claims in this area were limited by the fact that he did not have access to recent developments in grammatical theory. However, Vygotsky's analysis of "scientific concepts" (an analysis that assumes what Silverstein terms the "meta-semantic function" of language) led him to recognize some of the semantic relationships that guide an adult's use of language. This, in turn, led him to recognize that, when interacting with children, adults introduce a socially constituted set of interrelated linguistic categories. Thus, the child may gain entry into semiotically mediated social life through agreement on reference alone (i.e., without agreement on meaning). However, further progress occurs by mastering fully elaborated meanings embodied in the norms of the adult community.

We have seen that the speech of adults around the child, with its constant, determinant meanings, determines the paths of the development of children's generalizations, the circle of formations of complexes. The child does not select the meaning for a word. It is given to him/her in the process of verbal social interaction with adults. The child does not construct his/her own complexes freely. He/she finds them already constructed *in the process of understanding others' speech*. He/she does not freely select various concrete elements and include them in one or another complex. He/she receives a group of concrete objects in an already prepared form of generalization provided by a word. . . .In general, a child does not create his/her own speech, he/she masters the existing speech of surrounding adults. (1956, pp. 180–181; emphasis added)

This point by Vygotsky brings us back to our claims about his notion of internalization. The mastery of word meaning is an instance of what Leont'ev (1981) terms the formation of an internal plane of functioning. Notice that one must speak here of the *formation* rather than the transferal of something from an external plane of activity. The notion of transferal is inappropriate here since Vygotsky's claim is that it is precisely through the development of internal mental functioning that the child comes to master social (and hence external) sign forms. As Zinchenko (Chapter 4, this volume) notes, "Internalization is the activity-semiotic transformation not of tools, but of their meanings."

Vygotsky's account of the development of word meaning also provides insight into what he meant by his claim that mental processes retain a "quasi-social" character. His claim is not that full-fledged social interaction occurs internally. Rather, his analysis of the development of word meaning reveals that one aspect of his claim is that the concepts used in mental processes are provided by the speech community in which one has developed. Instead of viewing the meaning system of a language as mapping onto preexisting cognitive processes, it is viewed as a social formation that plays a much more active role in the creation of consciousness. As one of us has emphasized elsewhere (e.g., Wertsch, 1983), this does not mean that experience with physical environment plays no role in Vygotsky's overall argument. It does mean, however, that the social environment (in this case, the socially evolved meaning system of a speech community) will be an important determinant of the form of internal intrapsychological functioning.

The development of egocentric and inner speech

As we have seen, Vygotsky saw social interaction as playing an essential role in the development of word meaning. In his view it is through interaction with experienced members of the speech community that the child is exposed to linguistic norms. The primary reason for adults and children to participate in social interaction is not, however, to produce mastery of word meanings. Rather, it is to engage in communication and mutual regulation. It is in connection with speech functions such as these that Vygotsky proposed his account of egocentric and inner speech. This account grew out of his critical reinterpretation of Piaget's notion of egocentric speech. Piaget (1926) described the phenomenon of children's egocentric speech as "speech for oneself, speech which is not intended for others." According to him, egocentric speech is a manifestation of the child's solipistic understanding of the world, his or her, "egocentricity." He argued that as the child becomes socialized this peculiar speech form disappears. In contrast, Vygotsky argued that egocentric speech is the bridge between external interpsychological functioning and internal intrapsychological functioning. His claim was that the "scheme of development [is] first social, then egocentric, then inner speech" (1962, p. 19).

Vygotsky argued that the reason for the appearance of this intermediate speech form is that this new self-regulative function of speech is still not completely differentiated from earlier social functions. The failure to appreciate the existence of this new speech function leads the child temporarily to continue using overt, self-regulative speech and to produce such speech in potentially communicative settings. As the child comes to appreciate and master this functional differentiation, egocentric speech gradually disappears. However, unlike Piaget, who argued that egocentric speech dies out as a result of the child's socialization, Vygotsky argued that "it does not simply atrophy but 'goes underground,' i.e., turns into inner speech" (1962, p. 18). He explained the child's confusion over the differentiation of the communicative and self-regulative functions in the following terms:

Subjectively, from the child's point of view, egocentric speech is not yet distinguished from social speech ([hence] the illusion that others comprehend it). Objectively, it is not separated from the situation ([hence] the use of collective monologue). And in its form (vocalized) it is not distinguished or segregated from social speech. (1956, p. 350)

In support of these claims Vygotsky conducted a series of ingenious studies on the functional differentation of egocentric speech from social speech and concluded that "the child's egocentric speech is a functionally and structurally distinct form of speech. However, while it is emerging it is not definitively separated from social speech from which it has all the while been developing" (1956, pp. 353–354).

As the child recognizes and masters this functional distinction, egocentric speech begins to "go underground." The result of mastering and differentiating the self-regulative, planning function of speech as opposed to its social, communicative function is to recognize that the former does not require an overt form of a communicative context. The process of differentiation required to arrive at the stage where speech can become internalized goes on throughout the period when egocentric speech is used.

The structural and functional properties of egocentric speech grow with the child's development. At three years of age the distinction between this speech and the child's communicative speech is almost zero. At seven years of age we see a form of speech that is almost 100% different from the social speech of the three-year-old in its functional and structural properties. It is in this fact that we find the expression of the progressive differentiation of the two speech functions and the *separation of speech for oneself and speech for others out of a general, undifferentiated speech function* which, during the early years of ontogenesis, fulfills both assignments with virtually identical means. (1956, p. 346)

Among the claims that Vygotsky made about egocentric and inner speech is that they reflect their social origins.

Egocentric. . .emerges from its social foundations by means of the child's transferring social, collaborative forms of behavior to the sphere of an individual's psychological functions. . .children begin to converse with themselves exactly as they had earlier conversed with others. (1956, p. 87)

He also argued that inner speech is "quasi-social." This is implicit in his use of terms such as "inner *dialogue,*" and he occasionally emphasized it in statements such as the following:

[In inner speech] humans as it were preserve the "function of social interaction" even in their own individual behavior; they apply a social means of action to themselves.
　　In this case their individual functioning in essence represents a unique form of internal collaboration with oneself. (1960, pp. 450–451)

Thus, according to Vygotsky, inner speech clearly reflects its social origins. On the other hand, however, Vygotsky made it clear that the structure and function of inner speech are quite different from those of external social speech. For example, in contrast to Watson (1924), who understood inner speech as a subvocal copy of external social speech, Vygotsky argued that "even if we could record inner speech on a phonograph it would be condensed, fragmentary, disconnected, unrecognizable, and incomprehensible in comparison to external speech" (1956, pp. 355–356).

The dual claim that inner speech "preserves the function of social interaction" but is quite distinct from its social precursor brings us back to the contradiction outlined earlier. The reason for why this contradiction is apparent rather than real again can be found in Vygotsk's genetic analysis. In this case, the analysis focuses on egocentric speech because "the study of egocentric speech and its dynamic tendencies toward the emergence of certain structural and functional properties and the weakening of others is the key to the investigation of the psychological nature of inner speech" (1956, p. 354).

In order to explicate Vygotsky's claim that inner speech preserves the function of social interaction we will carry out a brief genetic analysis of one semiotic property of social and egocentric speech. This is the dialogical property of these speech forms. As one of us has argued elsewhere (Wertsch, 1980, in press), Vygotsky worked when there was a great deal of debate over the relationship between dialogic and monologic speech. The figure who had the most obvious and pervasive influence on him in this connection was Yakubinskii (1923), but our focus here will be on Bakhtin (1929), who also published under the name of Voloshinov (1929), since his ideas serve best to clarify Vygotsky's concept of inner speech.

One of Bakhtin's (Voloshinov, 1929) important contributions was his extension of the notion of dialogue beyond its usual interpretation. In addition to cases in which two speakers take alternating turns in discourse, he argued that speech that appears to be monologic often cannot be interpreted without taking into consideration its role in an implicit dialogue. As in the work of Yakubinskii, this reflects an interpretation of dialogicality in which the relationship and interpretation of utterances is the issue rather than whether or not one or two speakers are involved.

Bakhtin argued that, like external speech, inner speech is dialogic. In order to examine this claim within Vygotsky's framework, we must turn to the dialogic forms of social and egocentric speech. We will do this by examining the interpsychological and intrapsychological functioning of a 2-and-a-half-year-old girl as she worked with her mother on the task of completing a "copy" puzzle in accordance with a "model" puzzle. Our analysis will be concerned with three "episodes" of interaction between the child (C) and the mother (M). (An episode is defined as the verbal and non-verbal interaction that occurred in connection with identification, selection, and insertion of a piece of the copy puzzle.) In these three episodes the correct location of the piece in the copy puzzle could be determined only by consulting the model puzzle. In our present analysis we will be concerned with the initial phase of each episode. This phase involved the strategic substep of consulting the model puzzle in order to determine where a piece should go in the copy puzzle.

The first episode we will examine began as follows:

(1) C: Oh. *(C glances at the model puzzle; C looks at the pieces pile.)* Oh, now where's this one go? *(C picks up the black piece from the pieces pile; C looks at the copy puzzle; C looks at the pieces pile.)*

(2) M: Where does it go on this other one? *(C puts the black piece that is in her hand back down in the pieces pile; C looks at the pieces pile.)*

(3) M: Look at the other truck and then you can tell. *(C looks at the model puzzle; C glances at the pieces pile; C looks at the model puzzle; C glances at the pieces pile.)*

(4) C: Well. . .*(C looks at the copy puzzle; C looks at the model puzzle.)*

(5) C: I look at it.

(6) C: Um, this other puzzle has a black one over there. *(C points to the black piece in the model puzzle.)*

Although it is true that the child glanced at the model puzzle at the very beginning of this episode, it does not appear that she did so at that point in order to determine where a piece should go in the copy puzzle. The first time she consulted the model for some clear purpose was in response to the mother's utterances (2) and (3). That is, it was part of interpsychological functioning.

The initial segment of a subsequent episode between this mother and child proceeded as follows:

> (7) C: *(C glances at the pieces pile; C looks at the copy puzzle; C picks up the orange piece from the pieces pile.)* Now where do you think the orange one goes?
>
> (8) M: Where does it go on the other truck? *(C looks at the model puzzle.)*
>
> (9) C: Right there. *(C points to the orange piece in the model puzzle.)* The orange one goes right there.

In this episode we see that the child's action of consulting the model puzzle again occurred as a step in the interpsychological functioning between herself and her mother.

The next episode between the mother and child began as follows:

> (10) C: *(C looks at the pieces pile; C picks up the yellow piece from the pieces pile; C looks at the copy puzzle.)* Now where. . . .Now. . . .*(C looks at the model puzzle.)*
>
> (11) C: You. . .you. . .the yellow on that side goes. . . .One yellow one's right next there. *(C points to the yellow piece in the model puzzle; C looks at the yellow piece she is holding in her hand.)*
>
> (12) M: Okay.

Comparisons among these three segments of interaction reveal an important transition from interpsychological to intrapsychological and from external to internal activity. Recall that the first two episodes began with the child's asking where a piece was to go [i.e., utterances (1) and (7)] and the mother's responding by directing the child's attention to the model puzzle [i.e., utterances (2), (3), and (8)]. In the case of both of these episodes, the child's original question led to a response by the mother which, in turn, led to the child's response of consulting the model. All of these "moves" or "turns" were part of external, interpsychological functioning. The third episode began quite differently. First, the child did not produce a fully expanded question about where a piece should go [although it appears that she began to do so in utterance (10)]. Second, and more importantly, her gaze to the model puzzle after utterance (10) was not a response to an adult's directive. Rather than relying on an adult to provide a regulative communication, she carried this out independently using egocentric and inner speech. That is, in the case of some of the strategic steps required here, there was a transition from external social functioning to external and internal individual functioning.

Furthermore, the child's utterance [i.e., (11)] in this third episode is strikingly similar to utterances (6) and (9) in the first and second episodes, respectively.

First episode

   (6)   C: Um, this other puzzle has a black one over there. *(C points to the black piece in the model puzzle.)*

Second episode

   (9)   C: Right there. *(C points to the orange piece in the model puzzle.)* The orange one goes right there.

Third episode

   (11)   C: You. . .you. . .the yellow on that side goes. . . .One yellow one's right next there. *(C points to the yellow piece in the model puzzle; C looks at the yellow piece she is holding in her hand.)*

In all three cases the child makes a statement about the location of a particular piece in the model puzzle. In addition to the similarity in the structure and content of the utterances, an examination of the sequences of behaviors in the three episodes reveal that (6), (9), and (11) served the same function in the problem-solving stategy. In all three cases the statement served to advance this strategy in the same way (i.e., they all were concerned with the strategic step of consulting the model to determine where a piece from the pieces pile was to go).

However, there is an important difference between (11) on the one hand and (6) and (9) on the other. Utterances (6) and (9) were part of external social functioning. They were the child's responses to utterances by the adult. Utterance (11), on the other hand, was not a response to an adult utterance; that is, it was not part of an external social process. We would argue that the reason for the striking similarity between (11) and the other two is that (11) is part of a quasi-social, partially internalized, individual activity that reflects the patterns and processes seen earlier in external social activity.

The mechanism that makes this transition possible is again the emergence of control over sign forms. The full significance of the utterances (6), (9), and (11) derived from the fact that they were involved in a dialogue based on a particular way of defining the task setting and the appropriate strategy. By uttering each of these statements, the child was making a statement about where a piece should go in the copy puzzle if one is following this strategy. However, the child's utterances (5) and (6) in the first episode indicate that she did not realize the "dialogic import" of what she was saying. Her response to the mother's utterances (2) and (3) indicates that she viewed it as that and nothing more – a response to the mother. By the time she progressed to the third episode, however, matters had changed in an important way. The child now apparently understood and controlled the full significance of the utterance. Again we see that it was the external sign form that allowed the child to participate in social activity before being able to control all aspects of the sign on the intrapsychological plane and that the child is the last to become conscious of the full significance of the sign.

Conclusions

The major point which we have attempted to develop in this chapter is that for Vygotsky, the concept of internalization and the related question of the link between external and internal activity lie at the center of a broader concern with the acculturation of the child. Vygotsky's theoretical framework is constructed in such a way that the concept of internalization cannot be discussed independently of the social origins of individual activity. In the final analysis, as Vygotsky says, internal activity is quasi-social in nature. In order to appreciate the import of this claim, the social origins of internal activity must be examined.

We have argued that one way to construct an integrated account of these issues is to examine the child's emerging control of external sign forms. This process involves the mastery of socially defined activity through coming to appreciate the full significance of the signs one uses in social interaction. It is the importance of this mechanism in the internalization process that we attempted to illustrate with the examples in the second half of this chapter. Hopefully, we have made the potential power of this explanatory tool evident in tracing the origins of the new significance of old signs and new definitions of old settings for the child. As the example should indicate, the mechanism is a rich and varied one. Vygotsky laid the groundwork for our argument, but he left many aspects of it largely undeveloped. We would argue that future work in this area would contribute significantly to our understanding of the nature and origins of internal activity.

REFERENCES

Bakhtin, M. M. 1929. *Problemy poetiki Dostoevskogo.* [Problems of Dostoevsky's poetics.] Leningrad. (Translated as M. M. Bakhtin, Problems of Dosteovsky's poetics. Ann Arbor, Mich: Ardis, 1973.)

Furth, H. G. 1969. *Piaget and knowledge.* Englewood Cliffs, N.J.: Prentice-Hall.
Gal'perin, P. Ya. 1969. Stages in the development of mental acts. In M. Cole and
    I. Maltzman (Eds.) *A handbook of contemporary Soviet psychology.* New York:
    Basic Books.
Gal'perin, P. Ya. 1976. *Vvedenie v psikhologii.* [Introduction to psychology.] Moscow:
    Izdatel'stvo Moskovskogo Universiteta.
Janet, P. 1926 – 1927. "La pensée intérieure et ses troubles." Course given at the
    College de France.
Janet, P. 1928. *De l'angoisse à l'extase: Etudes sur les croyances et les sentiments.* Vol. 2: *Les
    sentiments fondamentaux.* Paris: Librairie Felix Alcan.
Kochurova, E. I., Visyagina, A. I., Gordeeva, N. D., and Zinchenko, V.P. 1981.
    Criteria for evaluating executive activity. In J. V. Wertsch (Ed.), *The concept of
    activity in Soviet psychology.* Armonk, N.Y.: Sharpe.
Leont'ev, A. N. 1972. *Problemy razvitiya psikhiki.* [Problems in the development of
    mind.] Moscow: Izdatel'stvo Moskovskogo Universiteta.
Leont'ev, A. N. 1975. *Deyatel'nost', soznanie, lichnost'.* [Activity, consciousness, per-
    sonality.] Moscow: Izdatel'stvo Politicheskoi Literatury. (Translated as A. N.
    Leont'ev, *Activity consciousness, and personality.* Englewood Cliffs, N.J.: Prentice-
    Hall, 1978.)
Leont'ev, A. N. 1981. The problem of activity in psychology. In J. V. Wertsch (Ed.),
    The concept of activity in Soviet psychology. Armonk, N.Y.: Sharpe.
Luria, A. R. 1981. *Language and cognition.* New York: Wiley.
Marx, K. 1959. Theses on Feuerbach. In L. S. Feuer (Ed.), *Karl Marx and Fredrich
    Engels: Basic writings on politics and philosophy.* Garden City, N.Y.: Anchor
    Books.
Mead, G. H. 1934. *Mind, self, and society.* Chicago: University of Chicago Press.
Piaget, J. 1926. *The language and thought of the child.* New York: Harcourt, Brace, and
    World.
Piaget, J. 1962. *Play, dreams, and imitation in childhood.* New York: Norton.
Rubinshtein, S. L. 1957. *Bytie i soznanie.* [Being and consciousness.] Moscow:
    Izdatel'stvo Akademii Nauk SSSR.
Sapir, E. 1921. *Language.* New York: Harcourt, Brace, and World.
Toulmin, S. 1972. *Human understanding.* Princeton: Princeton University Press.
Toulmin, S. 1979. The inwardness of mental life. Ryerson Lecture, University of
    Chicago.
Voloshinov, V. N. 1929. *Marksizm i filosofiya yazyka.* [Marxism and the philosophy
    of language.] Leningrad. (Translated as V. N. Voloshinov, *Marxism and the
    philosophy of language,* New York: Seminar Press, 1973.)
Vygotsky, L. S. 1956. *Izbrannie psikhologicheskie issledovaniya* [Selected psychological
    research.] Moscow: Izdatel'stvo Akademii Pedagogicheskikh Nauk.
Vygotsky, L. S. 1960. *Razvitie vysshikh psikhicheskikh funktsii.* [The development of
    higher mental functions.] Moscow: Izdatel'stvo Akademii Pedagogicheskikh
    Nauk.
Vygotsky, L. S. 1962. *Thought and language.* Cambridge: MIT Press.
Vygotsky, L. S. 1978. *Mind in society.* Cambridge: Harvard University Press.
Vygotsky, L. S. 1981a. The genesis of higher mental functions. In J. V. Wertsch
    (Ed.), *The concept of activity in Soviet psychology.* Armonk, N.Y.: Sharpe.
Vygotsky, L. S. 1981b. The development of higher forms of attention in childhood.
    In J. V. Wertsch (Ed.), *The concept of activity in Soviet psychology.* Armonk, N.Y.:
    Sharpe.

Watson, J. B. 1924. *Behaviorism.* New York: Norton.

Wertsch, J. V. 1980. The significance of dialogue in Vygotsky's account of social, egocentric, and inner speech. *Contemporary educational psychology,* 5, 150–162.

Wertsch, J. V. 1983. The role of semiosis in L. S. Vygotsky's account of human cognition. In B. Bain (Ed.), *The sociogenesis of language and human conduct: A multi-disciplinary book of readings.* New York: Plenum.

Wertsch, J. V. In press. *The social formation of mind: A Vygotskian approach.* Cambridge: Harvard University Press.

Yakubinskii, L. P. 1923. *O dialogicheskoi rechi.* [On dialogic speech.] Petrograd: Trudy Foneticheskogo Instituta Prakticheskogo Izucheniya Yazykov.

Zinchenko, V. P., and Gordon, V. M. 1981. Methodological problems in the psychological analysis of activity. In J. V. Wertsch (Ed.) *The concept of activity in Soviet psychology.* Armonk, N.Y.: Sharpe.

Extending Vygotsky's approach: semiotic issues

8

Language acquisition as increasing linguistic structuring of experience and symbolic behavior control

RAGNAR ROMMETVEIT

Introduction

Search for "the lost paradise of childhood" often takes within literature the form of an attempt at retrieving some forever-lost spontaneity of experience. Our adult knowledge is at times conceived of by the intuitively engaged artist as a filter by which "objectivity" is achieved via alienation.

Vygotsky's basic theory of symbolic regulation and control of behavior and Piaget's general notion of decentration may be interpreted as key notions in scientific investigations of the transformation of the paradise of childhood into mature adult thought. Decentration may indeed be interpreted as increased self-regulation via linguistic–symbolic structuring and control. Some of Piaget's central ideas appear to be complementary to those of Vygotsky and may in modified versions possibly be integrated into an expanded and explicitly "pluralistic" and "relativistic" outlook on cognitive development. An expansion of scope and inclusion of anthropological perspectives, however, seem required in order to account for socialization within variant cultural frames and man-made conditions of life.

The present chapter aims at an explication of the development of language and thought in the spirit of Vygotsky, but within the framework of a consistently pluralistic and social–cognitive approach to human communication. I shall proceed from the assumption that human discourse takes place in and deals with a pluralistic, only fragmentarily known, and only partially shared social world.

Vagueness, ambiguity, and incompleteness – but hence also versatility, flexibility, and negotiability – must for that reason be dealt with as inherent and theoretically essential characteristics of ordinary language. Paradigms based upon stipulation of invariant "literal meanings" of verbal expressions have to be abandoned in favor of an explicitly constructivistic approach to language and thought. And hitherto largely unexplored social–interactional features of verbal communication such as *states of intersubjec-*

tivity and social reality and *patterns of dyadic communication control* must be made the foci of renewed theoretical analysis.

I shall in the first part of this chapter present the preliminary results of such an analysis in the form of fragments of a general pluralistic and social–cognitive approach to verbal communication. Notions of particular revelance to Vygotskian perspectives on language and thought will in the second part of the chapter be illuminated by findings from a study of 6-to-8-year-old Norwegian children.

Fragments of a conceptual framework

Some of the underlying assumptions and focal issues of a dynamic, consistently pluralistic, and social–cognitive approach to verbal communications have been explored by philosophers of language such as Voloshinov (1973) and Wittgenstein (1968). The point of departure of Voloshinov's contribution is a radical critique of our major traditions of linguistic thought. The stronghold of the "abstract objectivism" of Descartes and Saussure, he argues, is largely due to the facts that "the first philologists and the first linguists were always and everywhere priests" and that "European linguistic thought formed and matured over concern with the cadavers of written languages." His own dialectical philosophy is based upon the assumptions that "the sign and its social situation are inextricably fused" and that "consciousness becomes consciousness only in the process of social interaction" (See Voloshinov, 1973, p. 11, 37, 48, 74).

Wittgenstein conceives of the incompleteness and inherent ambiguities of ordinary language as a necessary consequence of the fact that its semantic system borders on our fragmentary and imperfect knowledge of the world. Thus, any scheme of interpretation will have a bottom level and "there is no such thing as an interpretation of that." (Wittgenstein, 1962, p. 739) Utterances have meaning only in "streams of life." Linguistic communication must hence be examined as embedded in more inclusive patterns of human interaction, as moves within "language games." Ordinary language *is* "a form of life."

Wittgenstein's legacy to subsequent philosophical enquiries into ordinary language and empirical studies of verbal communication consists to a considerable extent of profound questions and suggestive metaphors. Aspects of particular "language games," however, may upon closer examination be systematically described as "interaction rituals" (Goffman, 1971), and the problem of the embeddedness of linguistically mediated meaning in more inclusive patterns of human interaction may be pursued in social scientific analysis of metacommunicative frames (Bateson, 1973).

Our intuitive mastery of the multiple social realities of everyday "streams of life," moreover, is made a recurrent theme in enthnomethodological research (Schutz, 1945; Garfinkel, 1972). And even the more narrowly defined linguistic study of presuppositions is currently expanding so as to cope with dialogically and temporarily constructed "possible worlds" of actual conversations (Karttunen, 1974; McCawley, 1978). Modal logic is thus today in part replacing classical propositional logic as an auxiliary in formalization of linguistic theory.

These philosophical and social scientific trends converge in a serious concern with dynamic, social–interactional features of linguistic communication. They constitute hence, together with the symbolic interactionism of G. H. Mead (1950), the theoretical framework for empirical semantics developed by Naess (1953), and the psychology of language and thought of Vygotsky (1962, 1978) and Piaget (1958), significant contributions toward the foundation of an interdisciplinary social–cognitive approach. And classical psychological studies of attribution by Michotte (1954) and Heider (1958) may indeed within such a novel, broadly empirically founded paradigm be reinterpreted as significant psychological contributions within a perennial search for semantic universals.

Piaget's very important contribution within such an interdisciplinary venture, I shall claim, can only be fully appreciated if we reject his own peculiarly narrow use of the term "language" in favor of the vague yet broader and more realistic conceptions of Voloshinov, Wittgenstein, and Vygotsky. A confessed lack of respect for traditional boundaries between and within the various academic disciplines dealing with language, thought, and human communication does not at all, however, imply lack of appreciation of the composite nature and complexity of the issues under investigation. On the contrary: There is hardly any more efficient way of *evading* the complexities of ordinary language than to disassociate it from actual use and explicate its syntactic and semantic rules under stipulated "ideal" conditions. It is only when we deliberately abandon such scholastic strategies that we are seriously challenged to capture conceptually – and hence requested to be precise about – its incompleteness, inherent ambiguity, and flexibility. What appears chaotic to the researcher who believes in invariant "literal" meaning, moreover, may possibly be accounted for as orderly variance when we adopt a consistently pluralistic perspective.

Imagine, for instance, a situation in which two persons who engage in conversation about some state of affairs S differ with respect to *what they believe S to be*. The person p_1 takes it for granted that S is A_i, whereas his conversation partner "sees" S as A_j. How can we *as linguists or psycho- or sociolinguists* in such a situation transcend the "private worlds" of p_1 and p_2 and pass verdict with respect to the "real" nature of the state of affairs S? And, granted that we form some carefully elaborated third epistemological–ontological position venture to claim that S *is neither A_i nor A_j, but A_k*, how can such a presumedly superior knowledge of the "real" world help us grasp what is being meant, understood, or misunderstood by p_1 and p_2 in that particular situation?

The only alternative seems to be to take the multiplicity of possible human perspectives on states of affairs for granted and assume (Moscovici, 1979, p. 11) that "la realité dans laquelle nous vivons. . .peut avoir des significations multiples, existant côte à côte." Thus Wittgenstein (1968, p. 212) maintains: "What I perceive in the dawning of an aspect is not a property of the object, but an internal relation between it and other objects." These "other objects," though, are an attribution of meaning to specific objects or events very often provided by the observer himself in terms of tacitly presupposed alternatives. Which aspects are focused upon by each of the two participants in any particular case of dyadic interaction are thus in part determined by the individual actor's engagement and perspective. How different, explicitly introduced referential domains of discourse affect linguistic encoding and decoding has been cogently demonstrated in psycholinguistic experiments by Olson (1970) and Deutsch (1976). Which of a set of possible verbal expressions will be used to refer to any particular object is clearly determined by *the range of objects from which the referent must be set apart*. And there is no reason to believe that such referential domains are of less significance when they are tacitly taken for granted – for instance, in a case in which two people are talking about the "same" state of affairs S as A_i and A_j, that is, as assimilated into frames or "schemes" representing different possible perspectives (see Rommetveit, 1980, 1981).

The major hazard of a consistently pluralistic paradigm is that we deliberately deprive ourselves of the opportunity to seek refuge in any unequivocal present-tense reality, uncontaminated by the repertory of possible human perspectives and the strategies of attribution and categorization inherent in ordinary language. The sign and its social situation are, as Voloshinov maintained, in some sense "inextricably fused." Our position is thus that any "real" state of affairs is enigmatic and remains so until it is viewed from a certain position (Hundeide, Chapter 13, this volume) and within some particular referential perspective (Wertsch, 1980). The enigma of "the real world as it is now" is then *subjectively* resolved in a process of comparison. We assume, moreover, that every single person has the capacity to adopt a whole range of perspectives on objects, events, and states of affairs and is in that sense *an inhabitant of many "possible worlds."* Which potential aspect(s) of a given object, event, or situation will be generated by any particular person attending to that state of affairs, moreover, is contingent upon his or her perspective and "private" domain of salient experiential alternatives at that moment.

What happens when a monistic outlook is replaced by a consistently pluralistic paradigm is thus a radical reformulation of assumptions and focal issues of research on human intersubjectivity and verbal communication. The problem of *what is being meant by what is said* cannot any longer be pursued in terms of stipulated unequivocal "literal" meanings of expressions. The basic riddle within a pluralistic approach is rather how states of intersubjectivity and shared social reality can be attained in encounters between different "private worlds." Orderly negotiability and variance in what is meant by what is said is clearly contingent upon some semantic invariance embedded in ordinary language. Some basic shared knowledge of the world appears indeed to be embedded as meaning potentials of ordinary words and expressions. Such potentials, we shall claim, reflect at a very abstract level some minimal commonality with respect to experientially founded perspectives on and categorization of our pluralistic social world and may hence be conceived of as a common code of potentially shared cognitive–emotive perspectives on talked-about states of affairs. What traditionally has been labeled "semantic rules," moreover, must within our social–cognitive paradigm be conceived of as linguistically mediated drafts of contracts concerning categorization of and attribution of meaning of states to affairs.

The attainment of states of *inter*subjectivity in verbal communication, we shall maintain, is contingent upon contextually appropriate specification and elaboration of such abstract drafts or contracts. And such a state may be tentatively defined as follows:

A state of intersubjectivity with respect to some state of affairs S is attained at a given stage of dyadic interaction if and only if some aspect A_i of S at that stage is brought into focus by one participant and jointly attended by both of them.

A dyadic state of perfectly shared social reality, moreover, may be described in the following way:

Some aspect of A_i of a given state of affairs S constitutes at a given stage of dyadic interaction a perfectly shared social reality if and only if both participants at that stage take it for granted that S is A_i and each of them assumes the other to hold that belief.

William James, being persistently intrigued by the varieties of human experience, was also seriously concerned with the conditions under which states of intersubjectivity and shared social reality are attained in encounters between different "private worlds." He maintained: *"You accept my verification of one thing. I yours of another. We trade on each other's truth."* (James, 1962, p. 197) And the currency par excellence in such trade is, of course, ordinary language. But what, more specifically, is implied by such "trading of truths"? How can it be specified in terms of social–interactional features, as a basic characteristic of ordinary language as "a form of life"?

Max Black (1978) has carefully examined the notions of *"form of life"* and *"language game"* in Wittgenstein's later work. He doubts whether Wittgenstein's choice of term "language game" to express one of his central notions was a really happy one. There is, Black tentatively concludes, in Wittgenstein's later works an uncompleted progress from a relatively formal and abstract conception of language games to more liberal and realistic conception. And Black continues (1978, p. 330):

Such a conception must importantly involve not merely analogues of "pragmatic" rules but also much that does not easily fit the rubric of "game–rule" at all. It is at such a point that reference to a "Lebensform," however, imprecise, is attractive. It is as if Wittgenstein were signalling that there is much more to be looked at, much important territory still to explore.

Some of this territory may be illuminated by investigations of very early mother–child interaction (see Bruner, 1978; Lock, 1978). The human infant is for a long period entirely dependent upon its caretaker, and some rudimentary, though basic, features of language as "a form of life" may hence possibly be revealed by careful examination of the ways in which the separate activities of mother and child are coordinated into a single social activity. Features of early child–adult interaction such as turn taking and convergence of gaze onto the same object have accordingly acquired saliency in recent enquiries into possible early precursors of verbal communication.

Vygotsky (1978, p. 29) maintains: "Signs and words serve children first and foremost as a means of social contact with other people." And a primitive but possibly "primary" form of intersubjectivity is according to Trevarthen and Hubley (1978) attained at a very early stage in the sense that infants "share themselves with others." What according to their observations seems to emerge at about the age of 9 months, moreover, is a "secondary" intersubjectivity in terms of a "deliberate, self-conscious and reciprocal sharing of focus with another." And Newson (1978, pp. 36–37) maintains about the prerequisites for such a development:

Someone who is trying to communicate with the infant. . .is bound to respond selectively to precisely those actions, on the part of the baby, to which one would normally respond *given the assumption that the baby is like any other communicating person*.

. . .It is. . .only because mothers impute meaning to "behaviours" elicited from the infants that these eventually do come to constitute meaningful actions so far as the child is concerned.

A state of "primary" or "secondary" intersubjectivity in early mother–child interaction – whatever else such a state may entail – is thus inconceivable without naïve, reciprocal faith in a shared experiential world. But this, I shall argue, is true of any state of human intersubjectivity and indeed a defining characteristic of ordinary language as a "form of life." How unreflectively taken for granted and essential such mutual confidence is in normal verbal communication can perhaps only be fully appreciated when we examine what happens when it breaks down under certain pathological conditions (see Rommetveit, 1974, pp. 53–56).

Intersubjectivity must in some sense be taken for granted in order to be attained. This semiparadox may indeed be conceived of as a basic pragmatic postulate of human discourse. It captures in a condensed form not only an insight arrived at by observers of early mother–child interaction and students of serious communication disorders, but also convergent conclusions from ethnomethodological enquiries into the routine grounds of everyday adult conversation and recent linguistic reflections on axiomatic features of normal speech. The linguist Uhlenbeck thus refers to the basic *"makes sense"* principle of ordinary speech. And he describes it as follows: (Uhlenbeck, 1978, p. 190)

It says that the hearer always takes the view that what the speaker is saying somehow makes sense. It is this certitude which makes him try to infer – on the basis of lingual and extra-lingual evidence available to him – what the speaker actually is conveying to him. This formulation implies that on occasion the hearer may be unable to do so or that he may make the wrong inferences. It is difficult to exaggerate the importance of this very general attitude. Awareness of its always being operative may keep us from entering into linguistically irrelevant discussions on the truth-values of sentences, or from participating in sterile debates about establishing a distinction between deviant and normal sentences.

The significance of this "makes sense" principle can perhaps only be fully appreciated in conjunction with Piaget's theory of decentration and the basic tenet of symbolic interactionism: An adult person's repertory of possible perspectives entails as experiential possibilities aspects that are immediately visible only from the position of her or his conversation partner, and an essential component of communicative competence in a pluralistic social world is the capacity to adopt the attitude of "different others." A mutual *commitment* to the same talked-about reality, moreover, is in ordinary discourse endowed with naïve confidence in "an intersubjective world, common to all of us" (Schutz, 1945, p. 534) on the part of communication partners.

Reciprocal commitment, moreover, implies reciprocal role taking. A significant dynamic feature of ordinary language as a social "form of life" is thus a peculiar circularity: The speaker monitors what he is saying in accordance with what he assumes to be the listener's outlook and background information, whereas the latter makes sense of what he is hearing by adopting what he believes to be the speaker's perspective. But what is actually being meant, then, and which potential aspects of the talked-about state of affairs are jointly attended to at any particular stage of a dialogue?

The mutual commitment and peculiar circularity inherent in acts of speech imply by no means, of course, that both participants in a dialogue assume equal or joint responsibility for what is being referred to and/or "meant" by what is said. The speaker – or, more generally, the participant who introduced whatever is being talked about at any given stage of the dialogue – has the privilege to determine which aspect(s) is/are to be jointly attended to at that moment. And this is the case even if she fails to make herself understood. Only she – not the listener – is in a position to pass final verdict with respect to what she herself intends to make known by what she is saying. Understanding (and misunderstanding) is in ordinary verbal communication by definition a dyadic and directional affair, and *vicious circularity is prohibited by reciprocal and intuitive endorsement of dyadic patterns of communication control*.

States of intersubjectivity are, in fact, contingent upon the fundamental dyadic constellation of speaker's privilege and listener's commitment: The speaker has the privilege to determine what is being referred to and/or meant, whereas the listener is committed to make sense of what is said by temporarily adopting the speaker's perspective.

This is, in essence, what has to be taken for granted in our intuitive mastery of dialogue roles in normal and symmetric dyadic interactions. Watching the other's face in search of additional information about *what is being meant* is thus in ordinary adult conversation an absurd act if performed by the person who is speaking at that moment. It may be a wise thing for his listener to do, though, and perhaps even necessary in order to find out whether what he hears is meant sarcastically.

Symmetry/asymmetry with respect to dyadic communication control may now be defined as follows:

An entire dialogue or a given stretch of discourse is characterized by a symmetric pattern of communication control if and only if unlimited interchangeability of dialogue roles constitutes part of the externally provided sustained conditions of interaction.

An entire dialogue or a given stretch of discourse is characterized by an asymmetric pattern of communication control if and only if the interaction takes place under sustained constraints contrary to the basic or "prototypical" dyadic regulation of privileges and commitments.

A pervading feature of infant–adult interaction is, of course, the overall pattern of dependency. The overriding constraints upon early adult–child communication, moreover, reside in the factual and reciprocally taken-for-granted adult superiority with respect to linguisitic competence and knowledge of the world. It is hence not at all absurd for a 1-year-old boy to watch his mother's face while uttering something in order to explore what is being meant by his utterance. And it may indeed be essential to observe her response if he is going to make himself better understood on subsequent similar occasions. Some of the most firmly established and significant findings in recent research on preverbal mother–child interaction and early language acquisition (Bates, 1976; Bruner, 1978; Lock, 1978) seem thus to converge into an apparently paradoxical conclusion: *Adult perfect interchangeability of dialogue roles can only develop out of adult–child interaction with an initial consistently asymmetric pattern of communication control.*

This insight is actually in full agreement with Skinner's general account of language learning as operant conditioning by adult social reinforcement (Skinner, 1957). It seems also to capture the essence of Vygotsky's thesis concerning ontogenetic transformation of "other-regulation" into higher-order symbolic self-regulative capacities (see Vygotsky, 1981; Wertsch, 1979). Skinner and Vygotsky would thus probably both – even though from different theoretical positions – endorse Newson's claim that the mother imputing "meanings" to her infant's preverbal communicative behaviors is indeed engaged in *self-fulfilling prophecy.*

The issue of coordination of activities and dyadic control of joint ventures becomes in early mother–child interaction to a considerable extent a matter of establishing *foci of joint attention.* The child's "protodeclarative" act of communication may indeed be conceived of as "a preverbal effort to direct the adult's attention to some object or event in the world" (Bates, 1976, p. 57).

Adult–child interaction at an early stage of language acquisition, however, is nevertheless necessarily asymmetric in the sense that the adult partner – not the child – is the one who is supposed to know both what talked-about states of affairs *are* and what words *"mean."* This basic asymmetry – the adult's overriding control of the emerging sustained shared social reality – is of central concern in Vygotsky's explorations of the profound and subtle impact of adult "meaning" upon the child's preverbal world. Human higher-order or "symbolic" self-regulation develops, according to Vygotsky and his followers, out of adult–child interaction with a clearly *asymmetric pattern of communication control.* This core thesis in dialectical Soviet psychology of language has been further clarified by Wertsch, who points out how Vygotsky's general approach fits with Wittgenstein's notions of language games and ordinary language as a "form of life." Sustained and goal-directed adult control of discourse and interaction, moreover, is cogently brought to our attention in his own detailed records of conversations between child and adult working on a puzzle (Wertsch, 1979).

The intuitively mastered capacity to switch roles, from speaker to listener and vice versa, is a basic interactional feature of adult communicative competence. The actual settings of adult conversation, however, are constrained by unequal distribution of knowledge, power, and prestige in our pluralistic social world. Habermas maintains that "pure intersubjectivity" is attained under conditions of unlimited interchangeability of dialogue roles, that is, "when there is complete symmetry in the distribution of assertion and disputation, revelation and hiding, prescription and following, among the partners of communication" (Habermas, 1970, p. 143). These conditions may be fulfilled, though, in a political discussion in which each of the two participants *qua listener and qua speaker* insists on making sense of an ambiguous word such as "democracy" on his or her own particular premises, that is, in a frozen ideological conflict in which both parties are engaged *solely in "prescription."* A conversation about the emperor's magnificent new suit between two of his obedient admirers, moreover, may indeed also be described as perfectly symmetric with respect to communication control. What the naïve child in Hans Christian Andersen's story tells them is that the emperor is actually naked. The two admirers of his nonexistent new suit may therefore start quarreling about *which one of them was actually responsible for what was being meant* in their serious conversation a little while ago.

Dyadic states of intersubjectivity in verbal communication as we have defined them are devoid of such bewilderment because they are by definition directional, *either $p_1 \rightarrow p_2$ or $p_2 \rightarrow p_1$*. States of intersubjectivity are hence also attained under conditions of definite externally provided constraints upon interchangeability of dialogue roles such as, for example, those unequivocally induced by assignment of complementary tasks in an experiment by Blakar and Pedersen (1980). Symmetric dyadic interaction, on the other hand, may consist solely in reciprocal prescription *or* exclusively in reciprocal following. A pattern of perfectly symmetric communication control is therefore in itself neither a sufficient nor a necessary condition for attainment of dyadic states of intersubjectivity. It may indeed, as suggested in our brief excursions into frozen ideological conflicts and Andersen's tales, under certain conditions lead to *fusion* rather than perfect *interchangeability* of dialogue roles.

Such fusion must be clearly distinguished from intuitively mastered *dyadic control of question–answer sequences* in everyday discourse (see Goffman, 1976; Rommetveit, 1979, pp. 154–161). The person asking a question has qua speaker the privilege to decide what is being meant, and the conversation partner is qua listener committed to make sense of it by adopting the interrogator's perspective. The latter's response constitutes an *answer,* however, only to the extent that the commitment made when making sense of the question is sustained while responding to it. Reciprocal acknowledgment of such sustained commitments is indeed a very important feature of dyadic communication control in ordinary discourse.

The "power of the question" in ordinary human discourse, we shall claim, resides precisely in such sustained reciprocal commitments. The issue of "shared meaning" must within a pluralistic, social–cognitive paradigm be rephrased in terms of dyadic communication control. It may indeed at times become a question concerning whose "private world" is going to be endorsed by others as well, accepted as a basis for collective action, and thereby in some sense made "publicly valid." The "power of the question" is thus at a maximum under conditions of unequivocal asymmetry such as, for instance, adult–child dialogues of the kind reported by Hundeide (1980) in his modified replications of Piagetian experiments.

What follows from our reanalysis of basic social–interactional features of verbal communication is hence a reorientation toward recurrent issues in studies of ontogenetic development of language and thought.

Questions concerning the relationship between comprehension and production in individual language acquisition, for instance, may very likely have to be posed in novel ways. Apparent lack of correspondence can hardly be satisfactorily accounted for at all without explicit reference to dialogue roles, the directionality of intersubjectivity, and dyadic communication control (see Hagtvet, 1980). Both Hundeide and Hagtvet are thus in their recent studies of adult–child communication seriously concerned with "other-regulation," that is, with asymmetric dyadic control. And Vygotsky's basic notions, I hope, may gain additional clarity and explanatory power when pursued and further elaborated within a general, explicitly pluralistic and social–cognitive paradigm.

Language mastery and symbolic behavior control: some empirical illustrations

Constructivist theories of individual cognitive development are based upon the assumption that states of affairs are assimilated into a subjectively meaningful reality by categorization, attribution, and "operations of thought." The child learns about significant features of his or her immediate surroundings in exploration and manipulation of material objects. What things "mean," however, cannot be revealed in solitary transaction with them. Even apparently very simple objects and events remain in principle enigmatic and undetermined as *social realities* until they are talked about (see Feinberg, 1965; Davidson, 1971; Menzel, 1978; Rommetveit, 1980).

Behavioral mastery of the external reality develops into active conceptual mastery under conditions of cooperation and social validation. Meaningful aspects of the adult world are brought into joint focus of attention in the child's interaction with "significant others," that is, in a trade upon adult "truths." The child's expanding repertory of possible cognitive–emotive perspectives on states of affairs is necessarily constrained by an adult, preestablished *"Interpretationsgemeinschaft"*, and in some respects linguistically structured. The operative nature of the resultant knowledge of the world is reflected in an increasing capacity to make sense of objects and events in accordance with drafts of contracts concerning categorization embedded in ordinary adult language.

Linguistic structuring of attention and symbolic behavior control are according to Vygotsky (1981, p. 194) complementary features of a "cultural development of attention," that is, of *"evolution and change in the means for directing and carrying out attentional processes, the mastery of these processes, and their subordination to human control."* His conception of higher-order, symbolic control of individual behavior, it seems, is thus in full accordance with our analysis of social–interactional features of verbal communication: Control of joint focus of attention, we claimed, is indeed a defining characteristic of dyadic states of intersubjectivity. And linguistically mediated individual control of attention may be examined in simple tasks of identifying reference – for instance, by asking a child to fetch or point out one particular target object located within a specific referential domain of other objects. The target object is referred to by an unequivocal identifying description. Lack of intersubjectivity – and hence deficient symbolic control of attention on the part of the child – is revealed if the child fetches or points out some object other than the one described by the adult.

All empirical illustrations below are based upon observations of children in such tasks of identifying reference. Altogether 90 tasks were included in two separate, though in some respects strictly comparable, "pointing games," and the latter were designed in cooperation with my wife, Sigrid Rommetveit. The practical–educational aim of the games is a mapping of the child's "zone of proximal development" at school entry so as to help elementary schoolteachers adjust educational activities to individual needs. The teacher is supposed to take an active part in the interpretation of the child's performance and share the responsibility for conversion of psychological theory into educational practice. An intended and significant by-product of such cooperation is a "consciousness raising" on the part of the teacher, that is, a demystification of educationally important Piagetian and Vygotskyian notions in the context of individualized teaching.

Nearly two hundred 6- to 9-year-old Norwegian children participated in the study, and a detailed statistical account of their performances has been presented by S. Rommetveit (1980). The findings and illustrative examples to be presented below stem primarily from her "core group" of 73 children in the age group 6–8 years, all of whom had participated in both versions of "the game." The child was in each task simply asked to point out one particular target object in one particular drawing. Each task of identifying reference consists thus of an identifying description of an object and a specific drawing within which that object has to be identified. The rules of the two games are identical and the tasks pairwise strictly equivalent, moreover, apart from the sequential order of the identifying description and the exposure of the drawing. A unique and sustained rule of the first game is that *the child is not shown the drawing until the target object has been verbally described.* The sustained rule of the second game, on the other hand, is that *the child is watching the drawing while listening to the identifying description.* The two different versions of the game may hence be described as verbal *preidentification* and verbal *postidentification* of target object.

Our present purpose is neither to give a complete account of S. Rommetveit's findings nor to present empirical, evidence bearing upon specific hypotheses concerning, for example, dyadic communication control, contextual specification of "word meaning," or linguistically mediated control of attention. The aim is rather conceptual clarification. We shall selectively focus upon findings that may illuminate the conceptual framework suggested above and, more specifically, its implications for prospective research on language acquisition in a Vygotskian spirit. Only a few representative tasks of identifying reference from the actual games will be used as illustrative examples, and the small sample of drawings in Figure 1 may hence hopefully serve as a visual anchorage for excursions from relevant observational data into significant theoretical issues.

The game is in an introductory explanation to the child presented as a game of "difficult adult talk" (S. Rommetveit, 1980, p. 88). The pattern of dyadic communication control is hence unequivocally asymmetric: The adult is the speaker and the one who is supposed to know precisely what is meant by what is said, that is, which particular object in the drawing is being referred to. The child, having accepted the rules of the game and the invitation to participate, is listening with a commitment to identify and point out that and only that object. The target object in drawing 1, for instance, is

(1)   . . .the one of the LADIES who has the SECOND SHORTEST way
      to the bus.
      (In Norwegian: ". . .den av DAMENE som har NEST KORTEST vei til
      bussen. The demonstrative "den" is translated into "the one" in
      English.)

This particular task is representative of the more difficult ones within a subset of tasks of identifying reference that may be said to tax mastery of Piagetian "concrete operations of thought." Identification of the correct lady, it seems, requires combined mastery of class hierarchy and ordering.

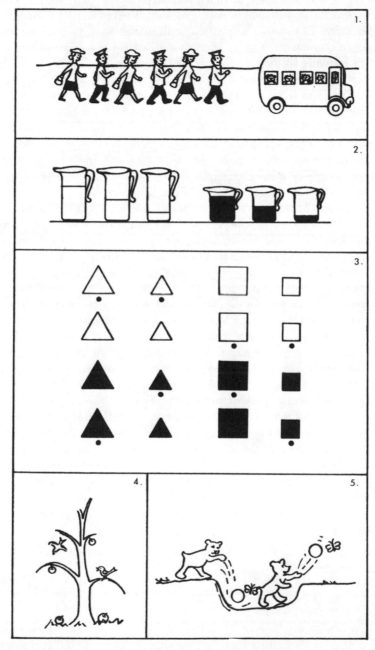

Figure 1. Drawings used in "pointing games."

Failure to attain intersubjectivity, moreover, is apparently due to a diffusion of the domain of the ordering operation on the part of the child (Rommetveit, 1978): The 6 1/2-year-old child, ordering ALL people with respect to distance from the bus, puts without hesitation his or her finger on the one of the LADIES who has the SHORTEST way. Tasks of type (1) differentiate thus very clearly between age groups. Extremely few 6 1/2-year-old but about half of all 7 1/2-year-old children manage to identify the verbally described target objects.

But what, more precisely, is involved in the diffusion of the domain of the ordering operation? Why cannot the empirically firmly established difference between age groups be accounted for simply in terms of developmental stages of concrete–operational thought and levels of language acquisition, that is, in traditional Piagetian and psycholinguistic terms? What, more specifically, is left unexplained by such an account, and how can that residual be demystified in terms of Vygotskian concepts?

What hardly can be accounted for in traditional Piagetian and psycholinguistic terms at all is, for instance, the fact that many children who fail in task (1) "comprehend" every word and expression in the identifying description *and* master all "operations of thought" required in identification of the target object. This is clearly demonstrated in their performances in other tasks. They can thus without any uncertainty or hesitation point out all LADIES in the drawing and also immediately, *if the three gentlemen are erased,* point out the one of the ladies who has the SECOND SHORTEST way to the bus. Quite a few of those who fail on drawing (1), moreover, succeed immediately when each *gentleman* in the drawing is replaced by a *dog*. And some succeed if we merely change the destination of the persons in task (1). They have apparently no problem in identifying the correct lady if "the bus" is replaced by "the toilet" (with door signs for ladies and gentlemen in the drawing).

Diffusion of the domain of the ordering operation is therefore by no means merely a matter of perceptual, spatial infiltration (of three gentlemen into a row of ladies). Nor is it a matter of general level of concrete–operational thought as such, uncontaminated by operative world knowledge and culturally provided perspectives. This may possibly be shown by employing modified versions of task (1) in systematic comparative studies. The *gentlemen* in the drawing may for instance be replaced by *black ladies* and the identifying description changed into ". . .the one of the WHITE LADIES who has the SECOND SHORTEST way to the bus." The average age level at which children in different societies master such a task, I venture to claim, will tell at least as much about prevailing patterns of discrimination and culturally determined distinctiveness of race as about general cultural enhancement of concrete–operational thought.

A failure in a task of type (1) can be safely interpreted as a diffusion of the domain of the ordering operation if and only if the child has shown that she or he "understands" every word and expression in the verbal description and can perform all "operations" involved in the identification of the target object. The failure can in that case hardly be *described* in any other way than as a diffusion, and it must accordingly be examined in terms of competing referential perspectives (see Wertsch, 1980, p. 16). Our demanded and linguistically mediated control of the child's attention is thus in task (1) played out against what in some sense is a "prelinguistic," perceptually sup ported and meaningful organization of a visually available referential domain. The child's immediate referential structuring of her or his visual experience is of course by no means "prelinguistic" in the sense that it is uncontaminated by operative world knowledge and ordinary language as a "form of life." On the contrary: The child can hardly make sense of the drawing at all without engaging in categorizations embedded in ordinary language and, hence, without attending to aspects of general cultural significance. It is precisely because *ladies and gentlemen* are *people, adults,* perhaps *parents*, potential *passengers*, and so on, that the 6 1/2-year-old cannot keep mentally apart while ordering distances to the bus in task (1).

Some such higher-order aspect (or, in Piagetian terms, superordinate class) of ladies and gentlemen alike is apparently a focal aspect in many 6- to 8-year-old children's making sense of the drawing. They are, in a way, imprisoned within a perspective that differs from that adopted by the adult in his or her identifying description of the target object. It is not enough, therefore, to be able to identify three of the persons in the drawing as LADIES. Such an "identity operation" must indeed override all other potential aspects and be sustained during the ordering of distances. This is actually a prerequisite for the attainment of a dyadic state of intersubjectivity. Linguistically mediated control of attention fails because the "LADIES-aspect" that is supposed to be brought into joint focus by the adult's referring expression is *not* properly attended to by the child.

Competition between a verbally imposed referential perspective and a perceptually supported way of making sense of the drawing is a recurrent feature in the guessing games. Since many of the tasks also may be said to deal with particular Piagetian "operations of thought," we are therefore in a position to attempt a synthesis of Piagetian and Vygotskian notions. Task (2) in our sample stems from the verbal preidentification game and may in a way be conceived of as a mirror image of tasks of type (1). The description of the target object of drawing 2 in Figure 1 may be translated as follows:

(2) You'll now see some jugs with milk and some jugs with cocoa. Point to the one of ALL the jugs containing the SECOND MOST.
(The actual referring expression is ". . .*den av ALLE muggene som det er*

NEST MEST i." This is – unlike the English translation – an ordinary and relatively simple description. A verbatim translation would read ". . .that of ALL the jugs that it is SECOND MOST in.")

A major challenge in this task is the verbally mediated request to ignore the spatial separation of the two sets of jugs as well as the striking differences between them both with respect to content and size. The target object is *the jug containing most cocoa,* but nearly half of all 6- to 8-year-old children fail to identify it. Some point out the jug containing *second most milk,* others the one with *second most cocoa.* The identification is often made hesitatingly, with oscillating gaze and hand movement. Quite a few of the 6 1/2-year-old children indeed use both hands, putting one finger on the jug with second most milk in it and another *simultaneously* on the jug containing second most cocoa. Deficient symbolic control may thus often be "externalized" in eye movement, pointing behaviors, and hesitant repetition of parts of the referring expression.

Statistical analysis of the performances of 6- to 8-year-old Norwegian children in tasks of type (1) and type (2) reveals rather consistent individual patterns (S. Rommetveit, 1980, pp. 107, and pp. 118). Immature preschoolers tend to fail on either type of task, whereas mature first-graders master both of them. From a Piagetian framework the two different types of tasks may be described as problems of class inclusion under strong perceptual resistance against, respectively, (1) formation of a *subordinate class* and (2) formation of a *superordinate class.* What captures the interest of a researcher adopting a Vygotskian position is the recurrent conflict between a linguistically imposed referential perspective and an immediately meaningful and "prelinguistic" organization of a visually available referential domain. What from a Piagetian point of view is interpreted as evidence of the child's increasing capacity to decenter is thus within a Vygotskian perspective explored in terms of an increasing linguistic structuring of experience and growing higher-order control of attention.

Whether an individual child will master particular formally defined "operations of thought" in identification of a specific target object is thus clearly contingent upon which of many possible referential perspectives is made a prerequisite for the attainment of intersubjectivity. And capacity to adopt a verbally imposed perspective is not merely a matter of language comprehension in the traditional sense, detached from symbolic behavior control. Most 6-year-old Norwegian children, for instance, understand apparently perfectly well the expressions "snowball" and "white circle." However, some of them can immediately identify the target object in a particular drawing when it is verbally described as a SNOWBALL, yet fail to attain intersubjectivity if the same object is referred to as a WHITE CIRCLE (Rommetveit, 1978). Some 6- to 8-year-old children moreover, are incapable of pointing out "the one of the TALL men who has the SECOND SHORTEST distance to run," yet succeed when the very same stick figure in that same drawing is referred to as "the one who wins SECOND PRIZE in the contest group of ADULTS" (S. Rommetveit, 1980, p. 100).

The problem of individual symbolic structuring of experience and behavior control is in our tasks of identifying reference explicitly posed in a context of unequivocally asymmetric adult–child communication about states of affairs that may be transformed into multiple social realities. The Vygotskian perspective is thereby expanded, and semantic competence becomes necessarily to some extent a matter of dyadic control of joint focus of attention. The two different versions of the task, moreover, represent different "stagings" of the potential conflict (or mutual support) between a linguistically mediated and a perceptually supported, "prelinguistic" perspective.

The adult's referential perspective is in the *verbal preidentification* game introduced without any support or resistance from a visually available referential domain of objects or events. A task requiring rather diverse contextual specifications of the members of a bipolar adjective pair seems under such a condition to demand a very high level of sustained symbolic control. The very abstract draft of a contract concerning categorization embedded in LONG/SHORT, for instance, may have to be endorsed in anticipation of contextual specifications tagged on to for example, *horizontal distances* and *vertical body height* (or stick figures) in the subsequently exposed drawing. Such tasks, it turns out, are more easily solved under conditions of *verbal postidentification* of the target object (Rommetveit, 1978; S. Rommetveit, 1980).

The sequential order between identifying description and drawing strongly affects very important temporal–sequential features of attention control. This is clearly demonstrated in pre- and postidentification of task (3) in our sample (see Figure 1). The target object is in this case

(3)   ...the one of the figures with a DOT beneath it that is SMALL, BLACK, and TRIANGULAR.
       (In Norwegian: ". . .*den av figurene med en PRIKK under som er LITEN, SORT, og TREKANTET.*)

This is a task of memory and mastery of sequential–spatial order. Four attributes must be kept in mind in order to point out the proper object. However, the attributes are made known to the child in a temporal order contrary to the systematic spatial organization of referential alternatives in the drawing. The most frequent error in the verbal *preidentification* condition, moreover, is simply that the child forgets about the first-mentioned DOT. Most of the children who fail in the equivalent *postidentification* task, on the other hand, point out the figure with a dot beneath it that is small, black, but a SQUARE. The eager and immature preschooler's gaze – and even her or his finger – may indeed be steered sequentially by the adult's description and already fixated at the moment the fourth attribute is made known.

The role of short-term memory in tasks of identifying reference is hence obviously strongly affected by sequential order between identifying verbal description and exposure of the visually available referential domain. And observation of overt, "externalized" manifestations of symbolic behavior control is an essential part of the researcher's task in the pointing games. A record of the finger's final destination may indeed be deceptive if we ignore the observable behavioral prelude.

Typical patterns of "errors," moreover, may serve as important clues to the nature of the child's failure to make sense of "difficult adult talk." Consider, for instance, tasks (4) and (5) in our sample. The primary challenge in both these tasks is of a syntactic nature. The target object of drawing 4 in Figure 1 is thus

> (4) . . .the APPLE right below the bird on the branch.
> (In Norwegian: ". . .EPLET *rett under fuglen på grense.*")

Some 6½-year-old children in this task put their fingers on the BIRD on the branch. This type of error occurs quite often when the target object is verbally identified by a nesting of prepositional phrases, and most often in the verbal *preidentification* version of the game. The nesting may be formally described in terms of bracketing, that is, as one set of parentheses enclosed within another. The child pointing to the BIRD is, in a way, imprisoned within the innermost brackets. The initially totally unspecified APPLE fades away as the child's attention is steered toward features of the drawing by which its final identity is to be established.

The target object in drawing 5, finally is

> (5) . . .the BUTTERFLY in front of the ball that is thrown in the ditch by
> the bear.
> (In Norwegian: ". . .SOMMERFUGLEN *foran ballen som blir kastet i*
> *gropa av bamsen.*

This is not only a difficult task but, indeed, a rather exceptional case of "difficult adult talk." Quite a few of the younger children are left in confusion, with their tip of the finger on some object other than the proper BUTTERFLY. Some point at the BALL right behind it (or the other ball), others put their finger on the BEAR throwing that ball, and still others signal the THROWING by tracing the course of the ball.

None of these errors has any immediate bearing upon the grammatical contrast suggested by the presence of the *two* butterflies in the drawing.

They are all of the "imprisoned-in-brackets" type. The number of "errors" of this particular type in all pointing tasks intended to tax mastery of "grammatical burden" is strongly negatively correlated with total performance on tasks of type (1) and (2) in the games. An immature preschooler may thus indeed often succeed in task (3) yet be hopelessly lost in some nonfocal aspect of the talked-about state of affairs in tasks (1), (2), (4), and (5).

Children who manage to identify the target object in tasks of type (4) and (5) must both solve the "bracketing" problem involved and master the salient grammatical contrast. And total performance in tasks involving "grammatical burden" *under conditions of verbal preidentification*, it turns out, is highly correlated with total performance in tasks of type (1) and (2) in either one of the two (pre- and postidentification) variants of the game. Mastery of "grammatical burden" *under conditions of verbal postidentification*, on the other hand, is indeed very weakly related to performance on the Piaget- and Vygotsky-inspired tasks (S. Rommetveit, 1980, pp. 118–124).

What do these preliminary findings suggest? May Vygotskian notions of linguistically mediated control of attention be pursued further and, possibly, even shed light on thoroughly mystified issues of children's syntactic competence? Can Vygotskian perpectives within an explicitly pluralistic and social–cognitive paradigm restore our respect for the holy *trinity* (as opposed to *trichotomy*) of semantics, syntactics, and pragmatics?

Time will show.

REFERENCES

Bates, E. 1976. *Language and context: The acquisition of pragmatics*. New York: Academic Press.

Bateson, G. 1973. *Steps to an ecology of mind*. Suffolk: Palladin.

Black, M. 1978. *Lebensform* and *Sprachspiel* in Wittgenstein's later work. In E. Leinfellner (Ed.), *Wittgenstein and his impact upon contemporary thought*. Vienna: Hölder-Pichler-Tempsky.

Blakar, R. M., and Pederson, T. B. 1980. Control and self-confidence as reflected in sex-bound patterns of communication: An experimental approach. *Acta Sociologia*, 23, 33–53.

Bruner, J. 1978. From communication to language: A psychological perspective. In I. Markova (Ed.), *The social context of language*. Chichester: Wiley.

Davidson, D. 1971. Agency. In R. Binkley, R. Bronaugh and A. Marras, (Eds.), *Agent, action, and reason*. Toronto: University of Toronto Press.

Deutsch, W. 1976. *Sprachliche Redundanz und Objekt Identifikation*. Marburg: Lahn.

Garfinkel, H. 1972. Studies of the routine grounds of everyday activities. In D. Sudnow (Ed.), *Studies in social interaction*. New York: Free Press.

Goffman, E. 1971. *Interaction ritual*. London: Penguin Press.

Goffman, E. 1976. Replies and responses. *Language in Society*, 5(3), 257–313.

Feinberg, J. 1965. Action and responsibility. In M. Black (Ed.), *Philosophy in America*. Ithaca, N.Y.: Cornell University Press.

Habermas, J. 1970. Toward a theory of communicative competence. In P. E. Dreitzel (Ed.), *Recent sociology*. London: Macmillan.

Hagtvet, B. E. 1980. Comprehension and production in a social psychological perspective. Paper presented at Conference on Language and Language Acquisition, Mons, Belgium.

Heider, F. 1958. *The psychology of interpersonal relations*. New York: Wiley.

James. W. 1962. Pragmatism's conception of truth. In W. Barrett and H. D. Aiken (Eds.), *Philosophy in the twentieth century*, (Vol. 1). N.Y.: Random House.

Karttunen, L. 1974. Presupposition and linguistic context. *Theoretical Linguistics, 1*, 182–194.

Lock, A. (Ed.) 1978. *Action, gesture, and symbol: The emergence of language*. London: Academic Press.

McCawley, J. D. 1978. "World-creating" predicates. *Versus*, 19–20, 77–93.

Mead, G. H. 1950. *Mind, self, and society*. Chicago: University of Chicago Press.

Menzel, H. 1978. Meaning – who needs it? In M. Brenner, P. Marsh, and M. Brenner (Eds.), *The social contexts of methods*. London: Croom Helm.

Michotte, A. 1954. *La perception de la causalité*. Louvain: Publications Universitaire de Louvain.

Moscovici, S. 1979. Paper presented at Colloque sur les Representations Sociales, Paris.

Naess, A. 1953. *Interpretation and preciseness*. Oslo: Dybwad.

Newson, J. 1978. Dialogue and development. In A. Lock (Ed.) *Action, gesture, and symbol*. London: Academic Press.

Olson, D. 1970. Language and thought: Aspects of a cognitive theory of semantics. *Psychological Review*, 77, 257–273.

Piaget, J. 1958. *The child's construction of reality*. London: Routledge & Kegan Paul.

Rommetveit, R. 1974. *On message structure*. London: Wiley.

Rommetveit, R. 1978. On Piagetian cognitive operations, semantic competence, and message structure. In I. Markova (Ed.), *The social context of language*. London: Wiley.

Rommetveit, R. 1979. On negative rationalism. In R. Rommetveit and R. M. Blaker (Eds.), *Studies of language, thought, and verbal communication*. London: Academic Press.

Rommetveit, R. 1980. On "meanings" of acts and what is meant by what is said in a pluralistic world. In M. Brenner (Ed.) *The structure of action*. Oxford: Blackwell.

Rommetveit, R. 1981. On "meanings" of situations and social control of such meaning in human communication. In D. Magnusson (Ed.). *Toward a psychology of situation: An interactional perspective*. Hillsdale, N.J.: Erlbaum.

Rommetveit, S. 1980. *Skolestart ut fra barnets egne forutsetninger*. Oslo: Tiden.

Schutz, A. 1945. On multiple realities. *Philosophical and Phenomenological Research, 5*, 533–576.

Skinner, B. F. 1957. *Verbal behavior*. New York: Appleton-Century-Crofts.

Trevarthen, C., and Hubley, P. 1978. Secondary intersubjectivity: Confidence, confiding, and acts of meaning in the first year. In A. Lock (Ed.), *Action, gesture, and symbol*. London: Academic Press.

Uhlenbeck, E. M. 1978. On the distinction between linguistics and pragmatics. In D. Gerver and H. W. Sinaiko (Eds.), *Language, interpretation, and communication*. New York: Plenum Press.

Voloshinov, V. N. 1973. *Marxism and the philosophy of language*. New York: Seminar Press.

Vygotsky, L. S. 1962. *Thought and language*. Cambridge: MIT Press.

Vygotsky, L. S. 1978. *Mind in society: The development of higher psychologcial processes*. Edited by M. Cole, V. John-Steiner, S. Scribner, and E. Souberman. Cambridge: Harvard University Press.

Vygotsky, L. S. 1981. The development of higher forms of attention in childhood. In J. V. Wertsch (Ed.) *The concept of activity in Soviet psychology*. Armonk, N.Y.: Sharpe.

Wertsch, J. V. 1979. From social interaction to higher psychological processes: A clarification and application of Vygotsky's theory. *Human Development*, *22*, 1–22.

Wertsch, J. V. 1980. Semiotic mechanisms in joint cognitive activity. Paper presented at Conference on Theory of Activity, Moscow.

Wittgenstein, L. 1962. The blue book. In W. Barrett and D. H. Aiken (Eds.), *Philosophy in the twentieth century* (Vol. 2). New York: Random House.

Wittgenstein, L. 1968. *Philosophical investigations*. Oxford: Blackwell.

9

The functional stratification of language and ontogenesis

MICHAEL SILVERSTEIN

There are many recognizable views on what is learned or acquired or achieved in performance in language ontogenesis. (The choice of participle is already, by connotation, an indicator of theoretical inclination.) The view that *functional stratification* of language is crucial to this process is closest in spirit to Vygotsky's understanding. I want here to explain what we mean by the italicized term and to contrast this concept with *formal stratification* (which is perhaps more familiar to readers, at least by silent assumptions). I can then illustrate how a close, functional study of language itself motivates fruitful hypotheses about ontogenesis in the spirit of Vygotsky.

It is possible to distinguish several "functionalisms" that have appeared in the linguistic and psychological literature, some reductionistic and others not. First, I offer a brief summary of what I see as the essentials of such approaches. Then I will be able more precisely to contrast formal and functional stratification. This will permit a presentation of the major areas of functional stratification of language, which broaden, but maintain the essence of, Vygotsky's attempt to explain the ontogenesis of "word meaning," as he called it. Results of syntactic work carried out in a functional framework yield several critical notions, which are then presented.

Functionalisms

Linguistics can be seen as a formal science in at least two ways, as a *science of form* in language and as a *science* of language *using formal methods and models*. The two views are not, of course, mutually exclusive in modern linguistics. Recent approaches to language, however, rest on certain "functional" assumptions that determine both what facts are to be explained, and what shall count as "explanation" of them.

There are many senses of the term *function* in the accumulated specialist literature about language, with more or less of the connotational baggage that derives from common parlance and from other fields, such as mathematics. Some functionalisms are reductionistic in intent. These seek

205

to "explain" linguistic forms by their role or "function" in accomplishing some psychological or social–communicative imperative that is postulated to be independent in principle from language itself. Thus, it has been argued that the alleged general psychological ability to process 7 ± 2 chunks (or bits) of information simultaneously accounts for the fact that, in any specific language, segmental sound units (phonemes) in their characteristic sequences can be characterized using about this number of specifications of their differential sound features, out of a larger set of possibilities. The distinctive linguistic form of phonemes in any language, then, is a function of, is reductively explained by, an alleged general psychological property (Miller, 1956; Jakobson, Fant, and Halle 1963; Jakobson and Waugh, 1979).

Other "functionalisms," by contrast, are fully structural–functional, that is, they seek to "explain" particularities of linguistic form by their place in the larger totality of grammar. Bloomfield's notion of function, for example, which he applied to lexical forms (elementary and complex) is an equivalent of privileges of occurrence or distribution within the total system of distributional possibilities for lexical forms in sentences. Thus, it has been claimed that in any language, certain linear orders of elements in one kind of syntactic construction (say, Adjective and Noun in a modifier–modified syntactic phrase) can appear (if and) only if certain orders of elements in another kind of syntactic construction (say, Pre-/Postposition and Noun in an adpositional syntactic phrase) also appear (Greenberg, 1966). The symmetric or asymmetric harmony of such structures as formal configurations within the larger whole of grammar can be taken as a fact about grammars as formal objects per se.

In this connection, it should be noted that with reductionistic explanatory intent, the particular aspects/features/elements of language *form* are directly motivated by their "function(s)" within some larger framework of essentially nonlinguistic cognitive/communicative imperatives. With a structuralist explanatory intent, the "function" of linguistic forms can be located within the particular structure of language itself, generalizing from specific instances. Of course, any one particular writer on the subject may not be consistent in the mode of explanation offered; but this is not a matter of principle, only of rhetorical as well as scientific strategy.[1]

There would seem to have been at least one major shift in approach over the last 30 or so years. Linguistics has shifted from being a positivist project of at least promissory explanation by reduction of language form to more elementary sufficient causes – for example, in communication and in cognition – to a structuralist project of explanation by discovery of necessary abstract principles of form itself that are manifested in specific linguistic systems, though sometimes obscurely so from the perspective of naïve phenomenal reality (as in manifest language use).

Thus formerly one might attempt to explain various universal facts about limited discontinuities tolerated in syntactic constituency directly in psychological processing terms, just as one might attempt to explain the number of simultaneously implemented axes of phonological distinctiveness in terms of "magical" quantification of information to be processed. Or one might even attempt to explain the seemingly arbitrary relationship between lexical sign and its denotatum on the basis of stimulus–response patterns, their generalization and displacement in the individual, combined with "historical transmission" of sign–denotatum relationships in the aggregate of individuals over time.

Such approaches to explanation by reduction of linguistic phenomena to general psychological ones have been unconvincing, at least partly because of the particular functional assumptions about language that, piecemeal, try relating a very specific linguistic fact about form to a very specific psychological or communicative regularity. They ignore the fundamental systematicity of linguistic structure, expressible as an interlocking set of rules and metacriteria, that has become the typical analytic tool of modern structuralism and the assertibly fundamental "explanatory" value of metacriteria on linguistic form as such.

Yet it must be observed that this argument between what we might term "substantivist" and "formalist" approaches to the explanation of language *form* can have taken place and can be taking place only because both views, as currently manifested, rest implicitly or explicitly on a view of language as a semiotically *unifunctional* symbol system. That is, both approaches see language as *essentially* (fundamentally to be explained) a system structured in its form by the criterion of reference-and-predication as the primary functional value of its signals. In the reductionist accounts, the attempt is made explicitly to relate various structures used in reference-and-predication (sometimes only statistically predominant ones in a survey of languages) to substantive mechanisms of cognition and communication. Thus, we find that the syntactic categories of (sentence) Subject and Predicate are (at least predominantly) found, respectively, in first or relatively prior structural position, and second or relatively later structural position, and relatable to (utterance) topic versus comment. This is, in turn, attributed to the "natural" psychological focus on, in order, first "old" then "new" information. (What to do with statistically nonpredominant orders of sentence-structural constituents is not quite clear, to be sure.) So the old-then-new information-processing strategy is the explanatory basis for the topic-then-comment preference in utterance, whence the explanation for the order of structural constituents in sentences.

In formalist accounts, by contrast, the equivalent structures are generally merely assumed at the level of linkage of utterance and sentence phenomena, so that universal formal metacriteria, once proposed, explain the various formal recurrences and are, in the most extreme accounts, said to be the (quasi-) biological basis for the formal structure itself. It is the formal structures, motivated by general metacriteria, that are primary in such accounts, and the referential-and-predictional values of these structures in actual languages that are secondary. Under such assumptions, it is no wonder that, eschewing any outward-looking functionalism, we must consider not only ontogenesis of language, but also phylogenesis to be exceedingly problematic as gradual processes.

As I have elsewhere discussed (Silverstein, 1980), there are at least three older traditions dealing with the problem of function in language within linguistics itself, each with its own special problems. The "formalist" approach to language, for example, is a kind of *structural functionalism*, with each aspect of linguistic form in a specific language at its proper plane of abstraction, finding its function as its place within the total formal structure, dictated by relevant metacriteria on grammars as formal objects. Bloomfield's (1933) notion of function, at a much less abstract level of consideration, is, as I noted above, of this type. Surface lexical forms, individually or in grammatical construction, have privileges of occurrence that, taken as a set, specify the "function" of the lexeme or expression in the total grammatical system of the language. But in Bloomfieldian as in modern formalist approaches, the delimitation of the totality of grammatical forms to be so analyzed is, implicitly, restricted to the referential-and-predicational view of language. Thus, from a semiotic point of view, there is a unifunctional assumption about the data to be explained.

One of the recognizable functionalisms that purports to be fully of a "substantivist" sort is *illocutionary* or *speech—act functionalism*, where each aspect of linguistic form in a specific language finds its function (sometimes unfortunately called its "meaning") in the system of conventionally understood communicative acts that it occurs in, or is implicated in as signal. Among such speech acts is reference-and-predication, though of course as Austin (1975, pp. 139–147) himself recognized, this never occurs as a "pure" (il)locutionary act. Indeed, as it turns out, at this level of analysis there is nothing in speaking that occurs as a "pure" illocutionary act, for a variety of reasons that ultimately undermine the analysis itself.

For the real basis underlying this whole assertedly functionalist and substantivist theory is the so-called explicit primary performative constructions in language, to which all else must be relatable as extension to prototypic core. Explicit primary performative constructions (e.g., in English, those of the general types *I* [VERB] *(to) you that* [SENTENCE] / *to* [VERBAL PHRASE] and their syntactic transforms) seem actually to comprise the intersection of illocutionary or speech – act function with complete propositional form; that is, they have at once the functional and formal characteristics of both functional views of language, and thus seem to be a very special case. The substantivist/functionalist account here, then, is based ultimately on deriving all illocutionary value of a language from its particular set of explicit primary performatives, or worse, from some purported universal set of underlying or abstract or ideal type ones, regardless of the specificity of the particular language under study. And unfortunately, referential-and-predicational structures must then be seen as outgrowths of illocutionary values, with no clear criteria for motivating these formal structures in any systematic way.

There is, thirdly, what we might call (broadly) *pragmatic functionalism*, which seeks to explain linguistic structures by their occurrence in, and hence by their serving as indexes of, particular presupposable communicative contexts of use. To be sure, any linguistic form can occur in a variety of contexts, whether these are contexts considered from the individual or social points of view. And indeed, the alleged essential *decontextualization* of reference-and-predication with linguistic forms has been a fundamental of formalist analysis, and the dominant trend in linguistics itself, since early in this century. This property has been pointedly reiterated in the last decades as argument enough against any form of behaviorist pragmatics in attempts at reductionist linguistic explanation. Nevertheless, the contextualization of language forms in usage does seem, contra such formalist claims, to show some regularity, and it is not implausible to seek explanation in terms of such facts, even, where promising, of "essential" features of language form.

For certainly, even with the unifunctionalist assumption that language is referential-and-predicational, there are substantive categories such as pronouns, tenses, anaphors, that, taken as individual language forms, are strictly context-dependent for their basic contribution to reference-and-predication, hence for their basic meaningfulness. Furthermore, when we consider the contextualization of language forms within the flow of discourse itself [the problem of textuality, or "texture," as Halliday and Hasan (1976) term it], we find that with very few exceptions, there are asymmetries of textual distribution that cannot be explained as merely epiphenomenal additions/happenstances from putting together units coded only up to and including the sentence as structural building block. Such central regularities show that text-building properties are locatable in schemata of cross-sentence interactions of linguistic categories, even where the categories themselves seemed at first blush to be locatable within single-sentence structures of reference-and-predication. It would seem that this interaction provides an important clue to the nature of the pragmatic–functional organization of language, should we seek to find it.

This pragmatic functionalism has not been without its difficulties in the way of psychological assertions about the internal states and so forth that linguistic forms are said to index in speakers/contexts. We therefore carefully distinguish between (1) context and contextualization as the partially structured and ongoing set of factors indexed/indexable by occurring forms in language, and (2) the specific psychological processes in the individual that are related, by complex processing strategies in both speaker and hearer, to the social fact of context. There is a tension in the philosophical accounts of language concerning the conventionality (in illocutionary realms) of language as social act in interpersonal and intersubjective contextualization, as opposed to the naturalistic basis of illocution and of indexical expressiveness in the individual psychology of the language user. This tension is, to be sure, manifested as much in the account of a Vygotsky as it is in that of a Grice (1957, 1975). But in Vygotsky's case, and in more modern accounts deriving from him, there is really no contradiction in the functionalism.

Of late, there has unfortunately been an essential identification of "functionalism" with individual psychological accounts and with the substantive requirements of such individual psychology for productive or receptive processing of the forms or signs of language. Contrariwise, there has been an essential identification of "structuralism" with the search for invariant metacriteria on abstract formalisms that are said to underlie regularities of the forms or signs of phenomenal language. Neither of these approaches treats of the kind of functionalism that takes the social event of communication as the explanatory groundwork. The functionalism that purports to, unfortunately, does so with a theory that is ultimately as individually and pseudopsychologically based (speech–act theory) as the others. We must then distinguish between the professed functionalisms within the recent tradition of (psycho)linguistics and true semiotic functionalisms.

Professed "functionalism" of various trends in linguistic study must be seen in terms of dichotomy of *formalist–structuralist* versus *substantivist–functionalist* approaches to explanation of linguistic forms. A psycholinguistic account of development based on these different modes of explanation must take account of the differences between them. The formalist account derives certain metacriteria on propositional formal grammars, a "universal grammar," presupposed to be an input to the developmental process as an individual's *faculté de langage*. The substantivist account interprets formal features of language as codings, or shapings, of language-independent properties of cognition/communication, seen as necessary – one could not at this point say sufficient – conditions on the acquisition of a language.

Both approaches seem to have been talking past one another, in interesting ways. The formalist account has tended to study the logic of achievement of the overall syntactic processes characteristic of adult grammars in their global abstract characteristics. The substantivist account has tended to study particular cognitive/communicative strategies and how they seem to be (en)coded in specific linguistic forms over a period of development. Thus, there have been wide levels of difference between the two approaches, both in method of work and type of contributory investigation.

For the formalist, the achievement of the proper, abstractly characterizable properties of the specific adult system at issue is the goal of explanation in linguistic ontogenesis. An initial state is invoked including a rich, language-specific and language-focused set of structural principles deemed necessary for this process by deduction. For the substantivist, by contrast, the continuity in prelinguistic-to-linguistic development of specific/cognitive/communicative characteristics is the goal of explanation. An initial state of otherwise nonlinguistic characteristics becomes in this process a linguistic encoding or formal consequence. The substantivist must demonstrate that the interaction of various principles of encoding produces the formal result attested. In a sense, then, the structure of interaction of such principles, if any, is a "formal" structure encompassing all specifics and determining ontogenesis.

Of course, in the latter view, there should not be any a priori reason to think that such overriding ontogenetic structures are recoverable directly from synchronic examination of adult grammatical systems themselves. But certainly, there is a relationship between adult grammatical systems, insofar as they are *functionally decomposable* and demonstrably *hierarchically functional*, and the course of ontogenesis. This is ultimately the only viable goal for such an approach, to which I return in conclusion. What will be essential here is the claim that there is a hierarchical nature to the functions of language, such that in the adult system, there are functional tensions serving as countervailing force of stability/instability of formal language structure. In the child, various functional claims on language form would appear to grow and become more differentiated and enriched partly as a function of formal mastery itself. This is the process that needs unraveling.

Formal and functional stratification

Under more simplistic assumptions about language, its *formal stratification*, in two senses, has long been a commonplace truth. First, the *double articulation* of language (Martinet, 1964, pp. 22–27; Benveniste, 1966, pp. 121–123), its *duality of patterning* (Hockett, 1977, pp. 152–155) into a phonological realization and a morphosyntactic organization, has been accepted as a basic structural characteristic. Units of sound structure – for example, phonemes – are themselves without fixed denotational value ("meaning"). Rather, they function in patterned combinations to differentiate and identify the higher, meaningful segments of words, phrases, and sentences. These second-level, meaningful units, in turn, function in patterned combinations that ultimately allow speakers to refer to entities and to predicate states of affairs of them. Thus, the three phoneme units of *cat* in English, k, æ, t, differentiate this noun stem each time it occurs from, respectively, *bat* (in the first unit), *cut* (in the second), and *can* (in the third), among others in the overall English lexicon. But the phonemes k, ae, and t in English do not themselves have any constancy of denotational value, as does their ordered concatenation, *cat*, occurring in such words as *catgut*, in such phrases as *the gray cat*, and in such sentences as *The cat was on the mat*.

Patterned combinations of these higher-level, denotational units how a second type of formal stratification involving *hierarchical constituency*. Morphosyntactic units are organized into regular groupings of more and more inclusive span. Each level of grouping is a constituent – continuous or discontinuous – of one at a higher or more inclusive level. Thus, in the phrase *the chagrin of the populace*, there are two immediate constituents, *the* and *chagrin of the populace*. The latter, in turn, consists of two constituents, *chagrin* and *of the populace*. The latter, in turn, consists of two constituents, *of* and *the populace*. And the latter, in turn, consists of two constituents, *the* and *populace*. A great deal of the study of modern linguistics is devoted to establishing the constituent types in an idealization of the language, the kinds of different hierarchical groupings in which they can occur, and the regularities (rules) that characterize the relationships of such groupings, for example, as so-called transforms of each other. Observe that referring and predicating constitute, by assumption, the unique function recognized for language relevant to this kind of systematic investigation. And the particular kinds of formal stratifications I mention are a consequence of the assumption (necessary, I would claim) for such analysis.

Such a unifunctional assumption about language permits the study of the entailed formal stratifications, both structurally, or *in potentia*, as in linguistics, and psychologically, or *in praesentia*, as in cognitive investigations of language production and comprehension. It also dictates that we formulate the problem of language acquisition in certain ways. For example, we would want to know if the first utterances of children are most like adult words, or phrases, or sentences, in formal and referential-and-predicational correspondence. We would want to trace how the distinct adult language levels and hierarchical constituencies are developed. We would want to know if there are regularities in the development of morphosyntactic structures of the various attested types. Given the role of phonological units in the double articulation of language, we would want to investigate developmental changes that start from a productivity undifferentiated (but probably receptively more differentiated) phonological inventory. And so forth.

These problems all depend on the assumption that the end point of linguistic ontogenesis is the adultlike, assumedly unifunctional system with particular types of formal stratification. These questions about the development of linguistic form can be asked in the manner indicated only when we assume that, from the beginning, the child's language system is unifunctional also, in a way corresponding to the adult's. The uniform measure of language acquisition is the range of forms and how they contribute to reference-and-predication, the function assumed to be constant, though only nascent, from the beginnings of language in the child.

Indeed, this referential-and-predicational (propositional) function of language (or "referential function," as it is sometimes called) has constituted, by more or less explicit design, the backdrop for essentially all modern theorizing about linguistic ontogenesis, even by those who question its primacy, but in ways that are seen to be extensions of the same view. A great number of studies have sought to explain the growth of denotational content of words, assuming that word units encapsulate or encode a categorization of the world in a basically unchanging denotational way from the beginning of their use. Again, a large number of studies have sought to document the seeming expansion of the child's repertoire of syntactic types, under the assumption of propositionality. Writers have, in fact, been able to argue for a stagelike development from "pivot-open" grammatical-class organization of utterance syntax through phrase-structure and transformational grammars implied by the range of attested, referentially interpreted syntactic types, viewed of course by comparison with their analyses in adult referential linguistic systems.

Others even see the "grammatical faculty" as being constant throughout development, and only certain peripheral processing factors undergoing enrichment, so as to yield growing productive and receptive capacity for differentiated syntactic types.

In the developmental literature, there has been the tendency either to assume the unifunctional propositionality of utterances throughout development and the isofunctionality of particular units and types of units from stage to stage or to ignore the problem altogether, thereby making the implicit claim that investigation of ontogenesis in a purely structural sense can nevertheless proceed, regardless of functional values from stage to stage.

By contrast, I want to outline here the *functional stratification* of adult linguistic systems, as understood by a more semiotically informed approach to language structure and use. Starting from the analysis of the contextualized use of language, we can motivate *levels of different sign phenomena,* that is, *semiotic functions,* all implicitly contained in seemingly one-dimensional (temporally unfolding) linguistic signals. Some "formal" aspects of the linguistic signal are functionally *indexes* of configurational factors in the linguistic or nonlinguistic context in which the form is uttered or otherwise instantiated; other aspects of linguistic signals are internally regulatory; yet others are uniquely used to *refer* to factors in the linguistic or nonlinguistic context; and so forth. Each of these functional criteria for linguistic analysis dictates its own formal segmentation, organization, and structural relationships encapsulated within the speech signal. The investigation of the integration of these different organizations into a coherent signal is exactly the task of a truly functional linguistics.

To be sure, such a view does not deny the validity of the regularities of formal stratification, gained under the unifunctional assumption. We must recognize that propositionality of adult language is one of its most important and "psychologically real" functional organizing principles. Indeed, through propositionality, language is probably to be considered functionally – and thence, structurally – unique among all semiotic systems in its representational capacity. There are good reasons for considering propositionality central to language in several ways in fully mature adult systems.

But the alleged importance and centrality of the propositional function in certain adult situations of language use is neither a necessary nor a sufficient reason to assume the same for all stages of language development, and certainly not to assume the relative invariance of functional values and relationships throughout development. It is interesting that a functional analysis demonstrates that even the most straightforward reference-and-predication is a complex of at least two levels of sign functions integrated in the event of using language. There are the *fully symbolic*-referential ("semantic" in the strictest sense) and the *indexical*-referential ("pragmatic" in the strictest sense). So, from a functional point of view even reference-and-predication is not a single unitary linguistic system, but the integration of distinct and analyzable functional systems, which points up the developmental problem, to be sure.

In the more simplistic, unifunctional view, the formal stratification of language is a general property of the system. The linguistic analysis of any specific *sentence* (note: this is already an abstraction from any actual utterances themselves) can be accomplished only by appeal to the systemic properties of hierarchical levels of units, as these are manifested in the particular sentence and all others that, by comparison, are relevant to its analysis. Hence the familiar notion of the potential "surface (formal) ambiguity" or "(formal) indeterminacy" of any utterance type being analyzed as a sentence in the referential-and-predicational structure as in the famous example *They are [flying planes]/They [are flying] planes*, both of which bracketed higher-order structures are potentially being instantiated in the same string of words.

Likewise, the functional stratification of language is a general property of the system. The semiotic analysis of any particular utterance-in-context into its different functional sign components in their hierarchical relationships can be accomplished only by appeal to the systemic properties of language in this respect. Hence, there is also *functional ambiguity* or *functional indeterminacy* of any utterance with respect to the full functional system. A simple and very obvious example of this is what in philosophical discourse would rest on the "use" versus "mention" doctrine about linguistic forms. Consider the old child's game: "*I* can spell the word *antidisestablishmentarianism*. *You* spell it!/. . . .spell *it*!" The last word of the first homophonous alternant is an anaphoric pronoun, a discourse indexical that appears to refer to whatever its antecedent, appositional noun phrase, *the word*[=] *anti*. . . ,does. The correct response to the imperativelike directive here is to spell out "*a-n-t-i-*. . ." The last word of the second alternant is the name of a word form, a metalinguistic referential term independent of any antecedently occurring noun phrases. The correct response here is to spell out "*i-t,*" as any child who knows the joke can recall. There are incredibly many more functional indeterminacies in actual uttered speech than we usually recognize consciously. For we impose functional interpretations on them (in not unexpected ways) in an automatic fashion, as receivers of messages, just as we resolve formal indeterminacies of referential-and-predicational structure by similar strategies. Speakers manipulate, often not very consciously, such indeterminacies as allow of creative interactional strategies depending on the functional systems of language.

Though evidence is suggestive rather than conclusive at this point, I would suggest an important empirical regularity about the functional overlap or semiotic plurifunctionality of signal forms in language: The kinds of overlaps of function in any particular, typologically controllable formal surface configuration are cross-linguistically recurrent and implicationally fixed, in the usual manner of linguistic universals. That is, there are recurrent functional overlaps across languages of how the equivalent multiple functions are located in equivalent forms. These networks of functional regularities form an anchoring system, or set of fixed formal–functional points, for the functional analysis of languages. To be sure, we know best the functional regularities of the various systems of sign relationships that go into reference-and-predication, since these have been the best investigated under the more simplistic assumptions. However, there are many such regularities to be located between referential and other functional systems.

We know, for example, that the ways in which reference is made in any language to those central participant roles of the presupposed situation of linguistic use ('speaker', 'hearer', etc.) is by a set of so-called personal pronominal forms that, from the abstract syntactic point of view (pure "semantic" function) have many of the same structural properties as whole noun phrases. Again, we know that whatever is the equative predicate or copula (as opposed to the existential one, if a difference is made) for stating referential identify will be used in the *metasemantic equation* or definitional specification in true "glossing" speech events: that is, the gloss and the occasional referential identity are nowhere formally distinct. Hence, in scientifically regimented, technical discussions it is necessary to flag actual definitions by extraordinary means, such as prefixed boldface "**Def.**" or formulaic nonverbal expressions like "$\equiv$" or "$=_{df}$." And so forth.

It is such fixed regularities of functional overlaps, which all linguistic systems exemplify in their respective formal terms, that anchor linguistic form to semiotic function(s) constituting use in communicational contexts. In particular, they anchor the seemingly abstract morphosyntactic system underlying referential-and-predicational capability to the functional systematicity of language use in regular ways. Thereby, such regularities explain how seemingly abstract morphosyntactic forms can be acquired using a mode of linguistic exposure to exemplars, or tokens, of the functional and formal systems in the context of ongoing communication.

For, if there are regular ways in which the various functional systems that make up language do in fact formally overlap with the central, referential-and-predicational structure of unifunctional morphosyntactic theory, we can see how this latter structure, the highest achievement of linguistic and cognitive capacity, can be made possible through an actual process of acquisition. In broad terms, we would agree with Vygotsky that the pragmatic or interactional substrate is "internalized" in language in the form of abstract referential-and-predicational capacity. For a child need not acquire the referential-and-predicational value associated with a form as the original one in the process; rather, this can emerge from a developmental process in which functional overlaps play a significant and indeed determining role. Thus, insofar as we can demonstrate the specifics of formal overlap of functionally distinct systems, we can formulate testable hypotheses about the gradual emergence of abstract referential-and-predicational structure as fully generative, infinitely propositional, and functionally dominant.

The most powerful demonstration of induced formal overlap as a possible mechanism of language acquisition is based on the occurrence of what I term *privileged zeroes* on the markedness structures of reference-and-predication. Such constructional configurations as have positive communicational content even in the absence of positive, segmentable categorial forms – "zero signs" that occur in certain privileged constructions – demonstrate the *structural telescoping* of many functions into reduced structures that preserve the multifunctional characteristics of several distinct and more elaborate forms in a configurational way. Such telescoped structures are ontogenetically pregnant foci for functional differentiation and enrichment. One such case I have elaborately demonstrated (Silverstein 1976, 1981) is in the area of overlap between (1) the topic-comment structure of discourse cohesion; (2) the signaling of case – relations, or propositional roles, within the referential-and-predicational clause structure of sentences; and (3) the inherently speech-situation boundedness of referents. Before we can give a general overview of the process, we must turn to an overview of the functional characteristics of language in the general sense and their hierarchical relationships in linguistic systems, their functional stratification.

The stratification of functions in language

It is useful to adopt the Peircean framework for presenting semiotic functions, since it comes closest to providing the degree of differentiations we must make for linguistic signs, in some explanatory fashion. It is, of course, impossible to review the entire basis for the classification of signs, as given in Table 1, but the outline of these functional distinctions should serve to call up discussions in other sources contributory to our full, modern understanding of language.

We must distinguish between two great classes of linguistic sign functions, the *pragmatic* and the *semantic,* used in rather narrow senses. In one sense, the pragmatic aspect of language, all that meaningfulness of signs connected with its ongoing usage in contexts of communication, always encompasses the strictly semantic, if we take the latter very narrowly. Seeing semantics as the kind of meaningfulness of linguistic signs that can be specified through their *senses* (or the modern, more adequate notion of systematic, presupposable syntacticosemantic categories plus stereotype attributes) then every use of language presupposes the existence of a system of semantics, and implements and instantiates at least certain relevant aspects of one, if there is any regularity and continuity to linguistic structure in a synchronic sense from use to use. Semantics is an abstract set of relationships concretely instantiated in the pragmatic act.

In a different way, however, pragmatics is opposed to semantics, rather than constituting its implementational encompassment in the event. Pragmatics in this second, more canonically Peircean view, concerns the *indexical* aspect of linguistic signs, their spatiotemporal, causal, and so on relationships with that which forms the presupposed or entailed context of their use in a communicative event. It is plausible that part of this is sys-

Table 1. *Functional analysis of language*

Functional realm	Functional characteristics	
	Pragmatic	Semantic
[a] True reference (dicent indexical Legisigns)	Presupposes existence and quantifiability (e.g., uniqueness) of entity picked out	
[b] Attributive reference, denotation (rhematic Legisigns)		Characterizability conditions on entity to be picked out: 1. Metapragmatic (rhematic indexical Legisigns), determining indexical denotation; 2. Other, determining nonindexical denotation
[c] Sense (rhematic symbolic Legisigns; Saussurean *signes*) [the valid domain of Saussurean and Chomskyan syntactic argumentation]	Presupposes the organization of the sign system into a Saussurean grammar, up to and including syntax of sentences	Characterizability conditions on denotata systematically describable according to a Saussurean grammar with underlying syntactic structure for the signs [generates arbitrarily complex sense structures by recursion etc.]
[d] Metasemantics: 1. Naturally occurring	Presupposes an equational sentence form within the Saussurean grammar	Analytic truths; definitional equivalences of surface expressions
2. Virtual [underlying cryptotype structure or "logical form"]		Semantic representation of lexical items and expressions under Saussurean assumptions, with appropriate formalisms
[e] Pragmatics (indexicals) [functions$_2$, or analytically isolable domains of indexicality]	Speech event–bound presuppositional and entailment relations between linguistic tokens and contextual factors (cf. Jakobsonian components)	

Table 1. *(cont.)*

	Functional characteristics	
Functional realm	Pragmatic	Semantic
[f] Metapragmatics [functions₁, purposive uses of language in events]	Denotes speech events and their components	
1. Naturally occurring	Explicit primary performatives, all indexical denotationals	Characterizability conditions always in terms of speech events as institutions of language
2. Systematic–virtual		

tematic, that is, abstractable as constant and regular, and hence instantiated in particular situations (cf. the first semantics/pragmatics opposition characterized above). Semantics, by contrast in this second view, is the realm of context-free meaningfulness of specific signs, the regularities of meaning that do not necessitate reference to the sign–context nexus for their specification. Therefore, semantic meaningfulness seems to be abstract, context-independent, and unconnected with actual usage. In actuality, it is instantiated in tokens of types just as are pragmatic aspects of meaning. But the constitution of such *symbolic* meanings is not logically– whatever the case historically, causally, and so on – dependent on rules of use for indexicals.

As we mentioned above, we must diminish the fact that most phenomenal linguistic signs overlap semantic and pragmatic meaningfulness in a single apparent formal stretch of signal. Nevertheless, we can take the analytic stance that these aspects of their meanings or functions can be distinguished in principle and in practice. Table 1 is such an analytic perspective on the sign functions of natural languages.

In the table, various commonly noted foci of treatments of language are displayed and are analyzed according to both pragmatic and semantic functional characteristics that, together, specify the particular linguistic phenomenon. The general order of presentation in the table is from most intuitively obvious realm of meaningful function in language (and hence most usually treated) to most recondite without careful analytic treatment. Thus, it starts with true reference and concludes with metapragmatics. In each case, we seek a general specification of the particular mode of signification in terms of characteristic sign functions that specify that phenomenon's distinctiveness, not, I should repeat, a segmentation of linguistic signs into exclusive formal categories.

From this point of view, then, *true reference* (dicent indexical Legisigns) indicate, or point to, entities of reference the existence and quantifiability of which are presupposed in the pragmatic act of referring. Thus, at the functional level of true reference, the sign purports to index (be in spatio-temporal – "real world" – contiguity, direct or indirect, with) at least one and perhaps more existing individuals. We claim nothing for the spatio-temporal continuity of such objects or their actuality independent of the act of true reference. We claim merely that such a functional sign *qua* sign presupposes the conditions at the moment of use, the Legisign (form) itself being a perduring virtual regularity evidenced by recurrent uses of "the same" form, tokens of the type, in distinct speech events. A recognizable, hence communicative, pointing gesture with lips or finger, or any linguistic equivalent, incorporates such a sign function, as do the variety of "definite" noun phrases in a language (now known to be of unbounded complexity of structure), regardless of whatever other sign functions they incorporate and instantiate. The idea of true reference should be carefully dis-tinguished from the manner of presentation of an object, the manner of characterizing it, in which notions of correct and incorrect descriptions come into play, and with them, arguments as to whether or not one has referred if one uses an incorrect definite description for some presupposed object of reference. But this is already a complex sign function, the components of which are at issue in our presentation; it involves the applicability of semantic characterizability conditions to a particular ob-ject or objects presented as the object(s) of reference, in addition to the pragmatic function of true reference *tout court*. Unfortunately, we know of no natural language in which these two functions are represented by totally formally distinct phenomenal (surface) signs. The closest we come in English, for example, is the sign opposition *a* (pl. *some*) versus *the* in just their function of differentiating presuppositions of uniqueness, abstract-ing away from their integral role in the discourse–topic maintenance sys-tems of the language, and other functions.

Indeed, virtually every elementary sign for reference in a language like English already is at the level of *attributive reference and denotation* (rhematic Legisigns, whether indexical or iconic or symbolic). In actual use, sign users unavoidably present objects of reference or predication as charac-terizable in such-and-such manner, that is, as having such-and-such qualities, being in such-and-such locations (with respect to speaker, for example), entering into such-and-such relationships (with other objects of characterization, for example). Even the simplest demonstrative pronoun of English, *this* or *that,* presents an object of reference as being in certain spatiotemporal locations with respect to the speaker and hearer of that token of the form. That is, reference with such a demonstrative presents the object as characterizable by its spatiotemporal relation to the speaker-hearer in the *hic-et-nunc* of its utterance. So if we understand pragmatics to encompass indexical relationships of sign to its context of usage, then such characterizability conditions for demonstrative pronouns are "meta-pragmatic" in nature, descriptive of pragmatic conditions as is discussed below.

Such indexical–denotationals, with metapragmatic characterizability conditions, contrast with other signs with attributive denotational content, as for example the (formally definite) phrase type *the* [NOUN] [RELATIVE CLAUSE] used in the sense of "whatever (possible) object of class [NOUN] that fits the characterization [RELATIVE CLAUSE]." It is easily seen that virtually every sign in English used in processes of reference, whether formally simple or complex, already has this level of characterizability function, metapragmatic or otherwise, attached to its use.

Hence there exists the possibility of using definite noun phrases of any form in either truly or attributively referential manner, as noted by Donnellan (1971). Interpreted functionally this means that every actual surface noun phrase has presuppositions of characterizability of its object of denotation – that is, has some descriptive content. But usage of such noun phrases in only certain syntactic, discourse, and situational contexts – canonically, in subject position, with topical value, after prior presentation of referent – constitutes a true referential application of them, where the additional presuppositions of existence and quantifiability are automatically satisfied (verifiable independent of the particular linguistic usage).

So far we have been dealing with the fact of reference, both as indexical "picking out" and as characterizability of objects so as to identify them, and hence "pick them out." We have said nothing of systematicity in the way these are accomplished. But natural languages include a further level of semiotic function, one that constitutes of them "sense" systems in the Saussurean–Chomskyan mode. The basic surface expressions of language are Saussurean signs, *signes* (rhematic symbolic Legisigns), the "sense" of which is generated by their formal organization into a Saussurean grammar, "*un système où tout se tient*," where the generative value of each element in the system is the structural relationships it enters into with other elements of the system. In such a genuinely symbolic sign system, the individual (token) usage depends on the characterization of the general (type) to which it is referred. Each usage in "performance" presupposes the constitution of the sign value in systematic "competence" of a specifically linguistic sort. Since we are dealing with rhematic Legisigns, we must encompass characterizability conditions of some sort. However, in such a symbolic system, it is only with the equivalent of a Saussurean grammar that we can specify the systematicity of characterizability conditions. Note, it is not that we exhaust the characterizability conditions; just that the necessary defining systematicity of such in this kind of sign system is essentially specifiable in this way.

Thus, in natural languages, the principal breakthrough in our post-Saussurean understanding, due to the work of Chomsky, is that characterizability conditions for reference and denotation may be arbitrarily complex, built in systematic fashion by syntactic structural principles of recursion. Specifying such structural principles is the domain of modern syntax. Here are laid out the mechanisms of creating referring noun phrases with internal relative clause formations – such relative clauses with the structural value of sentences – themselves of arbitrarily complex structure (that is, themselves having internal parts that are unboundedly complex in structure in the same way). The structure of such systems specifies the regularity specific to the infinite set of characterizability conditions that any speaker of a natural language can control; "sense" or semanticosyntactic meaning of signs is the precipitate of this structure.

Note then that each usage of a Saussurean sign presupposes the organization of the sign system of which it is a part *as* a Saussurean grammar. The characterizability conditions of such Saussurean signs cannot be specified in terms of the aggregate of such individual usages, however, by studying acts of denotation en masse. They are specifiable only by Saussurean grammar extended in the Chomskyan manner to provide for syntactic recursion in an abstract level of sign types, independent of properties of the instances of usage. Such is a semantic level of meaning achieved by functioning sense systems. Not that all the meaningfulness of the average noun phrase is exhausted by, or is unique to, this level. Rather, the average noun phrase of a language has "sense" to the extent that it participates in the systematic Saussurean grammatical system for its constitution qua recurring sign. "Sense" is thus a component of the total meaningfulness of any functioning noun phrase, whether this noun phrase is used in some particular referential way or not in actual discourse implementation. Other components of meaningfulness must obviously be specified as well in any full account of the typical noun phrase, since its typical usage will be with true or attributive referential value. Similarly, for verbs and other parts of speech, and all grammatical expressions systematically built from these, sense is a component of their meaningfulness to the extent that the abstract sign type underlying specific instances is constituted within a Saussurean system, regardless of whatever other kinds of meaningfulness can be attached to instances of usage in particular contexts, systematic or not.

Still within the functional realm centering on reference and predication, natural languages are Saussurean sign systems of a further specific type: They achieve a *metasemantic* capability and allow a metasemantic reconstruction. If semantics is the realm of abstract, syntactically evidenced sense function, then metasemantics is the system for describing the sense system. In this respect, natural languages seem universally to provide the mechanism for constituting their own metasemantic systems; that is, natural languages encompass their own semantic metalanguages, in the form of definitional equation. What such a capability presupposes, on the pragmatic level of usage, is an equational sentence form within the Saussurean grammar. Taken at the level of symbolic function, then, a sentence of the form $[A] = [B]$ (A and B are expressions of the language; $=$ represents the equation mechanism, e.g., English *be*), when definitional, is an analytic truth, an equivalence true by definition of the units A and B as sense expressions in a Saussurean system. Whatever disequivalences are characteristic of A and B by virtue of other levels of function – for example, their reference characteristics due to "connotational" range – are not of any relevance to the matter at hand. It is, of course, entirely true that no two expressions with any non-sense components of meaning can actually be universally substituted one for another *salva veritate* in the extensional truth–functional realm. Any metapragmatic characterizability conditions, therefore, associated with particular sense expressions – for example, usage levels of vocabulary expressed as situational restrictions on usage – will mean that sense-equivalent expressions are not totally substitutable in a language. But to the extent that we can construct equational sentences of sense expressions, to that extent, independent of other factors, do we have a metasemantic capability. Thus, *To kill is to cause to die, An ophthalmologist is an eye doctor,* and so forth, equating [*kill*] and [*cause* [*die*]], and so on, in English.

So far we have examined a naturally occurring, and, to my knowledge, universal capability of languages as metasemantic vehicles in actual function, though any particular metasemantic attempt in a natural language will be impure or mixed with other factors like pragmatic differences. There is another metasemantic function underlying natural languages as Saussurean sign systems of the sort they are. This is a sort of virtual metasemantics of underlying or cryptotypic structure or "logical form" corresponding to each formable surface expression. Such a Saussurean "semantic representation" forms a kind of metalanguage for describing the "sense" of any surface expression. We will not be further concerned with this virtual metasemantics, since it requires particular analytic assumptions and techniques to achieve, it being the domain of modern linguistics as a technical field.

The *pragmatic* conditions on sign function we have so far invoked are all in the form of presuppositions that must be satisfied in order for the sign to function in a particular modality. Thus, true reference presupposes the existence and quantifiability of the object of reference, the thing picked out. Use of any semanticosyntactic or "sense" symbol presupposes the membership of this sign in a Saussurean grammar. Metasemantic usage presupposes a Saussurean grammatical system with an equation-forming syntactic capacity. The particular modality common to these functional characteristics is referring and predicating. This is the conceptualization of language most common in linguistic and psychological discussions.

Less obvious is the fact that the pragmatic dimension of referring, based as it is on the particular indexical relationship of presupposition – presupposition about the object of reference, presupposition about the code for reference, presupposition about the code of sense – is just one of any number of functional dimensions of a similarly pragmatic character. These involve indexical relationships between the token of language and the context in which it can be said to occur in one of two ways, *independent of the function of reference* organized in natural language by the basically Saussurean nature of structure. Either the linguistic sign token presupposes some aspects of the context in which it is used or, by virtue of the use of the linguistic sign token, the context in such-and-such configuration is entailed as a consequence. For analytic purposes, we may conceive of context as an organized, intersubjectively available and socially maintained configuration of factors of potential indexical relevance to linguistic form and meaning. [See Jakobson's (1960) schema of speech context articulated into communication-theoretic components.] Language use in context is the everchanging dynamic of indexical presupposition and indexical entailment between specific linguistic signs and specific aspects of the context in the speech event. To the extent that there are regularities of such, pragmatics is a realm of indexical Legisigns, of which there recur instances or tokens in actual language use. To the extent by contrast that usage is unique to the instant, it cannot be comprehended by systematic study, only "interpreted" as in the manner of ethnomethodology (see Cicourel, 1974 pp. 28–33, 84–88, 112, 124).

Any kind of "politeness" phenomenon, any kind of referential deixis, any kind of marking of social categorizations through the activity of using language are instances of indexical or pragmatic phenomena in language, generally quite independent of the function of referring and predicating that is accompanying them. Or, more precisely, their interaction in the single continuous surface manifestations of language does not render them analytically unsolvable. For example, personal pronouns partake of the sense system of language to the extent that they have noun phrase properties of structural value; they partake of the referential system to the extent that they pick out a particular object of reference in actual usage, in particular, one of the participants of the speech event; they partake of the indexical system of interpersonal marking to the extent that the very usage of either a token of *I* or *you* is in intersubjective spatiotemporal contiguity with the social roles of speaker and hearer (or equivalent) in some speech situation, *I* relatively more presuppositional (its usage does not in and of itself, beyond the mere fact of speaking, create a speaker), *you* relatively more entailing (its usage specifically focuses on the existence of a hearer as a goal of a message). It should moreover be noted that as noun phrases of attributive reference, *I* and *you* have metapragmatic (see below) characterizability conditions; that is, the objects they pick out are characterized as parts of the speech situation indexed in and by the pragmatics of use, independent of the fact that these objects are also the referents of the expressions *I* and *you*.

The indexical or pragmatic realm of function is, in a sense, the most elementary sign function in language. It bespeaks the simple fact of the situatedness of language use as a social action in some context. To describe such situatedness, the facts of language signs occurring in speech events with dimensionalized context, we would need a language that took these facts as objects of reference and predication. We would need a metalanguage for pragmatics, that is, a *metapragmatic* function for our descriptive language. Natural languages themselves, to a certain extent, provide their own pragmatic metalanguage, that is, have the metapragmatic function built in. In particular, they seem to provide ways of talking about talk as a purposive use of language in events of speaking, at the very minimum simply by providing an agentive predicate (verb) equivalent to English *say* as used in the characterization, *He said* "_____", that is, he engaged in speech-as-action with the sign vehicle "_____". Clearly, "he" denotes the (agentive) speaker, and whatever is communicated between the quotation marks, so to speak, represents the sign vehicle of the speech event. "Said" indicates that such an event took place; it characterizes a relation between speaker and message. Similarly, there are more complicated indexical–denotationals, as noted above, that denote by virtue of instantiating an indexable configuration of speech–event components.

Such is the nature of the pronouns *I* and *you*, as also of certain so-called speech-act or illocutionary (Austin 1975; Searle, 1969) predicates in many languages. Such naturally occurring linguistic elements indubitably form part of the system of reference and predication; yet they refer-to and predicate-of objects and relationships that are constituted in their very use as linguistic signs. The characterizability conditions on what they refer-to and predicate-of, in short, can only be spelled out in terms of describing the social institution of using language in certain ways in certain types of speech events. That is, their characterizability conditions are metapragmatic, and we can term them irreducibly metapragmatic elements of language. Thus, when I use the explicit primary performative construction *I baptize you* [Name], each of these words presupposes certain things about the situation of speech, and the use of the formula entails certain things, and the predicate is a metalinguistic term for characterizing precisely the utterance of the formula under the presupposed conditions, with the entailed consequences. There is sense to these terms as well, to be sure, inasmuch as the pronouns are both nouns, generally animate and human nouns, and so forth in their semanticosyntactic categorizations evidenced in syntax, and the verb is a hyponym of *say* and an inherently punctual aspect (telic) agentive verb of transitive case governance, and so on. What we have been describing of the metapragmatic functional value of these terms is over and above this sense value, however. The senses of the terms are common to many, many more of the relevant categories of animate nouns and agentive verbs; the particular metapragmatic value is what differentiates these items from the others of the classes.

It should be noted that the systematicity of metapragmatic lexical items varies widely from language to language, and that such things as the set of explicit primary performative verbs in any language can be a rather helter-skelter historical accident as to which metapragmatic characterizations of speech events of particular sorts have entered into conventional lexicalization. There is a *virtual metapragmatics* implicit in language usage, however, the systematicity of which can be analyzed and described in terms of a theory of language function as purposive use of language in events of communication. It is such systematicity, as though described by a metapragmatic discourse, that we must assume underlies the ability shown by speakers of a language to interpret indexicals. In a sense, then, the problem of formulating and understanding linguistic communication is to use this virtual metapragmatic system as the backdrop to the sending and receiving of indexical signs, all simultaneous with the manifest function of language for reference and predication in the usual manner. It is clear that metapragmatics in natural language, being a species of reference and predication, is closely related to the latter manifest function; in a real sense, it must form the basis for the ability to refer and predicate, since it grows out of the propositional representation of the act of communication in its indexical (context-related) aspects, being, in fact, its propositional "regimentation." Indexicals in and of themselves are multiply ambiguous as to focus, and ambiguously are presupposing or entailing (creative), in any given instance; it is a system of virtual metapragmatic regimentation that allows of interpretability of complex (and frequently simultaneous) indexical messages one in terms of another.

We have, then, the beginnings of a schema for understanding the nature of functional stratification in language, in that just as phonemes function as a formal stratum only within the higher formal stratum of morphosyntax, indexicals are forms with functional value only within the regimented context of a metapragmatic functions, virtual or instantiable. Instantiable metapragmatics is most lucidly demonstrated in the indexical–denotationals of the referential system; indexicals are most lucidly manifest in the function of indexical or true reference. Thus, the pragmatic aspect of the systems of reference and predication rest on the functionality of indexicals and metapragmatics (the latter being, in a full linguistic system, formally a subpart of reference-and-predication insofar as there is a manifest or naturally occurring metapragmatics). Just as, for example, a lexical part of speech forms the "head" or phrase center of a syntactic unit in formal stratification, with various larger and larger constituents formed around the head, so also can we see indexical denotation as a basic level at the center of the system of attributive reference from a functional point of view, in a second type of functional stratification.

Further, from a functional point of view, attributive reference in terms of unboundedly complex referring noun phrases (the complexity built in by the equivalent of a restricted relative clause formation) is clearly at the center of the whole Saussurean grammar, from a functional point of view. For it is here and here alone that necessarily language manifests the particular evidence of its recursive syntactic potential for its most characteristic functional domain, the domain of sense. Recalling our earlier discussion, we can say that if a language has a naturally occurring true metasemantics in the form of definitional equation, this is equivalent to having a Saussurean grammar underlying the syntax of noun phrases used in attributive reference. Moreover, having a Saussurean grammar implies the existence of a virtual metasemantics.

Now, of naturally occurring metasemantic systems, manifested in definitional equation, there is an empirical regularity that the form of metasemantic equation is the same as the form of attributive classification of referents. (Note the disambiguation possible with the nonitalicized portions: *A* [certain] *dog is* characterizable as/is *a* member of the set of all *mammals*, etc.) It might be seen, from the functional point of view, that here is no fault of natural language; indeed, just the opposite. *An ophthalmologist is an eye doctor*, our exemplary definitional equation within the English sense system, is essentially a predication of attributive referential identity *just under the presupposition that the elements being equated have systematic attributive referential capacity from their values within a Saussurean grammar*. That is, we might say that metasemantic equation is a more restrictive metapragmatics than is necessary in the general case of indexical denotationals, since it presupposes that the signs used in (pragmatic) reference are organized in terms of a certain form of structural system of the now familiar Saussurean sort. Because, in a word, metasemantic equation is telling us that whatever can have the characterizability conditions of [A], the left expression, can have the characterizability conditions of [B], the right expression, given the way characterizability emerges from the structure of a Saussurean grammar (and nothing else). It is a metapragmatics of a particular type of speech event with a particularly structured code employed for attributive reference. In this sense, then, metasemantics is functionally subordinated to metapragmatics, as perhaps the characteristic central manifestation of metapragmatics of reference. And since metasemantics is equivalent to a semanticosyntactic system of grammar, this latter system too is the central manifestation of reference, though we cannot derive principles of Saussurean syntax from any other functional system (it is an independent *formal* principle of organization).

Looking at Figure 1, we might say that there are two types of relationships that ought to be encompassed under the rubic of functional stratification. One, represented in the diagram by lateral relationships, indicates that the functional realm diagrammed on the left is the *naturally occurring prototype for* what is then the more general functional realm on the right, the essence of which is the same as/is an extension of the prototype one. So for example, as naturally occurring metapragmatics, indexical denotationals and explicit performative predications are the prototype means of talking about speech events – in particular the very speech events that the forms constitute as messages. Again, given the full grammatical structure that determines sense, attributive and predicative denotational equivalences become the prototypic example of the general class of metapragmatic utterances or uses of language, because such denotational uses purport to order true reference achieved with a sense system, the "application" of denotational terms.

The second kind of functional stratification, represented in the diagram by vertical relationships, is *functional realization*, on the functional plane analogous to the formal realization of morphemes and other meaningful units ("pleremes") in an otherwise meaningless but instantiable system of units called phonemes (or, more generally, "cenemes"). Thus, indexicals are functionally vague and/or ambiguous and/or uninterpretable save as organized into a system that realizes a virtual metapragmatics of functions or speech–event uses of language. In particular, then, moving (leftward) to the prototypic (and occurring) metapragmatics, speech events can be seen as the instantiation of the metapragmatic order specifiable in terms of indexical denotationals and explicit primary performative predicates. And further, given the assumption of Saussurean syntactic organization, in its prototypic form, metasemantic equation is instantiated each time we speak

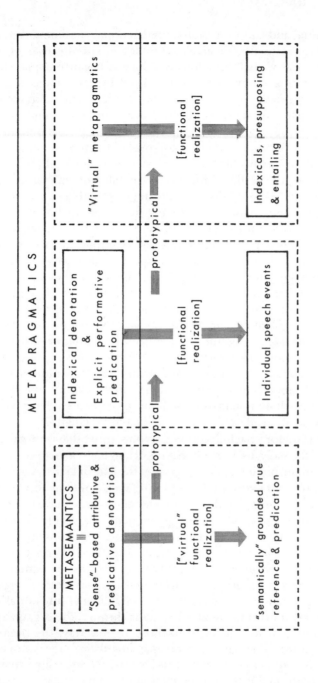

Figure 1. The organization of functions. Note that boxes enclose phenomenally realized functional realms; others are deduced through analysis of functional realms. See text for explanation of depicted relationships.

with referential and truth-functional predicational content. Given all the pragmatic factors involved in actual reference and predication, of course, this can only be a "virtual" functional realization, because actual reference and predication are then as much regulated by/instantiations of pragmatic–metapragmatic regularity as by/of metasemantics. But in natural human language metasemantics is the crucial differentiating factor from all other indexical systems. And the instantiation of metasemantics by reference-and-predication is the prototypic kind of functional realization in the naturally occurring full linguistic system, the universally functionally recognized one, the "official" functional modality of language.

In a sense, then, Figure 1 develops the notion that there is a nested set of relationships among naturally occurring functional realms of language, such that the prototypic exemplars, though included in the more general phenomena of which they constitute an example, are the seemingly regulatory functional subsystems with respect to the more general realms, for the language-using cognition. Thus, the schema of propositional regimentation that is the expression of the metasemantic principle is what organizes metapragmatics, as for example in such metapragmatic propositions as are explicit primary performatives. Explicit primary performatives, in turn, seem to be the mechanism for regulating the nature of indexical functions, since they provide schemata for representing the nature of systematic indexical presupposition and entailment relationships through language use. They seem to form the explicit or iceberg-tip-like part of the whole system of virtual metapragmatics in terms of which we would as analysts, describe the functionality of language.

It is important for what follows to stress once more that we are in no way dealing with formally discrete subsystems of language, akin to syntax, morphology (word formation), phonology, and the like, or akin to segmentably different words and expressions, or grammatical construction types, and so forth. Rather, a great number of such functions as we have reviewed are to be found in any particular language segment, analyzable formal structure, formal sign type, and so on in any language. Functions are laminated in linguistic forms in the most remarkable ways. Each distinct functional point of view determines a distinct kind of formal segmentation and organization of any particular linguistic message. Any formal segmentation and organization can be related to many distinct functional realms and to many distinct functional subsystems through the organization of prototypicality and functional realization. In this way, the notion that something "is the same sign" as it recurs in linguistic usage is strictly relative to the functional constancy of usage; strictly speaking, analysts of language, both linguists and psychologists, have been grossly presumptuous in this respect, generally relying at most on the constancy of presumed referential function.

Functional ontogenesis of linguistic form

If the mature linguistic system is a functional organization of many subsystems, we wish, of course, to be able to account for the gradual emergence of this capability in the child. Vygotsky, to be sure, perceived that this was the critical question, though he couched his investigation in what we now recognize as inadequate terms, centering on the ontogenesis of "word meaning," that is, semantically grounded true reference and predication with lexical elements such as words and expressions. What Vygotsky correctly perceived was the instrumental nature, the pragmatic function, of language as a communicative organization of external, public signs, on the one hand, as contrasted with the propositional nature of language as a cognitive organization for seemingly internal, private, rational thought, on the other. He posed the problem as the gradual intertwining of these two values of linguistic signs or, more precisely, as the gradual emergence of linguistic signs that have these indissoluble dual identities. In the mature system, language provides for the externalization of rational thought, so as to allow of communicability, and provides for the internalization of an individual's relation to the world of objects and other people as rational thought, so as to allow of propositional inference. Vygotsky did not assume that the *functions* of linguistic signs, as emerging *forms*, remained the same, either with this full mature functional complexity or otherwise. Rather, he maintained, the evidence suggested that there is thought before language, indeed, representational and computational processes independent of the existence of language, as would be currently phrased in cognitive studies. And there is instrumental implementation of linguistic signs as vehicles of dealing with the external world before these signs are grounded in a system of sense relations allowing of propositional representation and communication. "At a certain point," Vygotsky observes (1962, p. 44), "these lines meet, whereupon thought becomes verbal and speech rational."

With a more modern analytic apparatus, we can see that Vygotsky's account [e.g., in his remarkable chapters on the development of concepts (1962, pp. 52–118)] is really a logical reconstruction of the passage of words from being indexicals connected to the things they ultimately will truly denote, through an "egocentric" stage in which they serve as performatives of a sort, to their ultimate emergence as sense-valued elements of propositional schemata, each stage being a functional enrichment, not a replacement, of the cognitive utility of language. To be sure, Vygotsky's account is concerned exclusively with the single ontogenetic trajectory toward semantically grounded true reference and predication. But implicit in it is a more general theory of the development of the plurifunctionality of linguistic forms in all their varied manifestations in the adult linguistic system. For while the ultimate achievement is the endpoint system in which each lexeme and expression *can have* such a role in propositional function, Vygotsky clearly indicates that the developmentally more primitive functions are not lost in the adult system; indeed, they are manifested in all sorts of non-fully-"scientific" – i.e., propositionally functional – uses of language as a vehicle of adult communication.

We might trace the functional development of fully adult propositional ability in a general schematic way, by indicating what functional ability is to be reconstructed in the passage Vygotsky hypothesized. At the very earliest appearance of words, language has an indexical value as a property of objects (including people). A lexeme indexically presupposes the co-presence in the context of usage of some signaled phenomenal reality in the experiential field of the child (see Vygotsky 1978, p. 32). Whatever constancy is achieved in the relationship between lexeme and object allows for indexical entailment, with utterance preceding – at least in a logical sense – apprehension of object. Observe that this is entirely an episodic structure, a structure of events of utterance-and-perception, where utterance is, as it were, an extension of the apprehension of objects and the like. An episodic memory for objects and actions is all that is implicated in this phase of language function, regardless of the memory duration involved in achieving constancy of indexicality of words.

The pattern here is a means–ends structure, and the critical breakthrough is the achievement of the use of utterance as a means to an end or goal. For once a child is able to conceptualize entailment–indexicality as an action schema, that is, to abstract a concept of the speech event as an instance of entailment–indexicality, he has essentially gotten the means for a more complex type of linguistic event, the equivalent of the performative utterance. Naming the entailment event with the same term as the object entailed – naming it for the goal – achieves a metapragmatic capability. It is not only mnemonic, in the sense that it allows a context-independent means of calling up what has become a critical "property" of an object; it is, moreover, a mnemonic for a means–ends schema, *the instantiation of which is accomplished in the naming of which*. Here is the functional nature of so-called egocentric speech, according to Vygotsky, the function that ultimately is preserved in adult "inner speech" in the abbreviated, "comment"-only (as opposed to "topic–comment") propositional function and in adult external speech in performative predications (1962, pp. 142–151).

The primitive proposition, then, from a functional point of view has its origins in the metapragmatics of child discourse. It is a doubly mediated means–ends structure. In terms of the primitive "topic–comment" formal sequence of elements, the "topic" is essentially an indexical–denotational the utterance of which is a means to the object and a goal of the "comment," the performative. We should not be confused here by the logical analysis of the adult proposition in terms of truth-functional reference and predication. This is a later development. We are here concerned with a more primitive schema of the instrumental use of language for achieving relations to the language-external world. It should be noted then that the performative portion of such a lexeme sequence need not be of the class of the adult verb or other propositional predicate, as indeed is the case. This propositional regimentation of language into noun phrase = (unmarked) subject = (unmarked) topic = (unmarked) discourse theme versus verb phrase = (unmarked) predicate = (unmarked) comment = (unmarked) discourse rheme is emergent only when true reference and predication are achieved in terms of a sense system.

This achievement presupposes two things: (1) the functional ability to equate means toward a particular end, that is, to conceptualize the equivalence of two propositional-performatives as they could be used for a particular object; and (2) the ability to subordinate one means–ends schema to another. The first allows the speaker/hearer to differentiate a more presupposing-denotational in some given context and a more entailing-performative, *both* to be applied to some particular object of reference. The second allows the construction of the hallmark of true reference and predication, a sequence of constituents (manifested in surface expressions) of which one is itself split into an indexical denotational plus an attributive (would-be predicate) and the other is a predicate. At this point and this point only (see Quine 1973, pp. 82, 99–101) are the functional mechanisms for a sense system in the form we know it in place.

I must stress that this *Aufbau* does not purport to be an actual account of the real-time learning process, but rather a logical reconstruction of stages of achievement as they could follow one upon another to permit ultimately adult use of a propositional capability in language. In the adult system, as we described earlier, developmentally late stages are functionally the prototypic cases of developmentally earlier stages, such that they regiment, or formally constrain, the functional implementation of language forms in general. I have not here addressed the question of the learning process as to necessary inputs of an empirical or phenomenal sort and of a cognitively a priori sort. These questions have been rather inadequately addressed in a vast literature of the last 20 or so years, based as it has been on a view of child language both through and in terms of a unifunctional assumption about adult language and a principle of uniformitarian ontogenesis. On both these counts, I take strong exception to the utility of arguments both for structural "innateness" (e.g. Chomsky, 1975, 1980) and for radically reductionist alternatives for achieving *formal* structures of fully propositional language, when the necessary *functional* differentiations even for dealing with adult language systems have not been made. What must be assumed to be internal to the structure of the language-learning "machine," and what can be seen as a product of the interaction with the context in events of exposure to/use of external speech signals, has not yet been realistically considered beyond unifunctional and functionally homeostatic views of the emerging linguistic competence. We can, one hopes, now go beyond.

NOTE

1 Certain very prominent theorists of language or grammar, e.g., Chomsky (1975, 1980), clearly recognize both reductionist and structuralist possibilities for particular explanations of phenomena of language, as in the long-raging debate between speech–act substantivists and syntactic formalists. Yet Chomsky would insist that the very essence of language (or grammar) itself, not surprisingly, lies in those formal properties of linguistic systems, that are unsusceptible of reductionist explanation. From another point of view, this is at best a counsel of ignorance, and at worst tautological.

REFERENCES

Austin, J. L. 1975. *How to do things with words* (2nd ed.). Cambridge: Harvard University Press.
Benveniste, E. 1966. *Problèmes de linguistique générale*. Paris: Gallimard.
Bloomfield, L. 1933. *Language*. New York: Holt, Rinehart and Winston.
Chomsky, N. 1975. *Reflections on language*. New York: Pantheon.
Chomsky, N. 1980. *Rules and representations*. New York: Columbia University Press.
Cicourel, A. V. 1974. *Cognitive sociology: Language and meaning in social interaction.* New York: Free Press.
Donnellan, K. 1971. Reference and definite descriptions. In D. D. Steinberg and L. A. Jakobovits (Eds.). *Semantics*. Cambridge: Cambridge University Press, pp. 100–114.
Greenberg, J. H. 1966. Some universals of grammar with particular reference to the order of meaningful elements. In J. H. Greenberg (Ed.), *Universals of language* (2nd ed.). Cambridge: MIT Press, pp. 73–113.
Grice, H. P. 1957. Meaning. *Philosophical Review*, 66, 377–388.
Grice, H. P. 1975. Logic and conversation. In P. Cole and J. L. Morgan (Eds.), *Syntax and semantics*, Vol. 3, *Speech acts*. New York: Academic Press, pp. 41–58.

Halliday, M. A. K., and Hasan, R. 1976. *Cohesion in English*. London: Longman.
Hockett, C. F. 1977. Logical considerations in the study of animal communication. *The view from language*. Athens, Ga.: University of Georgia Press, pp. 124–62.
Jakobson, R. 1960. Linguistics and poetics. In T. A. Sebeok (Ed.), *Style in language*. Cambridge: MIT Press, pp. 350–377.
Jakobson, R., Fant, C. G. M., and Halle, M. 1963. *Preliminaries to speech analysis: The distinctive features and their correlates* (4th printing). Cambridge: MIT Press.
Jakobson, R. and Waugh, L. R. 1979. *The sound shape of language*. Bloomington: Indiana University Press.
Martinet, A. 1964. *Elements of general linguistics*. Trans. E. Palmer, London: Faber & Faber.
Miller, G. A. 1956. The magical number seven, plus or minus two: Some limits on our capacity for processing information. *Psychological Review*, *63*, 81–97.
Quine, W. V. O. 1973. *The roots of reference*. LaSalle, Ill.: Open Court.
Searle, J. R. 1969. *Speech acts: An essay in the philosophy of language*. Cambridge: Cambridge University Press.
Silverstein, M. 1976. Hierarchy of features and ergativity. In R. M. W. Dixon (Ed.), *Grammatical categories in Australian languages*. Canberra: Australian Institute of Aboriginal Studies, pp. 112–171.
Silverstein, M. 1980. The three faces of "function": Preliminaries to a psychology of language. In M. Hickmann (Ed.), *Proceedings of a working conference on the social foundations of language and thought*. Chicago: Center for Psychosocial Studies, pp. 1–34.
Silverstein, M. 1981. Case marking and the nature of language. *Australian Journal of Linguistics, 1,* 227–244.
Vygotsky, L. S. 1962. *Thought and language*. Cambridge: MIT Press.
Vygotsky, L. S. 1978. *Mind in society: The development of higher psychological processes*. Edited by M. Cole, V. John-Steiner, S. Scribner, and E. Souberman. Cambridge: Harvard University Press.

10

The implications of discourse skills in Vygotsky's developmental theory

MAYA E. HICKMANN

Vygotsky systematically investigated developmental processes by stressing the following three points: (1) the relationship between social interactive and higher mental processes, (2) the linguistic mediation of *both* kinds of processes, (3) the multifunctionality of language. Although some psychologists have looked at one or another of these issues, none has attempted as Vygotsky did to outline a developmental theory that would integrate them. This chapter first describes these three aspects of Vygotsky's contribution, highlighting in particular his notion of the "organizing function" of speech. It then extends some of Vygotsky's insights in order to account for the way speech comes to mediate sign-using activity itself. This notion is illustrated with some developmental trends in discourse skills that document different aspects of the developing ability to "use language as its own context": It is suggested that this general ability has implications for many aspects of the child's development in allowing him to organize his own use of signs.

Vygotsky always stressed that the development of higher mental functions must be considered in the context of the child's interactions with other social agents. In his view, a child's "developmental level" and his learning capabilities cannot be assessed without considering both his "actual" and "potential" levels of development: The actual developmental level "characterizes mental development retrospectively" by indicating which aspects of various psychological functions are consolidated and enable the child to perform in a given situation independently from other agents; the potential level of development characterizes psychological functions that have not yet matured enough to enable him to perform independently, but can be elicited by means of various "hints," "leading questions," or pieces of the solution provided by others (1978, p. 85). From these two "measures" of the child's developmental level, Vygotsky defines "the zone of proximal development" as:

the distance between the actual development level as determined by independent problem solving and the level of potential development as determined through problem solving under adult guidance or in collaboration with more capable peers. (1978, p. 86)

In this view, the "dynamic edge" of development consists of interactive processes that take place between the child and others. This is an important contrast to many other developmental theories that have considered the child as a self-enclosed unit of analysis and have not made interactive processes an *inherent* part of the developmental process. For example, although Piagetian theory has extensively considered the role of interactive processes in development (particularly in Piaget's early writings), they are either external to, or symptomatic of, the structural properties of children's operational thought that are defined independently and are seen as underlying both social interactive and cognitive processes. More generally, few have seriously considered the possibility that language may in fact be *constitutive* of both social and cognitive processes (Hickmann, 1980a).

The key to the relation between social interactive and internal processes in Vygotsky's writings is that the same sign system "mediates" both types of processes in development. Thus, the potential level of development involves the uses of signs, and particularly (although not exclusively) the uses of linguistic signs – for example, "hints" and "leading questions" in adult–child interaction. For Vygotsky, language is a specifically human sign system that plays a primordial role in development: It is socially constituted and historically developed, and it makes possible the child's participation in the surrounding intellectual and social life. Before the child uses language (or more precisely, speech), his development is characterized by "practical intelligence," or the ability to use tools to mediate actions in order to achieve goals. This ability is also present in some forms of animal behavior, but a fundamental change occurs in human ontogenetic development as the child begins to use the linguistic sign system to mediate his actions. Uses of speech take on "a specific organizing function that penetrates the process of tool use and produces fundamentally new forms of behavior" (1978, p. 24); for Vygotsky "as soon as speech and the use of signs are incorporated into any action, *the action becomes transformed and organized along entirely new lines*" (1978, p. 24; emphasis added).

The particular theory of language implied by Vygotsky's writings can be illustrated by his analysis of the relationship between "egocentric" and "inner" speech. Vygotsky views the ontogenetic progression of the uses of speech in terms of a gradual differentiation and integration of distinct functions of language. The result of this ontogenetic progression is that language eventually comes to mediate two major well-differentiated, but constantly interrelated, spheres of activity for the adult: Speech can be used to communicate and to establish or maintain social relationships among members of a culture; speech also becomes the primordial sign system that mediates the internal thought processes of individuals, the structuring of their conceptual and reasoning activities, and generally their reflective abilities (whether the object of such internal activities is social or nonsocial in nature):

The acquisition of language can provide a paradigm for the entire problem of the relation between learning and development. Language arises initially as a means of communication between the child and the people in his environment. Only subsequently, upon conversion to internal speech, does it come to organize the child's thought, that is, becomes an internal mental function. (1978, p. 89)

At first, ongoing actions and perceptions are fused: Speech is a functionally undifferentiated activity that simply accompanies the child's nonverbal actions. Between this phase and the adult's system, uses of "egocentric" speech correspond to an intermediary phase. In contrast to other theories that have viewed speech during this phase as "unsocialized" or "private," Vygotsky interprets them as showing that the child is experimenting with a *new* function of speech. During this phase, speech does not merely accompany ongoing actions but actually "transforms" them: The child begins to use speech to guide, organize, and plan them. This new emerging function is still undifferentiated from uses of speech in social interactions; for example, these egocentric utterances are produced externally, even though they are not addressed to anyone for *distinct* communicative purposes in interpersonal interactions. The following illustrates this framework:

A child of five and a half was drawing a streetcar when the point of his pencil broke. He tried, nevertheless, to finish the circle of a wheel, pressing down on the pencil very hard, but nothing showed on the paper except a deep colorless line. The child muttered to himself, "It's broken," put aside the pencil, took watercolors instead, and began drawing a *broken* streetcar after an accident, continuing to talk to himself from time to time about the change in his picture. The child's accidentally provoked egocentric utterance so manifestly affected his activity that it is impossible to mistake it for a mere by-product, an accompaniment not interfering with the melody. Our experiments showed highly complex changes in the interrelation of activity and egocentric talk. We observed how egocentric speech at first marked the end result or a turning point in an activity, then was gradually shifted toward the middle and finally to the beginning of the activity, taking on a directing, planning function and raising the child's acts to the level of purposeful behavior. (1962, p. 17)

The ontogenetic progression sketched in Vygotsky's writings is based on interpreting uses of signs minimally in terms of *two* macrofunctions: the interpersonal/communicative and the cognitive/representational functions. An important implication of this "multifunctional" view is that analyses of form–function relationships in children's and in adults' speech must take into account the relationship between linguistic signs and their context of use. Thus, Vygotsky's interpretation of egocentric utterances is based on the particular ways in which these linguistic signs occur in relation to various aspects of the immediate context: (1) the context of ongoing nonverbal activity, both in terms of how the activity is transformed as a result of speech and in terms of how difficult the activity is (i.e., the child produces more egocentric utterances as difficulty increases); (2) the context of interpersonal interaction (i.e., the child produces more egocentric utterances in the context of other agents).[1]

This relationship between speech and its context of use can be generally characterized in terms of the indexical properties of linguistic signs, that is, minimally a relation of direct copresence between signs and some aspect of the speech situation in which they are used, although these indexical properties can take many different forms (e.g., Peirce, 1931–5; Jakobson, 1957, 1960; Silverstein, 1976b, 1978). In general, indexicality and multifunctionality are inseparable aspects of linguistic signs from a functional/pragmatic point of view such as the one outlined in Vygotsky's developmental theory.

In his discussion of egocentric speech, Vygotsky focused on how the uses of linguistic signs affect the course of ongoing actions in the context of utterance. This analysis focuses on the relation between linguistic and nonlinguistic actions, showing how linguistic actions become the means of planning nonlinguistic ones. In his discussions of "scientific concepts," Vygotsky focused on how children can come to reflect on "word meanings" that become the mediating system for both interpersonal interaction and internal intellectual activity. This ability requires that the child differentiate linguistic signs from their uses to denote nonlinguistic reality in particular instances of referring, on the one hand, and their abstract semantic properties to categorize general classes and relations among them on the other hand. Before this point, linguistic and nonlinguistic reality are fused:

Simple experiments show that preschool children "explain" the names of objects by their attributes. According to them, an animal is called "cow" because it has horns, "calf" because its horns are still small, "dog" because it is small and has no horns; an object is called "car" because it is not an animal. When asked whether one could interchange the names of objects, for instance call a cow "ink" and ink "cow," children will answer no "because ink is used for writing, and the cow gives milk." An exchange of names would mean an exchange of characteristic features, so inseparable is the connection between them in the child's mind. In one experiment, the children were told that in a game a dog would be called "cow." Here is a typical sample of questions and answers:

"Does a cow have horns?"
"Yes."
"But don't you remember that the cow is really a dog? Come now, does a
dog have horns?"
"Sure, if it is a cow, if it's called cow, it has horns. That kind of dog has got
to have little horns."

We can see how difficult it is for children to separate the name of an object from its
attributes which cling to the name when it is transferred like possessions following
their owner....A child's ability to communicate through language is directly
related to the differentiation of word meanings in his speech and consciousness.
(Vygotsky, 1962, p. 129)

The inherent constitutive role of speech in the emergence of scientific concepts and the essential role of "consciousness" that it makes possible are
summarized below in Vygotsky's discussion on "spontaneous" versus
"scientific" concepts:

The child becomes conscious of his spontaneous concepts relatively late; the ability
to define them in words, to operate with them at will, appears long after he has
acquired the concepts, He has the concept (i.e., knows the object to which the concept refers), but is not conscious of his own act of thought. The development of a
scientific concept, on the other hand, usually *begins* with its verbal definition and its
use in nonspontaneous operations – with working on the concept itself. It starts its
life in the child's mind at the level that his spontaneous concepts reach only later.
(1962, p. 108)

The full-fledged development of inner speech requires that the child differentiate speech actions from other actions and that he be able to use
linguistic signs both in relation to nonlinguistic reality and in relation to
linguistically constituted reality. It is suggested that this differentiation is
made possible when "language becomes its own context", and that it
involves the uses of signs to organize and plan sign-using activity itself.

This notion of how language becomes its own context can be illustrated
by considering two ways in which the uses and interpretations of linguistic
signs are (at least partly) determined by other linguistic signs. First, linguistic signs can have an indexical relationship with other linguistic signs in discourse: Their uses and interpretations are then dependent on relationships
of co-presence between them and other signs in previous/subsequent
speech as discourse unfolds through time. These uses of signs involve
indexical relationships *strictly* within the linguistic context of utterance
(hereafter *intralinguistic indexical relationships*) and must be distinguished
from uses of signs that involve an indexical relationship with some aspects
of the nonlinguistic context (hereafter *deictic indexical relationships*). Inter-
linguistic relationships in discourse have been shown to contribute to the
"cohesion" of speech, or more generally to the "text-forming function" of
language (Halliday and Hasan, 1976), whereby linguistic signs are "linked"

to one another across clauses by being dependent on one another for their interpretation. Note that, although these two types of indexical relationships are distinct, they are continuous with one another: Linguistic context is but one aspect of the general context of utterance; in addition the *same* sign can often enter into both kinds of indexical relation.

Second, linguistic signs can be used not only to point to other signs in the immediate linguistic context, but also to point to, refer to, and represent in various ways the very properties and uses of signs. These cases correspond to some of the many "metapragmatic" uses of speech, such as when speech refers to speech – for example, when a speaker uses speech in one situation in order to represent speech that was uttered in another situation. Pragmatic and metapragmatic uses of speech are analytically distinct but formally continuous: for example, referring to linguistic entities and events is but one instance of referring. In addition, some signs can be used both in a pragmatic and metapragmatic way – for example, to simultaneously represent *and* effect aspects of the ongoing speech event in the immediate situation (Silverstein, 1976b, 1979, 1980).

For example, first- and second-person pronouns typically point to aspects of the nonlinguistic context of utterance, whereas third-person pronouns typically refer to nonlinguistic entities through an indexical relationship with other linguistic signs. Although both kinds of pronouns contribute to the referential content of the message, first- and second-person pronouns typically contribute to the "interpersonal" function minimally through deictic relationships,[2] whereas third-person pronouns typically contribute to the "text-forming" function through cohesive intralinguistic relationships. For example, in passage (1), below, "I" is interpretable (at least partially) through its indexical relationship with the particular person uttering the message in the immediate context. In contrast, although "he" refers to a specific nonlinguistic entity, this entity can only be identified through its indexical relation to previous (coreferential) noun phrases, such as the one that introduced it the first time it was mentioned in discourse ("a strange man").

> (1)   I saw a strange man in the street yesterday. He was wearing a black tuxedo and white tennis shoes. He was throwing rocks at people and even hit someone. Suddenly he fainted and was taken to the nearest hospital. I read in the paper that he died of a heart attack.

The properties of expressions such as "a strange man," as opposed to "the man" or "he," in fact make it possible for English speakers to introduce referents when they are not present in order for further discourse to proceed: they "create" referents linguistically so that presuppositions about their existence and specificity then become available, and more "presupposing" coreferential forms ("definite forms") can be used in subsequent discourse to maintain reference to these entities, thereby providing continuity in the content of speech. Note that "zero" forms (e.g., "...and ∅ even hit someone") are *maximally* presupposing: given the previous linguistic context, the referent is *so* presupposed that no overt signal need be used. In particular, zero forms in passage (1) are used when a coreferential expression in the previous clause occurs in a similar propositional role (subject or agent of active predicate), or, if a change to patient role occurs, the predicate is in the passive voice ("...and ∅ was taken to the nearest hospital"). Various properties of the unfolding linguistic context then interact in determining whether an "indefinite" or a "definite" form will be used, as well as how "presupposing" the "definite" forms can be at any particular point in discourse.[3]

Third-person pronouns clearly can be used deictically to refer to some entity, assuming it is present in the nonlinguistic context of utterance and can be identified by all participants. Similarly, first- and second-person pronouns can be used strictly within the linguistic context of utterance and thereby contribute to the text-forming function of language. For example, "I want your tie" in example (2) is a "direct quotation," whereby the narrator is reporting a speech event that occurred in another situation and involved people not present in the immediate context: In this case the first- and second-pronouns *inside* the quotation refer (through an intralinguistic relation) to the participants of the narrated event, whereas the first person pronouns *outside* the quotation refer (deictically) to the speaker in the immediate context of utterance:

> (2)   My brother told me a funny story. He met a strange man at a party last week. This man came up to him all of a sudden and said, "I want your tie." My brother refused to give it to him, so the man started screaming and had to be thrown out of the party.

In such cases the quotation must be preceded by a "frame" of some kind, typically a clause indicating linguistically a relationship between the message in the immediate context of utterance and the message reported in the quotation. For example, in (2) the frame for the direct quotation ("...and said, 'I want your tie.' ") consists of: (1) a "verb of saying" that refers to the speech event; (2) a "zero" form that refers to the speaker of the narrated event and that is coreferential with other linguistic elements in preceding and subsequent linguistic context (the addressee is also presupposed from linguistic context); (3) a tense form (past) on the framing verb that is different from the tense form (non-past) in the quoted message. All three properties indicate a distinction between the immediate message and the reported message it contains.

Example (2) also illustrates "indirect" quotations: "My brother refused to give it to him", represents the response given by the other participant in this reported speech event. In this case, rather than quoting exactly the particular utterance, the narrator has represented it as counting as an instance of "refusing." For example, the actual words uttered in response to "I want your tie" could have been utterances (3), (4), (5), or (6) or a number of other possible utterances (note that the response could have also been a nonlinguistic action, such as turning away and leaving without a word):

(3)   No, you can't have my tie.
(4)   No, this is mine.
(5)   What do you mean, you want my tie?
(6)   Don't you have your own tie?

The use of this particular verb of saying and of the construction that follows it has the effect of not only reporting and objectifying the words but of also representing in a particular way the relationship between the words and the context in which they are uttered. In particular, the previous utterance ("I want your tie") is assumed to count as an instance of a "directive," akin to an imperative (e.g., "Give me your tie") in contrast to other sorts of utterances (e.g., "This is a nice tie,") that would not necessarily be interpreted in this way. Finally, note that the first utterance in (2) ("My brother told me a funny story") constitutes a "frame" for all of the following utterances: All of example (2) is in fact a large quotation in story form, in which other quotations are embedded.

From a developmental point of view, one would expect both intra-linguistic and metapragmatic uses of speech to be late developments, considering the complexity of the indexical relationships involved in such examples. Thus, the available developmental literature suggests that it might be from earlier deictic uses of referring expressions that children learn to use the very same forms to organize discourse relationships when referring to entities and events that are not present in the nonlinguistic context of discourse. However, there are often large discrepancies in the results of various studies due to the fact that the data are collected in situations that are not always functionally equivalent (Hickmann, 1980a, 1982). In addition, the studies that tend to support this hypothesis are mostly based on "comprehension" (rather than production) data, in which children's interpretation of deictic and/or intralinguistic uses of referring expressions are analyzed, but no productions elicited. Studies that analyze children's productions of referring expressions often involve eliciting isolated forms; spontaneous uses of referring expressions in long stretches of discourse (e.g., conversations, narratives) are usually elicited in the presence of nonlinguistic context (e.g., pictures or objects) that often makes it difficult to differentiate deictic from strictly intralinguistic uses of these forms.

The following illustrations and discussions of children's uses of various text-forming and metapragmatic devices in discourse are part of a larger study (Hickmann, 1982) in which English-speaking 4-, 7-, and 10-year-old children (and adults) were asked to narrate "stories" in a number of situations. For the purposes of the discussions here, the illustrations below are based on narratives that were elicited in two of these situations: These will be referred to as the "film/narrative" and the "pictures/narrative" situations. The discussion focuses particularly on analyses of the intra-linguistic means used in discourse to "create" referents linguistically and to subsequently maintain reference to them, as well as the metapragmatic framing devices that were used to objectify speech events and transform them into cohesive texts.

In the film/narrative situation 10 children in each age group were asked to narrate short filmstrips for an interlocutor who had not seen them and who was then required to tell the stories back and to answer some questions about them.[4] Each film consisted of short interactions (1 to 1 1/2 minutes long) between two characters (common animals in the form of hand puppets) who appeared on the screen and immediately engaged in dialog using deictic first- and second-person pronouns. During this dialog, these characters (the "participants") talked about two referents (the "nonpartici-pants"), which were not present on the screen and which consisted of two objects in some films (inanimate nonparticipants) and two animals in other films (animate nonparticipants). An example of each type of film (type I and type II, respectively) is shown in this chapter's Appendix. When narrating these films, children had to objectify the dialog into a cohesive text, that is, report in narrative form the sequence of speech events that took place in the form of dialog. Since they could not assume that their interlocutor knew anything about the contents of the films, and since there was no extralinguistic context related to the contents of the films, children had to rely *strictly* on speech to narrate these films.

In the pictures/narrative situation, the same children were also asked to narrate two picture sequences (described in the Appendix) for an interlocutor who was blindfolded and could not see them. In this case, although nonlinguistic context related to the content of the narratives was present in the speech situation, text-forming devices were still necessary, particularly in order to create referents linguistically, since the listener could not see the picture sequences. This task was in many ways easier than the film/narrative task: The presence of the picture sequence during narration did not re-quire children to remember the content of the stories; it allowed them to use some forms deictically rather than strictly within the linguistic context;

the sequence of events did not necessarily involve speech events (although some could be inferred).

The referring expressions used to *first* mention referents in discourse were tabulated according to their relative presuppositional properties: They were grouped according to their relative effectiveness in establishing presuppositions of the existence and specificity of referents for the subsequent use of coreferential noun phrases in discourse. The expressions fell in three categories, "effective," "ineffective," and "mixed" forms. Effective forms consisted of conventionally effective means of introducing referents in discourse, such as the following: The indefinite article and the expression *this N* (e.g., "*a* dog came," "*this* donkey came"), sometimes in conjunction with an existential clause (e.g., "There was a dog," "There was this little dog") or a "topic" clause (e.g., "This story was about a frog"); possessive constructions, whereby a referent was effectively introduced in relation to another previously introduced referent [e.g., "a dog (1) came and then *his* (1) *friend* (2) came"]; the definite article in conjunction with sufficient descriptive content (e.g., He brought *the candy bar* and *the flower* he was gonna give to the frog for his birthday").

Ineffective expressions were those that presupposed shared background knowledge about the existence and specificity of the referents, and thus presupposed, rather than created, the referents on first mention. They consisted mostly of the following: the definite article (e.g., "*the* frog came"); pronouns (e.g., "*He* said, 'Hi' "); ineffective possessive constructions, whereby, for example, a referent *y* was introduced in relation to some other referent *x* that was never previously mentioned (e.g., "*Her* [*x?*]*friend* [*y*] had a box"). Mixed forms were those that could not be grouped unambiguously as effective or ineffective. They included, for example, "definite" articles used in conjunction with "topic" or existential clauses (e.g., "*this story was about the* elephant and a lion"); insufficient definite descriptions (e.g., "he had *the candy bar* and *the flower* that got too hot"); nouns without determiners (e.g., "*Chicken* came," "*Penny* was in the box"). There were relatively few mixed forms (mostly used consistently by a few individual 7-year-old children); they were combined with ineffective forms for the purposes of the discussions below.

The results in the film/narrative situation show a gradual increase in the uses of effective referent-introducing forms with age: 36% of the forms used to first mention referents in discourse were effective at 4 years, 59% at 7 years, and 89% at 10 years.[5] These data indicate that only the 10-year-olds used effective forms to create referents systematically and consistently more often than ineffective – mixed ones. The relatively high proportion of effective referent-introducing forms at 7 years (in comparison to 4 years) indicates the emergence of these linguistic skills at around this age in this sample. These results are consistent with studies suggesting that cohesive uses and interpretations of referring expression are a relatively late development (e.g., Warden 1976; Karmiloff-Smith 1977, 1979a,b). In addition, deictic and cohesive uses of referring expressions could not be confounded in this situation: the referents were not present and children could not assume that their listener knew anything about them.

Example (7) illustrates a 10-year-old's story of type I, in which all referents are effectively introduced (a donkey, a giraffe, a box, a penny):

(7)   A donkey and a giraffe. . .came out. (uh-huh) And. . .the. . .giraffe said, "Hi! Would you like to play with me? And. . .the donkey said, "No! I'm mad!" (uh-huh) And. . .she said, "What happened?". . . and. . .the donkey said, "Well, I made a box to keep my things in. (uh-huh) And I found a penny. And I put it in the blo−box but now I can't *find* the penny." (uh-huh). . .and. . .the. . .giraffe said, "Well, maybe it's at school! Remember? You took it to school." And the donkey said, "*How* do *you* know? I think *you*'re the one that took the penny!" (uh-huh) And. . .the gi-giraffe said. . .um. . ., "No I didn't." And. . .oh. . .she said, "How do *you* know?" He said, "Well . . .you know, I remember you took it." (uh-huh) And. . .then she thought about it for a while and she s− said. . ., "Well, friends don't steal! I'm sorry I was mad at you! Now let's go play." (Type I, 10 years)

Example (8) shows the beginning of a 10-year-old's type II narrative, where one of the (animate) nonparticipants is mentioned for the first time with a definite form (the cow):

(8)   This− this movie was about. . .a sheep and a owl. (uh-huh) The ow− the sheep has jus− had just came from the farm. . .and the cow. . . and a horse had got into a fight. (uh-huh) Because the horse hit the cow and the cow fell down. [. . .] (Type II, 10 years)

Examples (9) and (10) show two 7-year-old's type I narratives: in (9) the participants are both mentioned for the first time with definite lexical noun phrases (NPs) (the frog, the dog), in (10) with third-person pronouns (she, he). The (inanimate) nonparticipants are either effectively introduced in discourse with indefinite forms (a flower, a candy bar) or with a possessive construction (her penny). Note the child's uses of gender distinctions and stress in (10) to disambiguate pronouns. Similarly, example (11) shows the beginning of a 7-year-old's type II narrative where after a "false start" one of the participants (an elephant) is highly presupposed on first mention (him) and the other participant is introduced in relation to him (his friend); both (animate) nonparticipants are first mentioned with definite lexical NPs (the the tiger, the bird):

(9)   The frog came over to tell the dog that. . .He said, "Hi" that it was his birthday (uh-huh) and then the dog said he's sad because he

> bought a flower and a candy bar for his birthday. (uh-huh) The flower smelled good and the candy bar looked good, [. . .] (Type I, 7 years)
>
> (10) She was mad. . .because his – her penny. . .was lost. . .(uh-huh) and she thought *he* took it. . .(uh-huh) and *he* said, "Maybe you left it at school." (uh-huh) Then they went to school and got the penny. (uh-huh) And that's all. (Type I, 7 years)
>
> (11) His friend and the bird – the tiger was chasing after him and the bird made a lot of noise in the air so the tiger looked up and ran away. (uh-huh) And so his friend came long and said, "What's wrong?" [. . .] (Type II, 7 years)

Example (12) shows a 4-year-old's narrative [elicited with the same type I film as (7)]: with respect to first mentions this child only uses mixed or definite forms for the inanimate referents (*Penny* followed by *the penny; the box*) and a third-person pronoun for one of the participants ("*He* was mad at the giraffe"). Note also that this story begins with the objects, rather than with the participants, a pattern that occurred at this age:

> (12) Penny was in the box. (A2: Excuse me?) The penny was in the box (A2: Oh really? Oh, good) (pause) The next day it wasn't. (pause. . . He was mad at the giraffe. . .(A2: Uh-huh) (pause) 'cause he took the penny. (A1: He was mad at the giraffe because he took the penny.) Yeah, but he di – bu – but he – he thought he was *tricking* him. . . .(A2: Oh!) see b – because. . .bec – bec – he – he – he didn't know that he had the penny. (A2: Uh-huh) (pause) (A2: Very good, E.) (pause) They go play. (A1: Hm?) They went to go play. (Type I, 4 years)

The transcripts also showed some instances of "self-corrections," whereby children changed one type of referent introduction to another, for example, (13) to (15). These changes indicate that these uses were not fully "automatized" and that children hesitate among the presuppositional properties of various linguistic expressions in relation to their own previous or subsequent speech:

> (13) They. . .(A2: Uh-huh) the (pause) a cat (pause) the cat was playing with the. . .chicken. (A2: Oh) (pause) *Then*. . .a squirrel came by. [. . .] (Type II, 4 years)
>
> (14) A dog. . .and the – and a frog were. . .were wa – were um. . .a fr – a dog was there and looked sad. (uh-huh) An – and then a . . .dog came along and. . .(pause) (uh-huh) the frog came along and said, "Hi, today's my birthday." [. . .] (Type I, 7 years)
>
> (15) It's a story about the – the. . .a lion and an elephant. (uh-huh). The lion goes to the elephant, "You look tired." [. . .] (Type II, 10 years)

These particular corrections were more frequent at 7 and 10 years. In addition, at 7 years more corrections consisted of changing some expression (whether effective or not) to an ineffective one, whereas at 10 years more consisted of changing some expression to an effective one. Note the correction in the 10-year-old's narrative shown in (16): here, the child uses a definite NP to first mention one of the nonparticipants (*the chicken*) and proceeds to use a highly effective existential clause to create linguistically *both* nonparticipants at this point in discourse:

(16)   There's this littl– a hip– a li– a hip– a hippo and a cat. (uh-huh) The hippo said. . .to the cat, "You look sad today." (uh-huh) And then the cat said, "Cause I went to the park and. . .the chicken got mad at me. . ." (uh-huh) (lower pitch) and there is a chicken and um. . .a squirrel too in this. [. . .] (Type II, 10 years)

The same analysis was used for the referent-introducing forms in narratives collected in the pictures/narrative situation. Here, children narrated from a picture sequence that remained present throughout narration, although their blindfolded listener could not see it. Overall, the results are consistent across the two tasks for the 7- and 10-year-olds, indicating that in each age group, children tended to use effective and ineffective referent-introducing forms approximately as often regardless of the differences in these two situations. The data do show differences in the particular types of expressions that were used by the 4-year-olds. For example, the 4-year-olds used more highly presupposing and clearly deictic forms (e.g., "it," "this," "here," "there"), particularly in the context of explicit predicating constructions – for example, utterances in which an "indefinite article" was used to predicate the class membership of a referent that was denoted deictically (e.g., "it's a dog," "here's a dog"). In addition, during this task, the narratives of the 4-year-olds contained many utterances in which the linguistic elements did not explicitly form propositions (e.g., verb phrases without copulas or single NPs), such that propositions often had to be inferred across utterances. Examples (17) and (18) illustrate these tendencies at this age.

(17)   First a duck she's in her nest. . .(A2: uh-huh) here's Duck she's out of her nest. . .with a cat there. . .(A2: uh-huh) and here's a cat. . .sitting by the tree. . .(A2: uh-huh) here's a cat. . .climbing up the tree with a dog there. . .and here's a dog biting the. . .kitty-cat's tail . . .and *here's*. . .a dog who's chasing a cat and. . .and *that* thing is getting back into her next. (Sequence 2, 4 years)

(18)   Horse. A horse is running. (A2: A horse is running. . .go ahead). And a. . .horse and a cow. (A2: uh-huh) And a horse is. . .still running. (A2: uh-huh) Horse fell down. (A2: Oh. Oh my!) (A1 whispers: That's right) And a bird's. . .ca– and the bird came. (A1: The bird came) (A2: uh-huh) Cow. . .helped him. (Sequence 1, 4 years)

In these cases, although "indefinite" articles were used, these forms were not used in the same way as those of the 7- and 10-year-olds: they were often used to "name" referents whose existence and specificity were already presupposed from nonlinguistic context rather than to establish such presuppositions strictly through intralinguistic relationships in discourse.

In the film/narrative situation, the referent-introducing forms (first mention) and the coreferential forms that were subsequently used in discourse varied as a function of story types and referent types. Effective referent-introducing forms were systematically distributed as a function of whether the referents were participants, animate nonparticipants, or inanimate nonparticipants. This distribution can be summarized as follows: (1) the 4- and 7-year-olds tended to have difficulty introducing *all* animate referents (all participants and the animate nonparticipants of type II films), but not inanimate ones; (2) the 10-year-olds tended to only have difficulty introducing the animate nonparticipants of type II stories, systematically introducing the participants and the inanimate nonparticipants effectively. In general, then, children organized their narratives around highly presupposed and "topical" animate referents. However, the 4- and 7-year-olds tended to presuppose all animate referents from the first mention on, rather than using intralinguistic means to first create them in discourse, whereas this was only true of the animate nonparticipants in the 10-year-olds' narratives.

Overall, given the contents of the films, the great majority of coreferential noun phrases denoting all animate referents across clauses throughout discourse involved "actors" (subjects/agents), with two exceptions. First, the animate nonparticipants were mentioned in these roles from the very first mention on; in contrast, the participants were often first "presented as predicates" (e.g., with existential clauses), especially at 7 and 10 years, and only then were they represented as subjects/agents (e.g., "there was a dog, he. . ."). Second, the participants were also more topical than any of the nonparticipants. For example, although zero forms tended to denote mostly animate referents, reference-maintaining devices were more presupposing overall when they denoted the participants rather than the animate nonparticipants. In addition, when both a participant and a nonparticipant were mentioned in the same clause, children tended to "orient" their discourse toward the participant; for example, two 10-year-olds (and some adults) used passives in the case where a participant was mentioned in patient role in relation to a nonparticipant agent (e.g., "A tiger attacked me" reported as: "He said, 'I got attacked by a tiger' ") children at all ages (and many adults) tended to use constructions such as "X (participant) was playing with Y (animate nonparticipant)," even if the original dialogue contained "Y was playing with X"[6] (e.g., "A chicken was playing with me" reported as: "He said, 'I was playing with a chicken' ").

Finally, note that in many cases the 4-year-old's narratives required some adult "guidance" in the form of questions, such as those shown in example (19). In this example, the child uses highly presupposing expressions to first mention animate referents in discourse, shifting the referents of subject NPs across two adjacent utterances; for example, *he* in "He was tired," "And he was jealous" is used to first mention two different referents (the elephant and the lion, respectively). The child subsequently uses definite lexical NPs instead of pronouns [in (19c), (19e), and (19i)] only in response to the adult's requests to identify the referents with *who*-questions. Note the shift in the referents of subject pronouns across the question–answer sequence in (19f–19g) when the question was of a less "specific" type.[7]

(19) (a) He was tired. (A1 whispers: That's right, he was tired) (A2: He was tired?) And. . .he was jealous (A2: Oh!) (A1 whispers: That's right and he was jealous) And – and I don't. . .know – know what else. [. . .]

A1:   (b) (whispers) Now who was in the story? Tell her [A2] who was in the story.

Ch: (c) The lion. . .(A1: the lion. . .) and the – and the elephant. (A1: And the elephant, um-huh) I don't know what else.

A1:   (d) Who was tired?

Ch: (e) The elephant.

A1:   (f) The elephant was tired. Why was he so tired? (Ch: 'Cause. . .) What happened, tell T. [A2].

Ch: (g) C – 'cause – so he got – so he got so jealous.

A1:   (h) Because he got so jealous? Who was that?

Ch: (i) Uh-huh. The lion got at 'm – so jealous.

Further discourse analyses would be necessary to make general claims about these developmental trends, that is, analyses of the chains of co-reference throughout discourse with a wider range of materials. The data indicate that both animacy (animate/inanimate) and participation in speech events (participants/nonparticipant) played a role in the overall cohesive properties of children's narrative discourse. In addition, the distinction between participants and animate nonparticipants differs from the distinction between animate and inanimate referents in that it cannot be defined without reference to speech itself: by definition, participants were engaged in speech. The observations in the film/narrative situation are therefore not independent of the metapragmatic nature of the task that required children to objectify dialogues into texts in order to report the participants' speech.

The metapragmatic nature of this task can be demonstrated by examining the various ways in which children in different age groups reported speech. Overall, both the 7- and 10-year-old children used framing devices consistently when reporting the participants' speech. The great majority of these frames consisted of the verb *say,* followed by a "direct" quotation. Few indirect quotations occurred at any age in the children's sample. In comparison, although the majority of the adult's frames also consisted of the verb *say,* they used direct and indirect quotations as frequently; there was also a much wider range of metapragmatic verbs and frequent uses of more specific names of speech events, for example, *reply, ask, reassure, suggest, console, answer, refuse, agree, explain, remind.*

The 4-year-olds also often used *say* when they explicitly framed quoted speech, although their narratives show two different tendencies. First, these children tended in general to focus their narratives on the participants, rather than explicitly on their speech. Example (12) above illustrates this tendency with a story of type I, example (20) below with a story of type II (in which a hippopotamus and a cat were talking about a chicken and a squirrel): In these examples, there is not a single *explicit* mention of speech events.

> (20) The hippopotamus was there...(A2: uh-huh) and the hippopotamus...was...the hippopotamus was *happy*...but...(A2: uh-huh) the...but...the – but the *cat* wasn't – wasn't happy, *he* was *mad*. (A2: Oh, really?) 'Cause...'cause the squirrel was there and (pause) and (pause) the chicken was playing with...with the *cat*... and along came a squirrel...(A2: uh-huh) and...and the cat wanted to...play with the squirrel. (A2: Oh) And – and the – and the chicken...was – was...getting *mad*...(A2: uh-huh) and the squirrel was *crying*. (A2: Oh, my goodness) (pause) (A2: Ok) [. . .] And so they went out in the park...and he – and *then* (pause) and then the squirrel went away. (A2: Oh, ok) (pause) That's the end. (Type II, 4 years)

In some cases, this preference for focusing on the participants rather than on their speech involved inferences from speech and uses of predicates such as *think, know, want.* At this age, these types of predicates were occasionally accompanied by children's difficulties in shifting first- and second-person pronouns to third-person pronouns. For example, in (21) the original utterance "Maybe you forgot the penny at school" (giraffe addressing donkey) is reported as "the giraffe knows you left the penny at school"; similarly, "I think you're trying to trick me" (donkey addressing giraffe) is reported as "and the donkey thinks I trick." In (22) "You're trying to trick me" is reported as "He's trying to trick you"; in this case the child then spontaneously changes the second-person pronoun to a third-person pronoun. In (23), although the original "Do you want to play with me?" (giraffe addressing donkey) is reported as an explicit quotation ("he said that he wants to play with you"), a similar pronominal error occurs:

(21) [. . .] Then. . .he bring the box at school. . .the donkey. [. . .] And (pause) he lost his penny. And. . .he think. . .that it's at school. [. . .] And the – the giraffe. . .knows you left the penny at school. [. . .] And this (pause) and the donkey thinks I trick. (Type I, 4 years)

(22) [. . .] Then he said. . ., "How do *you* know?" Then he's trying to trick. . .you. . .(A2: Oh) trick him. (A1: Right) And. . .then. . .then they. . .and then they were looking for it. (Type I, 4 years)

(23) A – a donkey came by. (A2: Donkey?) (A1: Good job) Then the giraffe came. . .(A1: Then the giraffe came by. . .) Then. . .then it was. . .he said that. . .he wants to play with you. [. . .] (Type I, 4 years)

Second, when the 4-year-old children did focus on the participants' speech, they often used frames inconsistently or did not use them at all. This tendency is illustrated by the more extreme example (24), and can be summarized as follows: Generally, when objectifying speech events that occurred in another speech situation, these children tended not to indicate a clear separation between the reported message and the narrative message in the immediate speech situation:

(24) The donkey is angry. . .because "I put my toys in the box. . .Now I bring that to school. . .(A2: uh-huh) I think you're trying to *trick* me, . . ." "I'm not. . ." "*You* are – *you* h – *you*. . .took it. I'm very angry at you." "No. . .you don't understand me! (A2: uh-huh) W – well I. . .I'm your friend. Let's go and play." "OK." (Laughs) (A2: Is that the end?) (Child nods.) (A1: Very good. Who was in the story? The donkey?) And the giraffe. (Type I, 4 years)

For example, note in (24) how the child "slides" directly from narrative speech to narrated speech in the first- and second-persons ("The donkey is angry. . .because "I put my toys in the box. . .") and subsequently simply reproduces the dialogue in the first and second persons, without any third-person frames.

Framing devices involved using linguistic expressions to denote participants and to establish intralinguistic relationships with previous and subsequent coreferential expressions. The previous discussion showed that young children had difficulties "introducing" linguistically *all* animate referents (participants and nonparticipants) with effective forms that created a presupposition of their existence and specificity. In contrast, the 10-year-olds tended to consistently create such discourse presuppositions when mentioning the participants. Note that some 4-year-old and 7-year-old children sometimes began their narrative by reporting the speech of one of the participants without having ever previously *mentioned* (let alone effectively created) the other participant. Examples (25) and (26) illustrate this tendency in the 7-year-olds' narratives: In these examples, children begin their narrative by quoting the speech of one participant (e.g., "a lion. . .he said. . . ."), mentioning the addressee for the first time with a second-person pronoun inside the direct quotation (e.g., "*You* look tired today"); only subsequently do they mention this referent with a third-person form, as the dialogic speech roles are reversed:

(25)   A lion. . .he said, "You look tired today." And the. . .and the elephant said, "Yes, I was running." (uh-huh). . .And the. . .(pause) lion said, [. . .] (7 years)

(26)   The hippo came and he said, "Hi. (uh-huh) You – you look sad" and then the rabbit goes, "I was playing with the chicken and then the squirrel wanted to play with me. (uh-huh) So the chicken got mad and now the squirrel's crying and I don't know what to do." [. . .] (7 years)

Similarly, example (24) above shows this tendency for the 4-year-olds, although in this case the second participant was *never* mentioned throughout the entire narrative except through first- and second-person pronouns in the unframed direct quotations. Whenever possible, the children who only mentioned participants either with first- and second- or with third-person pronouns were asked questions after their narrative, as shown in (24). In the majority of cases, children had no difficulties answering these questions, indicating that the absence of mention in the narratives was not due to memory or comprehension difficulties, but rather to difficulties in using the intralinguistic devices and metapragmatic frames necessary to establish, maintain, or shift the interpersonal parameters of reported dialogic events. None of the 10-year-olds ever began reporting speech without having previously mentioned (and, in general, effectively created) both participants in the dialogues: at this age, children always first established linguistically the interpersonal parameters of the narrated speech events before reporting speech in narrative discourse.

In conclusion, these various observations indicate that the development of the intralinguistic and metapragmatic skills documented here is very gradual. The 4-year-old children's narratives indicate that the organization of linguistic signs in ongoing discourse is often not based *strictly* on the child's own speech but depends in essential ways either on nonlinguistic context (deictic indexical relationships) or on uses of signs in interactive processes between the child and an adult in the situation (e.g., their dependence on adult's questions). The 7-year-olds showed an emerging ability to rely strictly on linguistic means to organize their own discourse, and the 10-year-olds systematically used language as its own unfolding context and objectified dialogues into cohesive texts.

A few concluding remarks can be made about these observations in light of the previous discussion. Vygotsky's notion of the "organizing function" of speech can also be invoked in relation to children's ability to organize their own discourse. Thus, whereas egocentric speech takes on an organizing function with respect to nonlinguistic activity, uses of linguistic signs also take on an organizing function with respect to the very activity of using signs. In line with Vygotsky's framework, these skills have implications for both the child's social and cognitive development. Thus, framing devices used to report speech events not only are minimally necessary for the interpretability of ongoing narrative discourse, but they also encode culturally specific and salient information about how members of a culture interpret and represent interactive events (e.g., Voloshinov, 1973). The metapragmatic capabilities of language transform the child's developing ability to plan, organize, and interpret pragmatic uses of signs in interactive situations: They transform his ability to participate in gradually more complex interactive events with other agents, as well as his ability to reflect on, talk about, and reason about these interactive events.

In addition, this framework also allows us to further specify some of Vygotsky's insights about the developmental progression from egocentric to inner speech. Vygotsky's formulation of the nature of scientific concepts in relation to "word meaning" involves particular types of intralinguistic and metapragmatic abilities: The child must use speech to represent (linguistically) properties of linguistic signs that are detached from their indexical relationships in particular instances of use. This form of activity (whether "internal" or "externalized" in speech) is constituted by the uses of linguistic signs to point to and represent linguistically constituted reality: It is simultaneously dependent on the skills discussed here and distinct from them (also see Silverstein, Chapter 9, this volume).

The properties of language discussed here then allow the same sign system to mediate and transform many different aspects of the child's activities, and it is suggested that the development of inner speech takes the form of a gradual differentiation of language-internal functions. According to this framework, the child's social and cognitive activities are two aspects of the same sign-using processes that constantly interact with one another. Vygotsky's writings constitute a rich legacy in this respect, providing us with a way of specifying what is specifically human in ontogenetic processes.

Appendix: Materials used

1. Example of a type I film (inanimate nonparticipants)

(A dog appears on the screen, then a frog appears.)

Frog: "Hi, it's my birthday today. Do you want to come to my birthday party?"

Dog: "No, I can't go to your party. I'm very sad. I bought a candy bar and a flower for your birthday. The flower smelled good and the candy bar looked good. But now the candy bar is sticky and the flower is dead. I don't know what happened."

Frog: "It's very hot outside. Maybe the flower dried up and the candy bar melted."

Dog: "You're right. But now I can't give you the candy bar and the flower anymore and you won't be my friend anymore."

Frog: "Don't worry. I'm very happy because you remembered my birthday."

Dog: "Oh really? I'm glad you still want to be my friend. Let's go to your birthday party."

(The dog and the frog leave together.)

2. Example of a type II film (animate nonparticipants)

(A sheep appears on the screen, then an owl appears.)

Owl: "Hi, what are you doing?"

Sheep: "I'm thinking. A cow and a horse got into a terrible fight at the farm today. The horse hit the cow and the cow fell down. Now, the horse wants to fight some more. I am wondering how I can stop the fight."

Owl: "Well, what's the fight about? Do you think the horse is right or do you think the cow is right?"

Sheep: "The fight is about who is the most important animal at the farm. The cow gives milk. I think that's the most important. But the horse gives rides to people. What do you think?"

Owl: "Well, giving milk is important but giving rides to people is important, too. Everybody is important."

Sheep: "I guess you're right. Let's go to the farm. Maybe we can stop the fight."

(The sheep and the owl leave together.)

3. Description of each frame in picture sequences

Picture sequence 1:

1. A horse is running in a meadow. There is a fence in the background.
2. The horse comes to the fence. A cow is standing on the other side of the fence. A bird is standing on the fence.
3. The horse is jumping over the fence. The cow and the bird are watching him.
4. The horse has fallen down and is lying on his back. The fence is broken. The cow and the bird are watching him.
5. The bird is holding a first-aid kit. The cow is wrapping a bandage around the horse's leg.

Picture sequence 2:

1. There is a nest on the branch of a tree, a big bird on the nest, and three small birds in the nest.

2. The big bird is flying away. A cat is standing under the tree looking at the nest.
3. The cat is sitting under the tree looking at the nest. (The big bird has disappeared.)
4. The cat is climbing up the tree. A dog is approaching.
5. The cat is hanging from the branch of the tree and has almost reached the nest. The dog is biting the cat's tail. The big bird is flying back to the nest holding a worm.
6. The dog is chasing the cat away. The big bird is giving the small birds the worm.

NOTES

1 See Kohlberg et al. (1968) for some empirical observations about the effects of various factors on children's uses of egocentric speech in light of four developmental theories (Mead, Piaget, Vygotsky, and Flavell).

2 Note that the first- and second-person pronouns "I" and "you" are also related to the linguistic context in which they are used: e.g., "I" is the person uttering the linguistic message containing "I" (Benveniste, 1966). In this sense, their meaning is only partially determined by their (deictic) indexical relation with the presupposed nonlinguistic context of utterance. They are also metapragmatic in that the interpersonal roles of speech participants that they create are linguistically constituted (Silverstein, 1976b).

3 Many other aspects of the linguistic context not discussed here clearly interact in determining uses of referring expressions in discourse. In addition, a number of pragmatic effects can be accomplished when some of these processes are purposefully "violated" (e.g., see Silverstein, 1976a; Bolinger, 1977).

4 In the illustration below, *A1* refers to the person who presented the films to the children and *A2* refers to the "naïve" listener whom the children were addressing (in these cases, always an adult).

5 The total possible number of forms for the 7- and 10-year-olds was 240 (10 children × 6 stories × 4 referents) and 160 for the 4-year-olds (10 children × 4 stories × 4 referents). A few 7- and 4-year-olds omitted referents; referring expressions that were preceded by a specific question on the part of the adult (see below) were not included in these proportions. The total percentages of effective referent introductions can vary slightly as a function of how some "mixed" forms are interpreted.

6 Note that some of the original dialogues were slightly unnatural in this respect.

7 Different types of questions were systematically used when it was necessary to help young children proceed with their narratives and when "encouragements" did not suffice (e.g., "go ahead"). For example, questions varied in terms of their presuppositional properties, from the least "specific" type (e.g., "What happened?") to more specific types (e.g., *wh*-questions). Specific questions were always asked by A1 and never by the naïve listener A2. Note that when they had to be used, the situation became triadic, rather than dyadic. Brackets within some of the examples [. . .] indicate deletions where only a series of "encouragements" occurred.

REFERENCES

Benveniste, E. 1966. *Problèmes de linguistique générale.* Paris: Gallimard.
Bolinger, D. 1977. Pronouns and repeated nouns. Indiana University Linguistic Club, April.
Halliday, M. A. K., and Hasan, R. 1976. *Cohesion in English.* London: Longman.
Hickmann, M. 1982. The development of narrative skills: Pragmatic and meta-pragmatic aspects of discourse cohesion. Doctoral thesis, University of Chicago.
Hickmann, M. 1980a. Creating referents in discourse: A developmental analysis of linguistic cohesion. In Kreiman and Ojeda (Eds.), *Papers from the Parasession on Pronouns and Anaphora,* Sixteenth Regional Meeting of the Chicago Linguistic Society. Chicago: Chicago Linguistic Society.
Hickmann, M. 1980b. The context dependence of linguistic and cognitive processes, 1978. In M. Hickmann (Ed.), *Proceedings of a Working Conference on the Social Foundations of Language and Thought.* Chicago: Center for Psychosocial Studies.
Jakobson, R. 1960. Linguistics and poetics. In T. Sebeok (Ed.), *Style in language.* Cambridge: MIT press.
Jakobson, R. 1971. Shifters, verbal categories, and the Russian verb. In *Selected writings II: Word and language.* The Hague: Mouton.
Karmiloff-Smith, A. 1977. More about the same: Children's understanding of post-articles. *Journal of Child Language, 4,* 377–394.
Karmiloff-Smith, A. 1979a. Language as a formal problem-space for children. Paper presented at the conference "Beyond Description in Child Language," Max-Planck Institute for Psycholinguistics, Nijmegen, Holland.
Karmiloff-Smith, A. 1979b. *A functional approach to child language: A study of determiners and reference.* Cambridge: Cambridge University Press.
Kohlberg, L., Yaeger, J., and Hjertholm, E. 1968. Private speech: Four studies and a review of theories. *Child Development, 39,* 691–736.
Peirce, C. S. 1931–5. *Collected papers of C. S. Peirce* (Vol. 2). Edited by C. Hartshorne and P. Weiss. Cambridge: Harvard University Press.
Silverstein, M. 1976a. Hierarchy of features and ergativity. In R. M. W. Dixon (Ed.), *Grammatical categories in Australian languages.* Humanities Press.
Silverstein, M. 1976b. Shifters, linguistic categories, and cultural description. In K. H. Basso and H. A. Selby (Eds.), *Meaning in anthropology.* Albuquerque: University of New Mexico Press.
Silverstein, M. 1979. Language structure and linguistic ideology. In *Papers from the Fifteenth Regional Meeting of the Chicago Linguistic Society,* Chicago Linguistic Society.
Silverstein, M. 1980. The three faces of "function": Preliminaries to a psychology of language. In M. Hickmann (Ed.), *Proceedings of a Working Conference on the Social Foundations of Language and Thought.* Chicago: Center for Psychosocial Studies.
Voloshinov, V. N. 1973. *Marxism and the philosophy of language.* New York: Seminar Press.
Vygotsky, L. S. 1962. *Thought and language.* Cambridge: MIT Press.
Vygotsky, L. S. 1978. *Mind in society: The development of higher psychological processes.* Cambridge: Harvard University Press.
Warden, D. A. 1976. The influence of context on children's uses of identifying expressions and references. *British Journal of Psychology, 67,* 101–112.

11

Language viewed as action

DAVID McNEILL

No single system of description contains all the various aspects that we naturally and intuitively include under the term "language" (all that we include when we say, e.g., that humans – but not cats, butterflies, etc. – possess "language"). The perspective of this chapter is to regard the performance side of language as a type of action. The proper unit of analysis in this perspective is *one act* (not the sentence, phrase, word, etc.).

The action viewpoint contrasts with the more traditional perspective in which language is viewed as a system of objects – such as, for example, a system of sentences. The two points of view can be said to fit together, in the sense that language actions have language objects as their end products. If each token of a language object has its own individual life history, then the action and object viewpoints apply to successive slices of this life history. Regarding an utterance in a state of completion, after the language action has run its course (or pretending that an action has never taken place), is to see it as an object, assimilating it into a synchronic (hence static) system of objects. Watching the utterance while it is emerging is to see it as an action and to treat it as an aspect of individual psychological activity. Some of the features of the latter perspective are laid out in this chapter.

Dynamic and static perspectives are each valid, but are separate from each other; at least they have never been connected. The action and object axes cross in the development of any sentence, but there is no account given of how objects arise from actions – or rather, of how we can relate (as more than a simple succession) first seeing something dynamically and changing through time to later seeing it as a stable object.

In such a situation there is no "master science" from which the phenomena of other sciences can be deduced – for example, the internal structure of human linguistic performance deduced from restrictions on linguistic form; there is instead a division into neighboring fields between which relationships are cooperative but murky.

Properties of actions

In an action there is a sense of doing a single coherent performance through time. Language actions are like other actions in mediating between "stimulus" and "consummation" (Mead, 1938). They should be seen against the backdrop of the larger activity in which the person is engaged; they are part of this activity and cannot be taken out of it. An example of this embeddedness is the following. I was entering my building at the University of Chicago, bringing with me my bicycle (as one usually does around our neighborhood). As I wheeled it toward the elevator, I saw the door closing and inside the elevator another person, also with a bicycle, reaching toward the controls to reopen the door. It was obvious, however, that two bicycles in the same elevator would be one bicycle too much, so I said:

> that's okay, go on up.

[For later reference, the first clause of this utterance will be numbered (1) and the second (2); however, both clauses were part of a single utterance.] This utterance was used as a "psychological tool" to (in this case) influence the movements of the other person and through this the operation of the elevator, which was the larger activity in this instance. In other circumstances, the meaning of this utterance could be quite different – for example, quarreling. The language action was shaped by the activity and the external conditions. The action had to be fast, for example, and the greater articulatory efficiency (despite lessened elegance) of "that's okay" compared to, for example, "that's quite alright," is traceable to this aspect of the situation. That the second clause was "go on up" (rather than, for example, "stop") is traceable to the activity of trying to influence the operation of the elevator through the other person (I was saying that everything should continue on as before; please ascend). Probably details of pronunciation, had they been recorded, would also have shown influences of the external organization of the action. For example, the pitch declination during "that's okay" may have been flattened due to the influence of the soon-to-follow "go on up," since both clauses were part of a single action.

In language actions there is movement – actual phonation and movements of the hands in gesture. The action can be visualized as a space extended in two directions around this movement. In one of these directions is the exterior of the action: the physical layout of the setting, the "stimulus," and the new state of affairs to be produced that will permit the "consummation." In the other direction is the interior of the action, sometimes metaphorically called the "program" (though this brings with it additional meanings), having to do with instigation and control. In this image movement is the interface between the external and internal, a kind of resultant of these two [the image is from Bernstein (1967)].

Internally, an action is a synthesis of elements through time (time is a third dimension in the image above). There is not only a succession of elements but also a coordination of elements that are concurrent, and all of these elements are synthesized in the internal organization of the action. I reach out to pick up a pencil from the table; the trajectory, velocity, and orientation of my hand all must be coordinated; my fingers must extend and retract at the appropriate moments; closure on the pencil to the reversal of the arm movement; and so forth. All of these elements must be synthesized into a single smooth action.

In the case of psychological actions such as speaking, the action includes a synthesis of *thoughts* that come together in the process of controlling the action internally. Among these are thoughts that are themselves based on and readily expressible in actions. The following examples contain such elements:

(3) the story came to a halt (image of a moving object stopping);
(4) he held it [image of a manipulation of some kind, though the arrangement is in fact static; this example is from Whorf (1956)];
(5) weird out [image of leaving a space; this example is from Lindner (1981)].

In each case the image is of an action. The theory here is that these images are an aspect of the synthesis of thoughts that control the language action internally, or rather are the residue in linguistic objects (for that is what we see) of the internal structure of language actions (Lindner analyzes the movement imagery in a wide variety of examples connected with the verb particles "up" and "out").

In a concrete action the synthesis of elements is given by the factual requirements of the manipulation. That I am trying to pick up a pencil lying on the table at a certain angle settles how I synthesize the elements of the action – how I recruit, coordinate, and sequence my movements in order to lift up the pencil. In a language action the synthesis of thoughts is along the same lines.

Between language and other actions there is continuity internally as well as externally. This will be our dynamic view of language. The external functional equivalence of language actions and concrete actions (intervening between "stimulus" and "consummation") induces an internal structural equivalence as well. In both types of action the synthesis principle is given by the requirements, factual or imagined, of actions. In concrete actions these are the physical manipulations and movements of objects; in language actions they are thoughts of manipulations or movements. In a concrete action everything is held together by the factual requirement of physically picking up the pencil; in a language action the synthesis is given by the thought of an object moving ("the story came to a halt").

We are saying that psychological language actions and concrete physical actions are based on common concepts. In some utterances the internal structure of the language action can be seen to be modeled on the structure of a concrete action that might have been performed in the same situation. Speech acts of commands/requests are like this. For example, uttering "that's okay" had the external function *and* internal structure of a non-verbal action of pointing to the closing door and saying "okay." Uttering "go on up" had for its internal structure a hoped-for effect of this action (the elevator goes on up). The thoughts providing a synthesis in the internal structure of these language actions were thoughts of different aspects of the concrete action which, if it *was* performed, would have *had* the effect of sending the elevator on its way:

(1')   point at the closing door and say "okay";
(2')   elevator continues up.

Thought of the concrete action in (1') provides the synthesis of elements on which the utterance of (1) is based – that is, "that's okay" is internally modeled on pointing and saying "okay." Similarly, thinking of the effect of this action – that is, that the elevator continues going up – was the internal model of "go on up." The internal substitution of language actions for various aspects of concrete actions thus leads to deep structural similarities that give to "that's okay, go on up" (and other commands/requests) the power to show what concrete actions would be like, should these be performed.

The analysis of the internal structure of the action of saying "that's okay" as based on pointing and saying "okay" suggests a form in which this (virtual) action could be expressed – namely, as a pointing gesture. Such a gesture accompanying (1) would be regarded as a second manifestation of the internal action structure – the utterance of "that's okay" being the first (first in communicative importance). The same can be said of (2). The analysis of (2') suggests a gesture in which this outcome could be expressed – for example, a rising or lifting movement of the hand – which also should be regarded as a second manifestation of the language action structure, "go on up" being the first. The externalization of these structures in gestures offers a way of studying the internal organization of language actions that is separate from speech. The gesture and the speech can be compared in a relationship comparable in its ability to bring out details to triangulation.

To summarize this theory: Between language and other actions there is continuity both internally and externally in terms of function and structure, and this is our dynamic view of language.

Articulation can be viewed as the resultant of the external structure of the action (the attempt to control the elevator) and the internal structure (the thought of pointing and saying "okay"). Emerging from the interface of these structures is the series of articulatory movements carried out in uttering "that's okay." A conception of movement that lends itself to this form of description is the syntagma (Kozhevnikov and Chistovich, 1965). A syntagma is one meaning unit pronounced as a single output. Kozhevnikov and Chistovich did not define a meaning unit, but to equate this with a language action, as described here, does not seem to do violence to their idea. A meaning unit, then, is a (virtual) action, and a syntagma is a (virtual) action pronounced as a single output. For the idea of a single output, we can refer to phonetic conceptions of integrated speech contours (such as phonemic clauses and tone units).

Thus one language action will have an integrated phonetic profile, externally perform a function (mediating between "stimulus" and "consummation"), and internally synthesize thoughts of concrete actions [in the case of (1) and (2), actions that, if they could be performed, would have the same external effect].

Other actions, other contexts

From our viewpoint, other speech acts do not differ from commands/requests internally. The synthesis of thoughts that controls the language action is given by thoughts of concrete actions that the person or an object might have performed in the same situation. The language action is a substitution for this possible concrete action, which now appears as the language action's interior. The difference between speech act context lies in the relationship between "stimulus" and "consummation" that the language action achieves; rather than controlling the movements of another person, for example, there is achievement of the conclusion of an argument or presentation of an event plus some thoughts about it. These illocutionary effects are brought off with internal thoughts of actions – manipulations and movements of objects in the world – that seem to play a metaphorical role in the speech act. A concept or meaning is shown *through* a (virtual) action. In the following example the concepts of pursuit and inaccessibility are presented in a complex gestural image of moving but nonclosing objects. This image immediately presents a global and undivided picture of the conceptual content, while concurrently the content is segmented into words and arranged across time in the speech channel (the fact that the gesture image arises first shows that it is not a response to the words).

(6)   Speech: they um wanted to get where Anansi was
      Gesture: both hands held apart in the air; right hand flutters back and forth

(where the horizontal line shows the temporal extent of the gesture). The synthesis of thoughts on which this language action was based (as revealed in the gesture) was a (virtual) placement of two objects in motion but without closure. This image shows directly pursuit and inaccessibility. The utterance of "they wanted to get where Anansi was" is an expression of the same internal structure, as numerous and detailed parallels of form between the speech and gesture channels show. For example, the participants (referred to by the pronoun and proper name) correspond to the two hands that were held apart at spatial extremes, and in the sentence appear at temporal extremes (rather than together as would have been possible in a frame such as "the sons [coreferent of "they"] and Anansi couldn't get together"[1]); one participant is not in motion, and in the sentence is referred to in a stative locative construction ("where Anansi was"); the other group of participants is in motion, and in the sentence is referred to as the subject of a verb of motion ("they wanted to get"); and the motion of these participants in the gesture was of small scale and ineffectual, and in the sentence this group is the subject of the verb "want." All of these parallels show that the gesture and utterance were joint manifestations of the same internal structure – a synthesis based on the idea of placement and movement of objects. In this case, however, the speech act was one of representation rather than command/request [as in (1)–(2)]. (It is well to remind ourselves of the opening remarks of this chapter. The relationship between the structure of language action and that of language objects – these being two separate perspectives – is anything but clear; therefore, it is not a particularly interesting question to ask how thoughts based on these actions translate into deep structures or other underlying linguistic object configurations.)

Other metaphoric examples

Gesture evidence reveals a very widespread use of metaphoric thinking in performing language actions in which thoughts based on actions are used to show meanings of a nonaction kind.

Mathematics discussions are accompanied by a flow of gestures that show mathematical ideas in the form of actions. The mathematical meaning of a dual is that each concept is replaced by its converse; for example, the dual of upward is downward. The following examples (7)–(9), taken from nonconsecutive places in a technical mathematics discussion, each contains a gesture in which a hand rotates through the air from one orientation to the opposite orientation; the gestures therefore show the concept of a dual in the action realm.

(7) Speech: this gives complete duality

Gesture: right-hand palm rotates upward

(8) Speech: when you dualize

Gesture: right-hand palm rotates downward

(9) Speech: the powers of x kind of give a dual

Gesture: right-hand palm rotates front to back

Another mathematical concept is that of a limit (either direct or inverse), and in the following examples the hands move toward some boundary marked by the other hand or a sudden stop; thus these gestures also show an image of a mathematical concept in the action realm.

(10) Speech: it's an inverse limit,

Gesture: right hand flattens left hand moves up to the right hand

(11) Speech: the inverse limit of, . . . (trails off)

Gesture: right hand goes down, then up as to a boundary

(12) Speech: which is a limit, a direct limit

Gesture: right hand moves down, then up as to a boundary

Example (10) also included a second gesture that showed the mathematical concept of an inverse.

(10′) Speech: it's an inverse limit,

Gesture: right hand moves in a tight loop

The concept of finiteness is shown by the action of enclosing or pinching down on a space with the fingers and hands; thus here too is a mathematical concept in the action realm.

(13) Speech: through the finite pieces,

Gesture: fingers curl inward

(14) Speech: to get the finite group scheme

Gesture: fingers curl inward

(15) Speech: you have to define some finite group functor

Gesture: forms a two-handed bounded shape with palms facing and fingers curled

A rule of gesture production is that new movements indicate *changes* of meaning; and so a gesture often indicates the emergence in the discourse of a new element of meaning (information focus). Thus in (7), for example, the new element of meaning in the context was the concept of duality, and the other examples can be interpreted in a parallel way. The point of the following examples is to see where the subject would produce gestures; these are deliberately produced gestures to go with specific sentences. In each case, it turned out that the gesture was made with the element of the sentence that the subject had been told to regard as salient (nontopical). These examples thus confirm the rule that gesture movements indicate changes of meaning. The sentences (i.e., 16 and 17) themselves are from Prince (1980).

(16) Speech: my girlfriend   it sickens (topic = being sickened)
     Gesture: right hand   holds this position
              moves to
              chest;
(17) Speech: my girlfriend   it sickens (topic = my girlfriend)
     Gesture: right hand in   right hand moves up and opens
              lap;

Gestures thus are able to indicate new elements of meaning in the context of speaking. Utterances are structured in such a way as to make salient the same elements of meaning, and this is another parallel that suggests a common source for gesture and speech. In (7), for example, "that gives complete duality" was structured and pronounced to achieve the same effect as the gesture: Reference to the concept of duality was held off until the final sentence position (the position of the rheme; Halliday, 1967) where it was given main stress, and was introduced in full lexical form. On the other hand, the sentence topic was announced first with pronoun, which was weakly stressed. The transitive sentence form also enhanced the information focus on duality. In other words, the details of (7) can be regarded as end products of an action in which duality was the focus. Internally the model for the utterance could have been something (the sentence topic) pushing forward an example of duality (hence the use of "gives").

Other gesture uses

The examples of gestures in (6)–(15) can be called "iconic," by which is meant that the form and manner of execution on the gesture depict a meaning relevant to the proposition being expressed verbally at the same time. Other gestures indicate changes in the structure of discourse itself, and of these there are two important types – "beats" and cohesive uses.

These gesture types are direct evidence that language actions must be considered to have an external structure that is continuous with their internal structure. For these gestures are images of the external action structure. Just as iconic gestures show the interior of utterances, beats and cohesive gestures show the external scaffolding of the discourse.

Beats tend to have the same form regardless of the accompanying semantic content (McNeill and Levy, 1982). They are rapid, low-energy pulses of the hand that lack structure, and often are made at the rest position or are superimposed on another iconic gesture. Although beats fail to depict propositional meanings, they emphasize statements structuring the discourse, those introducing new characters into a narration, commenting on the narration, summarizing it, and so forth, but not adding new elements to the story itself. We found that iconic gestures emphasize statements that do add new elements to the story.

In addition, there are subpropositional beats – equally formless movements – that emphasize single words or syllables. This emphasis on subpropositional components also, of course, reveals discourse structure.

An example of a beat accompanying a discourse structuring statement is this:

(18)   Speech: right okay this one actually wasn't a Bugs Bunny cartoon
        Gesture: beat with right hand

An example of beats accompanying single words or syllables is this:

(19)   Speech: you see him drawing up lots   of   blueprints
        Gesture: beat   beat   beat

The statement in (18) was part of the introduction of the narration of a cartoon; that in (19) part of the narration of the story itself. In both cases, however, the gestures emphasize not the propositions conveyed in the sentences, but something off from these propositions (in two directions). In (18) the gesture indicates the idea of *this* one rather than *that* one, *this* story (to be related) rather than some other story; in (19) the gestures indicate the element of quantity within the proposition. Both examples show in their gestures that the statement is connected to the external structure of language action, which is emphasized.

The second kind of discourse structuring is cohesion, a term that refers to the linking of separate parts of the discourse. Halliday and Hasan (1976) describe a great many linguistic "devices," which have the effect of adding to discourse cohesion. For example, anaphoric (nondeictic) third-person pronouns presuppose coreferences that are anterior – over possibly quite large distances – to the pronoun. This presupposition connects the two places – where the pronoun is to where the coreference is. There is a form of gestural cohesion as well, performed with iconic gestures. For example,

(20)   Speech: the network of wires that hooks up the cable car

        Gesture: both hands meet at the fingertips, showing wires
                  crossing

Speech: um you know the trolley
Gesture: left hand remains in position; right hand swings back
          and forth next to head, showing a pantograph
Speech: (listener: oh a c–)

          right and there's a whole network of these wires
Gesture: resumes original arrangements of hands meeting at the fin-
          gertips

In this example, the speaker interrupts herself to make a side comment. At the same time, she breaks off the gestural depiction of the network of wires and makes a new gesture that shows the operation of a pantograph on a streetcar. When she returns to the narration proper, she also resumes the first gesture of depicting the wires. In the verbal channel there is also a cohesive item, "these wires," which has the same reference as the gesture. (That the cohesive gesture arises first shows that it is not a response to the linguistic item.)

The examples in this section (18) – (20), show that action-based images are possible evidence of the external structure of language action, of the discourse scaffolding, as well as of the internal structure of language actions.

Units of action

Our unit of analysis, we said at the start of this chapter, is *one act* (not the sentence, phrase, word, etc.). Units of analysis differ in form of analysis that produces them. What ends up in a given unit may be superficially the same as the contents of a different unit, but units cannot be equated if they are reached through different forms of analysis. (A unit is reached when there is resistance to carrying the form of analysis any further.) This conception ensures that units express the theoretical analysis of which they are the product. Thus when a single language action results in a sentence (a linguistic object), there are two units – the action and the sentence – reached over quite different routes; similarly when the language action results in other kinds of language objects (phrases, words), these all are different units.

An action unit is a product of analysis that retains the basic properties of actions and beyond which further analysis would result in the destruction of the action. Thus there is a limit beyond which reduction to smaller elements is not tolerated. Like other emergent properties, the properties of actions are legitimized, not by reducing them to such and such, but by connecting them to each other (Sober, 1980).

Vygotsky (1962) concluded that the units of the speech–thought complex could be conceptualized as words. However, words are only part of the fundamental unit of language action. The step we must take is to conceive of a unit of action that is more complex than the word. Then in this unit words will appear as elements.

Gestural evidence shows there are global-synthetic meanings that arise immediately in language actions. The example in (6), in which the concepts of pursuit and inaccessibility were shown in the placement of two objects (one moving), illustrates this. From such global-synthetic images segments are removed that are codable as words, and these segments are synthesized into a stream of words in time along the lines of original global-synthetic image. Thus several of the detailed surface properties of "they wanted to get where Anansi was" could be traced to the global meaning from which the word segments had been taken; given this meaning, there were very few degrees of freedom for arranging these words in other ways. The important step is to regard words and the linear combination of words as one in-dissoluble action unit that starts out from a global-synthetic meaning and ends up with a succession of elements through time. Systems of word meaning and grammar are but two sides of a single process – the temporal subdivision of undivided meanings. This process provides a unit of language action in which all of the elements of an action can be found. (This, rather than saying that sentences are constructed *out of* words, which conceives of two actions and moves from parts to whole.)

Sources of meaning

According to the view taken in this chapter, language actions have within them images that are thoughts of other actions (the virtual actions, or syn-theses of thoughts, that can be observed as gestures). These images are detected in the imagery that arises from language objects and in the con-nection of language actions to gestures. Such images based on actions come from the substitution of language actions for concrete actions as interventions between "stimulus" and "consummation." Ideas, no matter how abstract and noncorporeal, if they are clear, also can be shown in the form of actions and images;[2] the examples were mathematical concepts and the pursuit of inaccessibility. These concepts are shown through their images (e.g., the concept of pursuit and inaccessibility through the non-closure of two objects).

Such images enable speech to *show* its meaning directly. Insofar as there are images built into language actions, these actions show their meanings. From the viewpoint of the speaker, producing speech is to act to show the meaning in the action. The speaker does not *map* symbols onto meanings (regarded as something not in the language action from the start) but *exhibits* the meaning within the language action itself. Thus we have a sim-ple situation in which speech needs *nothing else* (neither "ideas" nor "representations") to mean what it means. A speaker does not think of an idea and then find a sentence which expresses this; he acts in a way that is appropriate to the situation, and all of the meaning is already in this act (including an act that contains a concept, such as pursuit and inaccessibility). This account has the advantage of reflecting the intuitive simplicity and directness of acts of speech (rather than being forced to posit unconscious processes of arbitrary complexity to accommodate "representations"). [This account obviously owes a lot to Wittgenstein (1961).]

NOTES

I am grateful to Catherine Greeno for hunting down and cataloguing mathematicians' gestures; to Joan Bowman, Mitsuko Iriye, Elena Levy, Laura Pedelty, and Debra Stephens for analyzing other gestures; and to Nobuko B. McNeill for commenting on several versions of the chapter. Financial support of the gesture research was provided by the Spencer Foundation.

1   That (6) was produced rather than this frame undoubtedly reflects the discourse topicalization of the sons and not Anansi at this point in the narration. This frame could be used to introduce the conjunction of the sons and Anansi as the joint discourse topic (Levy, 1982).
2   I am grateful to Jonathan Schwartz for getting me to see this.

REFERENCES

Bernstein, N. A. 1967. *The co-ordination and regulation of movements*. Oxford: Pergamon Press.
Halliday, M. A. K. 1967. Notes on transitivity and theme in English, I. *International Journal of Linguistics*, *3*, 37–81.
Halliday, M. A. K., and Hasan, R. 1976. *Cohesion in English*. London: Longman.
Levy, E. 1982. Towards an objective definition of "discourse topic." Paper presented at the 18th Regional Meeting of the Chicago Linguistic Society, University of Chicago, April.
Lindner, S. J. 1981. A lexico-semantic analysis of English verb particle constructions with OUT and UP. Doctoral dissertation, Department of Lingusitics, University of California at San Diego, La Jolla.
Kozhevnikov, V. A., and Chistovich, L. A. 1965. *Speech: Articulation and perception*. Publication No. 30543. Washington, D. C.: U.S. Department of Commerce, Joint Publication Service.
McNeill, D., and Levy, E. 1982. Conceptual representations in language activity and gesture. In R. Jarvella and W. Klein (Eds.), *Speech, place, and action*. Chichester: Wiley.
Mead, G. H. 1938. *The philosophy of the act*. Edited by C. W. Morris. Chicago: University of Chicago Press.
Prince, E. 1980. A functional syntax approach to text analysis: Left dislocation and

topicalization. Paper presented at the Symposium on Approaches to Text Analysis, University of Chicago, Oct. 10–11.

Sober, E. 1980. Language and psychological reality. *Linguistics and philosophy*, *3*, 395–442.

Vygotsky, L. S. 1962. *Thought and language*. Cambridge: MIT Press.

Whorf, B. L. 1956. *Language, thought and reality*, Cambridge: MIT Press.

Wittgenstein, L. 1961. *Tractatus logico-philosophicus*. Translated by D. F. Pears and B. F. McGuinness. London: Routledge & Kegan Paul.

PART III

Extending Vygotsky's approach: issues in education, cognitive development, and language development

12

Diagnosing zones of proximal development

ANN L. BROWN and ROBERTA A. FERRARA

Suppose I investigate two children upon entrance into school, both of whom are ten years old chronologically and eight years old in terms of mental development. Can I say that they are the same age mentally? Of course. What does this mean? It means that they can independently deal with tasks up to the degree of difficulty that has been standardized for the eight-year-old level. If I stop at this point, people would imagine that the subsequent course of mental development and of school learning for these children will be the same, because it depends on their intellect. . . . Now imagine that *I do not terminate my study at this point, but only begin it.* [Emphasis is ours.] These children seem to be capable of handling problems up to an eight-year-old's level, but not beyond that. Suppose that I show them various ways of dealing with the problem. Different experimenters might employ different modes of demonstration in different cases: some might run through an entire demonstration and ask the children to repeat it, others might initiate the solution and ask the child to finish it, or offer leading questions. In short, in some way or another I propose that the children solve the problem with my assistance. Under these circumstances it turns out that the first child can deal with problems up to a twelve-year-old's level, the second up to a nine-year-old's. Now, are these children mentally the same?

When it was first shown that the capability of children with equal levels of mental development to learn under a teacher's guidance varied to a high degree, it became apparent that those children were not mentally the same age and that the subsequent course of their learning would obviously be different. This difference between twelve and eight, or between nine and eight, is what we call *the zone of proximal development. It is the distance between the actual developmental level as determined by independent problem solving and the level of potential development as determined through problem solving under adult guidance or in collaboration with more capable peers.*

Vygotsky, 1978, pp. 85–86; emphasis in the original

Introduction

There are many implications of Vygotsky's theory of a zone of proximal development, not least of which concerns the design of the diagnostic tests to which we subject children. In this chapter we will concentrate on the

273

implications of Vygotsky's theory of a zone of proximal development for the dynamic assessment of learning potential. We would like to emphasize, however, that Vygotsky's theory is not just a testing philosophy but rather it is a rich theory of socialization (Laboratory of Comparative Human Cognition, 1983), and this point is demonstrated impressively by the diversity of topics discussed in this volume. Given our charge, however, we will restrict ourselves primarily to a description of existing work on learning potential assessment. We will concentrate primarily on current Soviet work (Lubovskii, Rozanova, and Egorova, pers. comm.) and our extension of that work, but we will preface our discussion with a brief consideration of some other approaches to assessing learning potential, notably that of Feuerstein (1980) and Budoff (1974). We will also examine briefly other attractive features of the zone of proximal development, noting its relevance to theories of intelligence based on concepts of access and use of knowledge (Brown and Campione, 1980; Campione, Brown, and Ferrara, 1982). First, we will consider standardized IQ testing, the existing state of the art.

Static nature of IQ tests

One of the traditional definitions of intelligence is the ability to learn. If this is so, then "estimates of it [intelligence] are, or at least should be, estimates of the ability to learn. To be able to learn harder things, or to be able to learn the same things more quickly, would then be the single basis of evaluation" (Thorndike, 1926, pp. 17–18). Despite this early claim that intelligence tests should measure learning potential, in general, relatively static measures have been used to assess intellectual functioning. Such measures reflect the end result of prior learning but they do not necessarily provide a sensitive index of the potential for improvement over current performance levels. They are good predictive but poor diagnostic tools. There are strong reasons to believe that for many people, particularly those from disadvantaged homes, the static test scores represent an underestimate of ability. In addition, static IQ measures do not provide direct information concerning the optimal level of performance of which the testee is capable, an optimal level that is of considerable interest for those who wish to design instruction.

Having stressed the static nature of traditional IQ testing, we think it is informative that even here an important ingredient is the dynamic interaction between tester and testee. Standardized test procedures for measuring IQ were explicitly designed to provide the same environment for each testee. Examiners are trained to remain neutral, not to question or add to the child's response, not to help the child in any way. But recent work by

Mehan (1973) and others has shown that the testing environment is by no means constant for each child. Testers often question a child's response so that the child, in response, will self-correct. Testers may inadvertently provide prompts such as indicating, verbally or otherwise, that an answer is correct (the responsive child then terminates her search) or incomplete (the responsive child uses these hints and continues searching). Even the simple practice of just waiting for a response elaboration gives time for the child to amend an inadequate first reply. Scoring the test protocols according to the strict criterion of considering only the child's unaided responses provides a quite different picture of her ability than the lenient criterion of accepting the child's responses as modified by the inadvertent aid. As much as a 27% increase of aided over unaided scores has been reported (Mehan, 1973).

The effects due to tester–testee interactions are not trivial. And there is considerable evidence to suggest that such biasing effects are more likely to benefit the middle-class child. A form of self-fulfilling prophecy operates whereby the tester expects the middle-class child to do well and therefore treats inadequate first responses as hasty mistakes rather than indices of stupidity – leeway is inadvertently given and the child scores higher than the strict procedure would permit. Such leeway is not usually afforded the lower-class child.

The substantial improvement over initial response that is achieved via the interaction of the adult and child is precisely what learning potential methods aim at measuring. By offering graded hints to all participants, the tester is able to evaluate if, and how much, the child can improve over initial performance. We will consider three such programs that have specifically addressed the problem of dynamic assessment of learning potential: Feuerstein's Learning Potential Assessment Device (LPAD), Budoff's Learning Potential and Educability Program, and recent advances in Soviet clinical assessments of the zone of proximal development (Brown and French, 1979; Vygotsky, 1978) together with our experimental examinations of their claims (Brown and French, 1979; Campione et al., 1982; Ferrara, Brown, and Campione, 1983; Bryant, Brown, and Campione, 1983).

Learning potential and educability

During the 1960s and early 1970s, Budoff developed a series of procedures for assessing the learning potential of educably retarded individuals. Convinced of the unsuitability of static tests, particularly for low-achieving children, he introduced a basic test–train–test procedure to all his assessment measures. Budoff regarded pretraining scores on any psychological test as reflecting the "present functioning ability of the child." Pretest scores, not surprisingly, correlate with IQ and with socioeconomic indicators such as family size, degree of intactness of family, English language competence, and so on. Posttest scores were seen as a composite measure reflecting (1) the initial starting level of competence, (2) an effect due to practice, and (3) an effect due to specific training. Budoff reported that although low-IQ children tend to gain little from mere practice,

following *suitable training*, many low IQ children will function at a level similar to the child from more privileged circumstances. This posttraining score, regardless of pretraining level, represents the child's optimal level of performance following an optimizing procedure. It permits a comparison between his *presently* low level of functioning, as indicated by his IQ and his *potential* level of functioning. . . .A third score is the posttraining score adjusted for pretest level. This residualized score indicates the child's responsiveness to training, and by extension to the classroom regardless of his pretraining level. It is hypothesized to indicate the student's amenability to training given suitable curricula and school experiences. (Budoff, 1974, p. 33)

Budoff's learning potential approach is based on a conceptualization of intelligence that stresses trainability, or the ability to profit from learning experiences directly related to the task at hand. Improved performance after training indicates problem-solving capability not evident when instruction is not provided as part of the test administration. Of interest is how these training sessions were devised. Budoff concentrated on IQ type tasks such as Raven's matrices and block building. We will describe Budoff's work with Koh's blocks in some detail to provide an example of his general approach.

Following a pretest on several block designs, the subjects enter into the training phase of the test–train–test assessment procedure. In the initial stage a problem is presented without aid and the tester waits until the children solve it or fail to solve it on their own. If a child fails, a series of more and more explicit prompts are given until a solution is reached. A series of prompts for a Koh's blocks problem is illustrated in Figure 1. The first prompt is to present only one row of the design. Initially the blocks composing the row are not outlined. On succeeding presentations, if the subject fails to align the blocks correctly, the design is progressively outlined; for example, see the progression in Figure 1. On the prompt cards where the blocks are given in outline (B_3, C_2, F_3) and on the final card (H), the subject is required to check whether each block in her design corresponds exactly with the comparable block on the card. Throughout the training period the child is urged to check her construction block by block against the design card, thereby encouraging the child to be more "planful" and "systematic" in her work approach.

Following training such as this, on a variety of IQ-like test items, Budoff

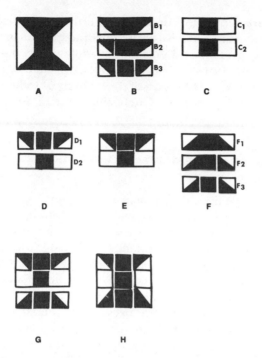

Figure 1. Learning potential assessment for Koh's blocks: illustration of coaching procedure. A. Initial design card. B. Stimulus cards for top row of design. C. Stimulus cards for middle row of design. D. Card showing relationship of upper two rows of design. E. Card showing the two rows placed together. F. Stimulus cards for lowest row of design. G. Cards showing the relationship of upper two rows and lowest row of design. H. Final card with all blocks outlined. (From Budoff, 1974).

found three classes of children within his educable retarded population: (1) subjects who demonstrate little or no gain following instruction (*nongainers*), (2) subjects who show quite marked gain (*gainers*), and (3) *high scorers,* those who performed quite adequately on the pretest. There are some problems associated with Budoff's approach, notably the concentration on product rather than process. For example, a gainer might be one who improved over pretest by four items while a nongainer improved one item or less. Budoff was aware that this was difficult to interpret as the child who solved no blocks on pretest and five on posttest is difficult to compare with a child who solved four on pretest and five on posttest. But despite the difficulties, Budoff reported interesting correlates of the gainer/nongainer status. For example, middle-class children in special education classes tend to be nongainers, while lower-class children have a much higher incidence of gainers. Budoff also claimed that learning potential status predicted performance on a variety of laboratory concept learning tasks and a specially constructed math curriculum. Furthermore, learning potential status was said to be predictive of successful adaptation to mainstreaming, the ability to get and hold jobs during adolescence, mother's perception of the child, and a variety of positive personality characteristics. Despite the somewhat vague specification of these effects of training, the importance of considering gainers and nongainers seems to be well justified.

Feuerstein's Learning Potential Assessment Device and Instrumental Enrichment Program

Feuerstein's theory of cognitive development is very similar to Budoff's and even more similar to Vygotsky's, as we shall see. According to Feuerstein, cognitive growth is the result of incidental and mediated learning, with the latter being by far the more important: "Mediated learning is the training given to the human organism by an experienced adult who frames, selects, focuses and feeds back an environmental experience in such a way as to create appropriate learning sets" (Feuerstein, 1969, p. 6).

These mediated learning experiences are an essential aspect of development, beginning when the parent selects significant objects for the infant to focus on, and proceeding throughout development with the adult systematically shaping the child's learning experiences. This is the principal means by which the child develops the cognitive operations necessary for learning independently. Thus, Feuerstein's theory is an internalization theory. By interacting with an adult, who guides problem-solving activity and structures the learning environment, the child gradually comes to adopt structuring and regulatory activities of his own.

Feuerstein believes that the principal reason for the poor performance of many disadvantaged adolescents is the lack of consistent mediated learning in their earlier developmental histories, either because of parental apathy, ignorance, or overcommitment. Quite simply, parents in disadvantaged homes may themselves have been disadvantaged children and cannot be expected to teach what they do not know. Similarly, large family size and the need for a working mother do not leave a great deal of time for Socratic dialogue games. In addition, these interactive styles of continually questioning and extending the limits of knowledge are typical of middle-class social interaction patterns and may even be alien to some cultures (Au, 1980).

But mediated learning activities are exactly what occur in schools, and the middle-class child comes well prepared to take part in these rituals. Not only do disadvantaged children lack prior exposure, but there is some evidence that teachers give less experience in this learning mode to those who, because of their lack of familiarity, need it most. For example, data from microethnographic studies of reading groups (Au, 1980; Collins, 1980; Gumperz, 1980; McDermott, 1978) suggest that good readers are continually questioned about the meaning behind what they are reading, asked to evaluate and criticize material, and so forth. The teacher adopts the procedure of asking every child questions and everyone gets a turn to read. In contrast, in the poor reading groups, precious little time is spent reading, a great deal of time is devoted to discipline, turn taking is at the teacher's request, and the poorer children are not called upon to perform to save everyone embarrassment. When poor readers do receive attention, it is focused on correct decoding and pronunciation (Au, 1980). Thus good readers receive continual practice with the kinds of questions one would like them to internalize: hypothesis testing, predicting, evaluating, bridging, and mapping (Brown, Palincsar, and Armbruster, in press). Poor readers rarely experience these questioning games and therefore can scarely be expected to internalize them.

In addition to the teacher–child pact to spare poor readers from these activities, there is growing evidence that children themselves conspire to reduce learning demands to a minimum. Witness the learning-disabled child (Archie) stuied extensively by Cole and Traupmann (1980). Archie spent considerable ingenuity circumventing situations where he would be called upon to read, or indeed perform any academic task unaided by his peers.

Feuerstein believes that the inevitable result of the lack of consistent mediated learning experiences is poor performance on a wide range of academic tasks, and the levels of performance displayed by *retarded performers* is an underestimation of the level they could achieve if subjected to intensive remedial mediated learning experiences. Like Budoff (1974) and Campione, Brown, and Ferrara (1982) in the United States and Lubovskii and his colleagues in the USSR, Feuerstein predicts that those retarded performers, who do poorly because of inadequate early learning environments, will be gainers or show a wide zone of proximal development.

To test his theory, Feuerstein developed two assessment packages: the Learning Potential Assessment Device (LPAD) and the Instrumental Enrichment (IE) intervention program. In the LPAD, Feuerstein also adopted the test–train–test procedure as a measure of the child's current status and potential for learning. And again, the LPAD tasks are variants of common IQ test items such as matrices, analytical perception, memory span tasks, and embedded figure problems. Feuerstein reports dramatic improvement as a function of brief training exposure to these items (Feuerstein, 1979; Haywood et al., 1975; Narrol and Bachor, 1975). The LPAD, however, lacks a fine-grained description of the prompts or aids given to the child in the "training" session of the test–train–test sequence. The approach is essentially clinical, with the examiner adding hints as needed.

The clinical approach of aiding the child traverse her zone of proximal development is also a feature of Feuerstein's (1980) Instrumental Enrichment (IE) intervention program. The IE program has been widely cited as a successful intervention program both in Israel (Feuerstein, 1980; Feuerstein et al., 1979) and in the United States (Haywood and Smith, 1979). Others, including Feuerstein, have described this instrument in detail and we will not repeat this here. (See Bransford et al., in press; Feuerstein 1979, 1980.) We will concentrate on the "training" aspect of the problem rather than the materials per se (which are very similar to IQ test items).

Feuerstein's training program is designed to overcome the systematic problems he regards as characteristic of the cognitive processes of retarded performers. Feuerstein's description of the problem solving of disadvantaged Israeli adolescents is reminiscent of the type of cognitive deficits that we and others have diagnosed as *metacognitive problems* (Brown, 1975, 1978, 1982a; Brown and Campione, 1978, 1981; Campione and Brown, 1977, 1978; Campione et al., 1982). We have described retarded performers as lacking a variety of systematic data-gathering, checking, monitoring, and self-regulatory mechanisms – in short, they are deficient in "autocritical" skills (Binet, 1909). They tend to follow instructions blindly (Brown, 1978), lack adequate question-asking skills (Brown et al., in press), and do not seek to overcome comprehension problems with remedial strategies (Baker and Brown, 1984b; Brown 1980; Brown et al., in press). They have a greater tendency than most to treat each problem as if it were a new problem, regardless of relevant prior experience. They generally develop learning sets slowly, transferring the effects of past learning reluctantly (Brown and Campione, 1978, 1981; Campione, et al., 1982) They have considerable difficulty learning from experience, as Feuerstein also notes:

The culturally deprived child does not internalize problems as they occur. . . .In his trial and error stabs at coming to grips with a situation, whichever resolution is finally hit upon is not insightfully incorporated into his behavioral schema with the result that upon a fresh recurrence of the situation, he must start from scratch. Every problem is a new problem. Internalization leads to the building of learning sets which the culturally deprived notably lack in their conceptual repertoire. (Feuerstein, 1969, pp. 8–9)

Given this diagnosis, it is not surprising that Feuerstein concentrates on self-control and self-regulation (Brown, 1982a) in his IE training program. The essential aim of Feuerstein's program is inherently Vygotskian. Through the mediation of a supportive teacher the child will be made aware of the significance of her learning activities and will come eventually, via internalization, to perform cognitive regulatory functions for herself that she has originally experienced in collaboration with an adult (Brown, 1982a; Brown and French, 1979; Brown et al., in press). This aim is explicitly stated:

The salient characteristic in Instrumental Enrichment is its consciously intentional, focused and volitional nature. The student is made aware that a certain concept is to be taught; he is made to focus on that concept and gradually to perfect his abilities with relationship to it. It is deemed of the utmost importance that his awareness and cooperation in this effort be enlisted and it will not be left to chance that perhaps he will come to understand the purpose and logic behind the disparate exercises. (Feuerstein, 1969, p. 18)

The essential aim of insightful learning in the IE program is to facilitate transfer of training, or access and use of information, that is potentially available to the learner (Brown and Campione, 1978, 1981; Campione et al., 1982). In Feuersteins's words:

Transfer of training is most observable in instances where learning is based on insightful processes. In order to achieve such insight (e.g., to provide the learner with skills, attitudes, problem solving behavior, category labels, etc.) the learner must be able to perceive the general characteristics and applicability of a given concept. Furthermore, one has to present the learner with a number of varied situations to which the newly acquired skills are applicable. (Feuerstein, 1969, p. 21).

The zone of proximal development

Our initial interest in learning potential assessment was triggered by a visit (on the part of the first author) to the Institute of Defectology in Moscow in 1978. There we were privileged to examine the materials and discuss the clinical assessment battery being developed by our Soviet colleagues, notably, Professors Lubovskii, Rozanova, and Egorova. Our program of research was initially an attempt to develop parallel batteries to those being used in the USSR and to test them with American children. As both our own and the Soviet work was influenced by Vygotsky's theory, we will discuss that next.

Vygotsky's theory of cognitive development rests heavily on the key concept of *internalization*. Vygotsky argues that all higher psychological processes are originally social processes, shared between people, particularly between children and adults. The child first experiences active problem-solving activities in the presence of others but gradually comes to perform these functions independently. The process of internalization is gradual; first the adult or knowledgeable peer controls and guides the child's activity, but gradually the adult and the child come to share the problem-solving functions, with the child taking initiative and the adult correcting and guiding when she falters. Finally, the adult cedes control to the child and functions primarily as a supportive and sympathetic audience. This developmental progression from other-regulation to self-regulation is the essence of mother–child learning dyads (Wertsch, 1978; Wertsch and Stone, Chapter 7, this volume), but age or the nature of the social agent are to some extent irrelevant. Teachers, tutors, and master craftsmen in traditional apprenticeship situations all function ideally as promotors of self-regulation by nurturing the emergence of personal planning as they gradually cede their own direction (Brown and French, 1979; Cole, Chapter 6, this volume).

It is within this context of the gradual internalization of cognitive activities that were originally shared, interactive processes that Vygotsky introduced his concept of the zone of proximal development. From Vygotsky's viewpoint it is essential to consider a child's problem-solving abilities in situations other than traditional testing milieux, and his essentially interactive theory of learning had an important effect on the development of clinical testing in the Soviet Union. For a variety of historical and social reasons, standardized intelligence tests have been widely criticized in the USSR (Brożek, 1972; Wozniak, 1975) but, at the same time, an essential feature of Soviet social policy is a major commitment to special education (Vlasova, 1972). In recent years there has been a growing interest in the development of reliable methods for the differential diagnosis of learning disabilities or temporary retardation and more serious and permanent mental impairment (Vlasova and Pevzner, 1971; Zabramna, 1971). Given the unfavorable climate for the establishment of standardized testing, the Soviets have concentrated on the development of clinical batteries of diagnostic tests to serve the purpose of evaluating differences in learning potential.

One particularly interesting suggestion from the Soviet work is that dynamic measures are especially sensitive to differences between learning-disabled (developmentally backward or temporarily retarded) and truly retarded children. Of prime importance for the diagnosis of the cause of school difficulty is the Soviet claim that whereas learning-disabled and mildly retarded children tend not to differ greatly in terms of their starting competence on a variety of cognitive tasks, the two groups differ dramatically in terms of their ability to benefit from the additional cues provided by the tester. Learning-disabled children need less aid than truly retarded children before they arrive at a satisfactory solution. They are also said to be more proficient at transferring the result of their brief learning experience to new variations of the task within the testing situation and in subsequent independent class performance. In Soviet studies, where comparisons with normal children were included, the average children were even more effective at initial learning and subsequent transfer than were the two clinical populations (Egorova, 1973; Lubovskii, pers. comm.).

As stated earlier, our research program was initiated in an attempt to replicate the Soviet findings. Our original point of departure was based on our observation of the type of tasks used by our Soviet colleagues. A typical testing session consisted of the initial presentation of a test item exactly as it would occur in an American IQ test, with the child being asked to solve the problem independently. If the child failed to reach the correct solution, the adult progressively added clues for solution. By these means it is possible to assess how much additional information the child needs in order to solve the problem. The child's initial performance, when asked to solve the test item independently, provides information comparable to that gained with standardized American IQ testing procedures. The degree of aid needed before a child reaches solution is taken as an inverse indication of the width of her proximal zone. Once a solution on a particular test item was reached another version of the original task was presented, and transfer to the novel item was considered by determining whether or not the child required fewer cues in order to reach a solution.

The following is a concrete example of the testing materials and procedures. We were struck by the similarity of the problem and procedure to that developed by Budoff (see Figure 1). The problem presented to the child is a common IQ test item, usually referred to as pattern matching or geometric design. Such items occur on many standard tests, including the Binet, the WIPPSI, and the WISC. The child is given a silhouette shape and is asked to copy this model by combining a subset of wooden geometric forms. In the Soviet version of this task, however, there is an interesting trick; some of the requisite shapes are not included in the set of available wooden pieces but must be constructed by joining two wooden pieces together.

The first step in the testing procedure is to present a small model picture and ask the child to copy it with wooden shapes; if she fails, she is given a series of additional prompts, including a model that has one of the composite geometric shapes (corresponding to one of the wooden pieces) clearly delineated in the picture. If this does not lead to solution, the child is given a further detailed model that clearly shows the join (trick) necessary to create the missing form. If all else fails, the tester constructs the figure and then encourages the child to go through the construction with her.

Of particular interest are the "transfer" tests. Following solution of problem 1 (provided by the tester if all else failed), the second problem is immediately presented, with the same series of aids if so needed. In problem 2 it is necessary to construct *two* of the composite forms. One of the required joined shapes is identical to that required in problem 1, the other is a new construction. Specific transfer would be measured by the recognition that the subpart constructed to solve problem 1 was again required for problem 2's solution. More general transfer would be the knowledge that joining shapes in general would be a requirement of the pattern-copying task, and this knowledge should be reflected in the facility with which the child attempts to construct the new joined subpart (Rozanova, pers. comm.).

The Soviet diagnostic testing method provides invaluable information concerning the child's starting level of competence, an estimate of the width of her zone of proximal development, and the level of competence she can reach with aid. In addition, we gain information concerning the child's ability to profit from adult assistance, her speed of learning, and the facility with which she transfers the new skill across tasks.

Quite explicit in the Soviet description of their program is the role of Vygotsky's theory of a zone of proximal development; the Soviets emphasize the place of graduated aids in uncovering the "readiness" of children to perform competently in any task domain. Also entailed by this position, and at least as important to contemporary theories of cognition, is an implicit theory of task analysis and transfer of training. We would like to argue that testing the zone of proximal development as a means of diagnosis requires a detailed task analysis of a suitable set of cognitive tasks and detailed task analysis of possible transfer probes. Without this information it would be difficult to select either the series of graduated aids for the original learning task or suitable methods for assessing the speed and efficiency of transfer. In the Soviet diagnostic sessions, what is being measured is the efficiency of learning within any one task domain. The assessment of the width of a child's zone of proximal development empirically translates into the assessment of how many prompts she needs to solve problem 1, versus problem 2, versus problem 3, and so on (i.e., how quickly she learns and how far she transfers). A child judged to have a wide zone of proximal development is one who reduces the number of prompts needed from trial to trial, that is, who shows effective transfer of a new solution across similar problems.

In summary, the three clinical programs of research concerned with the dynamic assessment of learning potential (Budoff, Feuerstein, and Lubovskii and colleagues) have many features in common; furthermore, these features are not dissimilar to the current position of many experimental psychologists interested in training studies and intelligence (Brown and Campione, 1981; Campione et al., 1982). All of these programs can be readily interpreted within a general theory of development based on Vygotsky's notion of a zone of proximal development.

The three programs agree that static measures of intelligence provide an indication of current performance that may be depressed for a variety of reasons and that it is informative to consider how children respond to training if one is interested in diagnosing learning potential. All agree that such training should be interactive, with a supportive adult providing hints or prompts to aid the discovery of problem solutions. All put forward, at least implicitly, an internalization theory of learning that follows a prototypic path from other-regulation to self-regulation. And finally, all pinpoint self-regulatory or autocritical skills as essential determinants of adequate learning and flexible transfer of training.

This emergent clinical literature, together with experimental studies of learning difficulties in aberrant populations (Campione et al., 1982), lends credence to traditional theories that identify important components of intelligence as the speed and efficiency of learning in the absence of direct or complete instruction (Resnick and Glaser, 1976) and the extent to which flexible transfer or use of information is achieved (Brown and Campione, 1981; Höffding, 1982; Thorndike and Woodworth, 1901; Gagné, 1970). The methodologies being developed to measure zones of proximal development within academic domains are ideal vehicles for uncovering learning potential in children that could be masked by their ineffectual performance on static standardized tests.

Experimental studies on the zone of proximal development

Inspired by the Soviet approach to testing learning potential as a means of differential diagnosis, we have begun a series of studies to examine the experimental reliability of their clinical claims and to investigate the feasibility of standardizing what is essentially an interpersonal situation (Bryant et al., 1983; Campione et al., 1982; Ferrara et al., 1983). Two of the test items we selected initially are variants of the letter series completion task and the Raven's progressive matrices. We chose these tasks because of (1) their demand for active processing strategies that could be acquired in a learning session, (2) their frequency of occurrence on common IQ tests, (3) their similarity to the material used by the Soviets (Lubovskii, pers. comm.), and (4) the existence of detailed task analyses on the problems to aid our design of learning and transfer tests (Jacobs and Vandeventer, 1972; Kotovsky and Simon, 1973).

Our primary concern was with the relation between dynamic measures and traditional IQ scores. Do indices of proximal zone width within a domain (zone of proximal development measures) relate to IQ; that is, are high-IQ children fast learners and far transferers and low-IQ children slow learners and narrow transferrers? If this were the case, then both the IQ and the zone of proximal development (ZPD) measures would be validated and we would add credence to a process theory of intelligence that defines it as speed of learning and efficiency of transferring. Alternatively, IQ status may not predict ZPD status, suggesting that different indices of efficiency are measured by each approach. If this were so, then it would be imperative that the predictive validity of ZPD scores be compared with IQ measures; that is, does knowing a child's ZPD score tell us more (or less, or something different) about how she will perform in a domain than knowing her IQ score? Or we could find a combination of the two alternatives just specified, that is, a combination of IQ and ZPD scores, which is the most informative. Without a great deal of careful empirical work the status of the ZPD concept cannot be rigorously evaluated. It was as a preliminary attempt to address these issues that our work began.

Letter series completion task

We will be discussing our work on the letter series completion task in some detail (Ferrara et al., 1983). The task was based on Kotovsky and Simon's (1973) analysis. Using this as a starting point we developed an instrument to estimate the zone of proximal development. Basically, there are three alphabetic rules employed in these problems: *identity*, the repetition of letters; *next*, the occurrence of letters in alphabetical sequence; and *backward next*, the occurrence of letters in reverse alphabetical sequence. The period refers to the number of letters that occur prior to the appearance of regularities. For example, in the very simple series A D A D A D A D, the period is two and the rules are both those of *identity*. In the series A M A N A O A P, the period is again two and the rules are *identity* in the first case and *next* in the second. In the string P A O A N A M A, the period remains two; and the rules are *backward next* followed by *identity*. Thus, a given series is defined by one or more rules and a certain periodicity.

The particular problems learned initially in our study involved *next* and/ or *identity* relations and a periodicity of either two or four letters. Examples of these two patterns are given at the top of Table 1. As a result of extensive pilot testing, these problem types were selected as ones that few, if any, third- and fifth-graders (the age of our subjects) would be able to solve initially on their own. In other words, in a standard IQ test situation, 95% of the children would have failed on these items.

Each problem was presented initially for the child to solve independently. Standardized prompts were then provided by the tester as needed in a graduated series of increasing explicitness. They began with subtle hints that directed the child to look for patterns and then became more explicit

Table 1. *Examples of test items*

Original learning (two pattern types)
   Pattern type:
   NN – (Next relations between letters; period = two)
                      N G O H P I Q J – (Answer: R K S L)
   NINI – (Next and Identity relations between letters; period = four)
                      P Z U F Q Z V F – (Answer: R Z W F)
Maintenance (learned pattern types; see above)

Near transfer (learned relations and learned periodicities, but in different combinations):
   NI   D V E V F V G V – (Answer: H V I V)
   NNNN   V H D P W I E Q – (Answer: X J F R)

Far transfer (Addition of Backward Next relation, "B," or period of three letters):
   BN   U C T D S E R F – (Answer: Q G P H)
   NBNI   J P B X K O C X – (Answer: L N D X)
   NIN   P A D Q A E R A – (Answer: F S A G)

Very far transfer (Secret code items; Backward Next as well as Next relation; "period" of two letters, but relations must be sought between rows of letters rather than within a row).
   Example:
   Pretend that you are a spy. You want to send the message on top in a secret code that only your friends will understand. Someone has begun coding the message for you on the second line. Try to figure out the secret code and finish coding the message by filling in the blanks with the letters that follow the code.
      S I X   S H I P S   G O N E
      T H Y   R I H Q R   __ __ __ __ (Answer: H N O D)

---

as they directed the child's attention to the important features of the problem. The final hints essentially gave the solution to the child [see Ferrara et al. (1983) for details].

Following training to a criterion of six independently solved problems, transfer was assessed. Some of the transfer problems were of the pattern types learned in training (maintenance items), whereas others deviated in systematic ways. Examples of these problems are given in Table 1. Near transfer items involved the rules (*identity* and *next*) and periodicities (two and four letters) already learned but displayed them in new combinations. Far transfer items incorporated either a new rule, *backward next*, or a new period of three letters. Two additional problems were given at the end of the transfer session, that is, very far transfer items shown in Table 1. These problems required the child to finish coding a brief message. In order to do so, the child had to employ the *backward next* and *next* rules, but the relationships existed *between* rows of letters, rather than within a row. All sessions were videotape-recorded.

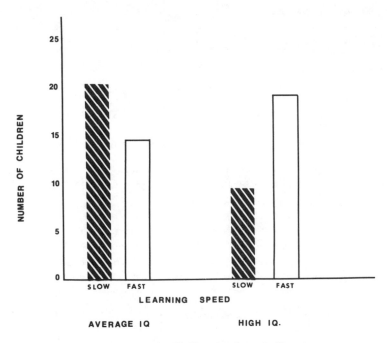

Figure 2. Number of children classified by IQ and speed of learning.

The total number of standardized prompts needed to reach criterion in original learning was selected as an index of speed of learning. Using this index, we found that fifth-graders learned more quickly than third-graders, that is, they needed less than half as many hints as the younger children to reach criterion. Similarly, the children with above average IQs (mean 122) tended to require only around three-fourths the number of hints needed by the average children (mean IQ 101).[1]

Within each grade we classified the children on the basis of the median number of prompts given, which resulted in the designation of children as either slow or fast learners (i.e., above or below the median, respectively). Because the patterns in the two age groups were very similar, we collapsed across grades to form Figure 2. For approximately two-thirds of the children, IQ scores predicted speed of learning. However, a good third of the children had learning speeds not predictable from their IQ scores.

The performance on the transfer test is shown in Figure 3. Few, if any, prompts were needed to solve the maintenance and near transfer problems, and neither grade nor IQ differences were found. However, significantly more prompts were needed to solve the far transfer items, and, of greater interest, there was a divergence in the number of prompts needed by third- and fifth-graders. Third-graders tended to require much more

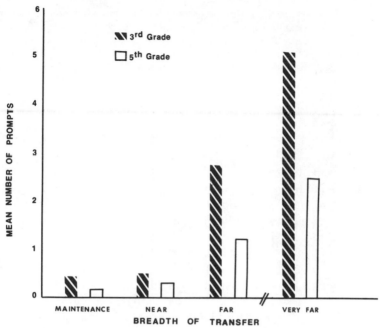

Figure 3. Mean number of transfer prompts as a function of grade level and breadth of transfer item.

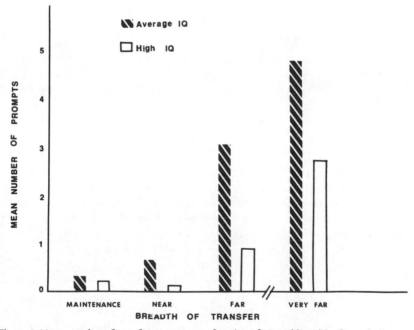

Figure 4. Mean number of transfer prompts as a function of IQ and breadth of transfer item.

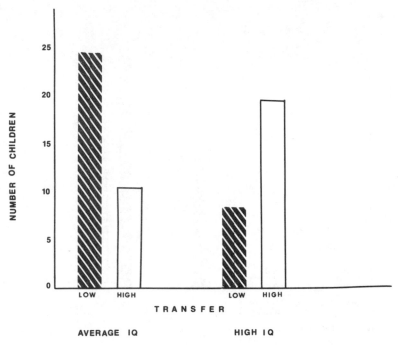

Figure 5. Number of children classified by IQ and degree of transfer.

assistance than fifth-graders as problems departed more drastically from the ones originally learned, and there was similar interaction between IQ and breadth of transfer that is shown in Figure 4. Mimicking the grade effects, farther transfer items were also increasingly sensitive to differences in IQ.

Within each grade, a median split was made on the total number of prompts needed during transfer, and the children were classified into low- and high-transfer groups on this basis. Because the results were very similar in the two grades, we again collapsed across this factor, which produced the pattern shown in Figure 5. IQ predicted degree of transfer for over two-thirds of the children. That is, most of the average-IQ children transferred relatively poorly and most of the high-IQ children transferred relatively well. However, a significant number of children fit neither of these profiles, as can be seen from the middle bars in the figure.

Let us now consider the relationship *between* degree of transfer and speed of learning. There was significant correlation between these two variables as delineated in Figure 6. Once again, however, almost a third of the children did not conform to the consistent slow-learning/low-transfer and fast-learning/high-transfer profiles. Figure 7 shows the breakdown of these

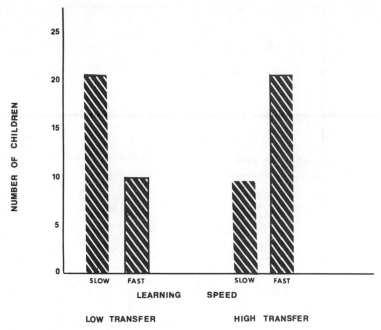

Figure 6. Number of children classified by speed of learning and degree of transfer.

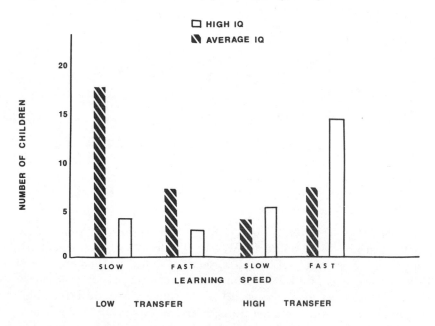

Figure 7. Number of children classified by speed of learning, degree of transfer, and IQ.

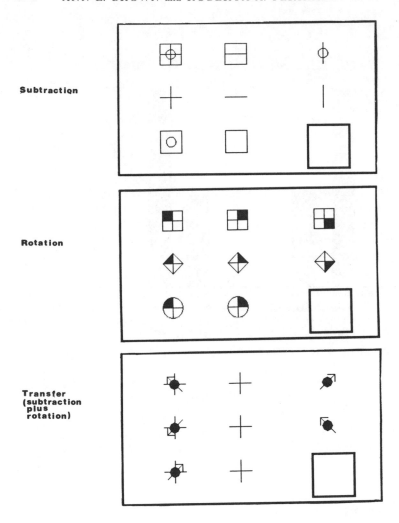

Figure 8. Illustration of two matrix problem types from the original learning session (subtraction and rotation) and a transfer problem (subtraction plus rotation).

profiles by IQ level. Overall, the IQ of almost 50% of the children did not predict learning speed and/or degree of transfer. Thus, from this fairly wide range of "normal" -ability children (IQ range 88–150) a number of different learning profiles have emerged, including (1) slow learners, narrow transferrers, low IQ *(slow)*; (2) fast learners, wide transferrers, high IQ *(fast)*; (3) fast learners, narrow transferrers *(context-bound)*; (4) slow learners, wide transferrers *(reflective)*; and (5) fast learners, wide transferrers, low

IQ (somewhat analogous to Budoff's *high scorers*). All of these profiles are hidden when one considers only the child's initial unaided performance.

Raven's progressive matrices task

We have already developed a second test instrument to use in establishing zones of proximal development in grade school children. The problems are similar to those on the Raven's progressive matrices tests, but we have reduced the number of solution rules and systematized their order of occurrence. Each problem consists of a 3×3 matrix of geometric figures following certain transformational patterns across columns and/or rows. The child's job is to figure out the pattern and to generate the missing figure in the lower-right hand corner. We have developed a computerized situation in which the child can construct the missing figure using a touch-sensitive panel and can receive hints from the computer by pressing a button.

We are using the same general paradigm developed for the letter series completions. Specifically, this entails a session in which the child first becomes thoroughly familiar with the computer and then learns three rules (rotation, superimposition, and subtraction of figures). As needed, she receives a gradated series of animated hints one by one on the computer (for full details, see Ferrara et al., 1983). In subsequent sessions, maintenance and transfer are assessed, again with hints given when requested. Transfer matrices involve a combination of two of the rules initially learned in the context of separate matrix problems. In Figure 8 we give examples of a subtraction problem, a rotation problem, and a transfer problem that combines rotation and subtraction.

The pilot data we have collected to date are encouraging. We will describe the high points briefly. First, samples of average and above average fourth-graders have been tested on the Raven's task. Second, a sample of educable mentally retarded students (IQ=70) have taken part in the learning stages of the program. All of the children learn how to interact with the terminal quite readily, enjoy the "game," and respond well to the hints. We are seeing clear indications of individual differences in the initial protocols. Although the data have not been completely analyzed, learning profiles very similar to those found for the letter series completion task are emerging.

Stability of profiles over tasks

How stable are these learning profiles across tasks? To begin to answer this important question we considered children's performance on the matrices

Table 2. *Learning and maintenance/transfer status of children across two task domains*

	Maintenance/transfer		
	Narrow	Borderline	Wide
Matrices			
Slow-learning	Douglas – CLT	Cliff	Lucie – CL
	Jack – CLT		Conrad
	Scott – CLT		
	Jeanette – CLT		
	Marcia – CL		
	Stuart – CL		
	Daniel – CL		
Borderline-learning	Mark		
Fast-learning	Curtis – CL	Margie – CLT	Sandra – CLT
			Audrey – CLT
			Sally – CLT
			Eddie – CL
			Joshua – CL
			Andrea – CL
			Melissa – CT
			Lizette
Series Completions			
Slow-learning	Douglas		Marcia
	Jack		Stuart
	Scott		Daniel
	Jeanette		
	Lucie		
Borderline-learning	Conrad		Melissa
	Lizette		
Fast-learning	Eddie	Margie	Sandra
	Joshua		Audrey
	Andrea		Sally
			Curtis
			Mark
			Cliff

Note: Slow/Narrow > (median number of hints +.99); borderline = (median ±.99); fast/wide < (median −.99). CLT, consistent in both learning and transfer status; CL, consistent in learning status only; CT, consistent in transfer status only. All names are pseudonyms.

task as well as the series completion task. Both involve inductive reasoning and are believed to share some common underlying operations. Thus far we have collected data from 21 normal fourth-grade children, who were classified on the basis of their speed of learning and breadth of transfer in the two task situations. These data are shown in Table 2.

The results of this investigation were somewhat mixed. Relative learning ability was highly correlated across the task domains. A Pearson product-moment correlation between the hints required to reach the original learning criteria of the matrices and series paradigms was .66 ($p <$ .001). Furthermore 76% of the children displayed the same learning status in both situations. (Children labeled "CL" or "CLT" in Table 2 were consistent in learning status across tasks.) An additional 19% of the subjects showed only a slight inconsistency in learning performance. That is, they shifted to or from a borderline status. Only one child (Cliff) changed from one extreme status to the opposite (from slow to fast learning). Efficiency of learning was thus highly stable across the task domains.

Maintenance/transfer performance, however, appeared much more task-specific than did learning ability. The Pearson correlation for hints in transfer across the two domains was significant although much reduced, $r = .39$, $p < .05$. Of more importance, whereas performance status on transfer within the matrices paradigm was identical to that within the series completion paradigm for 43% of the subjects (those labeled "CT" or "CLT"), an even larger percentage of the children (52%) shifted from one status to the opposite.

Finally, 38% of the subjects yielded profiles that were consistent in *both* learning and transfer status across the two tasks. (See children labeled "CLT" in Table 2.) Most of these fell into the typical slow/narrow or fast/ wide categories of ability in both domains. One child, however, (Margie) displayed a slightly more interesting profile. Within both task situations she was a fast learner but only average in transfer ability. One might say that she was consistently more *context-bound* than most of the other fast learners. We are currently trying to extend these results by conducting a similar study with a mildly retarded population. On the basis of our initial pilot data we expect to find less stable profiles for the aberrant children than we have found with children from within the normal IQ range.

It should be noted that the very far transfer items (secret code problems) that most of the children solved in the series completion study were adapted from the adult Binet scale. And the difficult "combination of rules" transfer problem on the matrices task does not occur until the adult superior version of the actual Raven's tests. With a little prompting a great deal of learning is occurring. Children's zones of proximal development on these tasks are indeed broad. Finally, we point out that different learning profiles such as we have discovered are not only found when children are the learners. Adults, too, display varying zones of proximal development (Fattu, Mech, and Kapos, 1954).

Extensions to young age groups

The success of our initial studies with grade school children is encouraging. The ZPD measures were related to IQ as one might expect, but they provide a better diagnosis of what it means to have a low IQ. Furthermore, if the learning profiles that emerged continue to be stable, it will be possible to consider whether these profiles provide a more sensitive prognosis of a child's particular problem-solving difficulties or strengths than does the simple static measure.

Our particular concern, however, is with the potential utility of ZPD measures at an age when static IQ scores do not act as good predictors, let alone diagnostic aids; that is, we are particularly interested in extending our work to younger children. We think this is not just nice but necessary. U.S. Public Law 94-142 mandates that special education be provided for children at risk for mental retardation from 3 years of age onward (from birth in some states). Compulsory cognitive screening programs are being established. But unless the cognitive deficit is quite severe, we have few reliable tools for detecting early forms of retardation. Basic research into normal cognitive development below age 4 is sparse (although getting better; see Gelman, 1978) and existing infant/preschool IQ tests are unfortunately less informative than one would like concerning mild retardation. The two principal problems are that (1) existing tests tend not to be theory-based, and therefore their diagnostic power is limited; for example, if a child cannot thread beads or indicate a body part at the "correct age," what does this mean in terms of general cognitive status? and (2) the preschool IQ tests are discontinuous with those used at age 6 and above; they tap different processes, contain different types of items, and therefore it is not surprising that their predictive validity is low. A good example of this is that even the "baby" Raven matrices test is discontinuous with the older versions, relying on perceptual matching rather then transformational rules like rotation, superimposition, and subtraction.

As existing IQ tests do not prove to be especially useful for predicting mild retardation or learning disabilities, diagnosing possible causes, or suggesting means of remediation, we sorely need a substitute. Dynamic learning profiles within a domain, such as those found with older children, could be very useful. What we need for preschoolers is a task domain that lends itself to the systematic gradation of prompts and controlled tests of transfer such as in the Ferrara et al. (1983) series completion study. We are currently piloting a variety of such tasks. For example, in a recent masters thesis, Bryant (Bryant et al., 1983) has found a pattern of learning profiles that is essentially similar to those reported in the Ferrara et al. (1983) series completion task. Bryant's subjects, however, were 4- to 6-year-olds, and the task was a very simple Ravens-type puzzle where the child must supply a missing piece that matches in terms of size, color and/or shape. The major profiles of slow, fast, context-bound, and reflective were replicated with the younger children. The stability and predictive validity of these profiles remains to be tested.

Advantages of zones of proximal development indices

Zones of proximal development have many advantages over standardized IQ or achievement scores. First, the whole concept of a zone within a domain suggests a clearly diagnostic function. Unlike the concept of IQ, a zone of proximal development invites the inference that a given child will have differing zones across a variety of domains. For the learning-disabled or mentally retarded child, a diagnosis of, for example, IQ 80 or reading scores three years depressed suggests not only a static estimate of ability but also a general estimate of dullness throughout the cognitive arena. But a description of the child's zone of cognitive operations within a particular sphere does not necessarily imply level of competence in any other arena. It is quite conceivable for a child with a narrow zone of proximal development in one domain to have a broad zone within another. Interest, knowledge, and ability all contribute to the learning potential shown by any one child in any one domain (Brown et al., 1983).

In our studies we have preliminary data to suggest that individual profiles found on one inductive reasoning task are likely to be duplicated on others. This is not surprising since the tasks share so many common factors. We do not predict, however, that the same learning profile would necessarily dominate learning in all situations; indeed, we expect differential readiness across divergent domains as a function of such factors as prior knowledge.

We have interpreted zone of proximal development mapping to include estimates of both efficiency of learning and breadth of transfer – hence, learning profiles such as fast learning–wide transfer. We would like to emphasize, however, that no claims are being made for wide transfer across disparate domains as we have concentrated on range of understanding within a severely restricted territory. Indeed, there are serious reasons for doubting that truly general transfer is the rule in mature learning (Brown et al., 1982b; Brown et al., 1983; Campione, 1982; Laboratory of Comparative Human Cognition, in press). Nevertheless, this does not invalidate the use of transfer as a sensitive individual difference metric.

Learning in some sense must always be context-bound. But contextual binding permits of degrees; generalization and flexibility are not all-or-none phenomena but continua. It is the range of applicability of any particular process by any particular learner that forms the diagnosis of maturity or bounds the zone of proximal development. The less mature, less experienced, less intelligent may suffer from a greater degree of contextual binding, although even the expert is bound by contextual constraint to some degree (Brown, 1982a).

The process of estimating learning and transfer is the process of mapping a particular child's zone width. This provides not only a clear diagnosis of the range of competence that one can expect, but also a rich prescription for remediation. The procedures being developed, both in the Soviet Union and the United States, to map zones of proximal development, have the potential for providing diagnostic tools with prescriptive significance. In order for this potential to be realized we need (1) *theoretically*, close attention to the thorny problem of what constitutes a domain and (2) *practically*, extensions of this work to academic tasks (reading, writing, arithmetic, etc.) so that the diagnostic and prescriptive promise of the zone of proximal development theory can be more fully realized.

Upper versus lower zone boundaries as estimates of cognitive readiness

Formerly, it was believed that by using tests, we determine the mental development level with which education should reckon and whose limits it should not exceed. This procedure oriented learning toward yesterday's development, toward developmental stages already completed. . .learning which is oriented toward developmental levels that have already been reached is ineffective from the viewpoint of a child's overall development. It does not aim for a new stage of the developmental process but rather lags behind this process. Thus, the notion of a zone of proximal development enables us to propound a new formula, namely that the only "good learning" is that which is in advance of development. (Vygotsky, 1978, p. 89)

Here Vygotsky clearly states a new twist on the old readiness problem. For many years it has been axiomatic in psychology and education that instruction should be aimed at the level of competence of the child. But what is meant by the level of the child? Vygotsky clearly warns against estimates of readiness based on the child's existing "unaided" level of performance. As an example of this fallacy, he criticized contemporaneous educational plans for the retarded. Based on the assumption that retarded children were incapable of abstract thinking, special curricula for the retarded were developed using "concrete, look-and-do methods"; that is, educational practices were designed to fit in with the retarded child's putative "inability" to deal with the abstract. Vygotsky denigrated such thinking:

It turned out that a teaching system based solely on concreteness. . .not only failed to help retarded children overcome their innate handicaps but also reinforced their handicaps by accustoming children exclusively to concrete thinking and thus suppressing the rudiments of any abstract thought that such children still have. Precisely because retarded children, when left to themselves, will never achieve well-elaborated forms of abstract thought, the school should make every effort to push them in that direction and to develop in them what is intrinsically lacking in their own development. (Vygotsky, 1978, p. 89)

A zone of proximal development is a map of the child's sphere of readiness, bounded at the lower end by her existing level of competence, but at the upper end by the level of competence she can achieve under the most favorabled circumstances. Vygotsky's insistence that education should be aimed at the upper bound, rather than fettered by the lower, has profound implications for the diagnosis and instruction of all children. But it is particularly important for the retarded child.

Special education in this country provides a good background in a static concept of readiness, and suggestions for instruction based upon estimates of the lower bounds of ability are still all too prevalent. Vygotsky's comments on special curricula for the retarded would not be totally out of place today. Indeed, Feuerstein (pers. comm.) claims that one reason for the dramatic success of his IE program is that teachers for the first time really believe that the retarded adolescent can learn. Demonstrations of the dramatic improvements shown by retarded children after only minimal prompting are exactly what is needed in order to create a more optimistic attitude toward their learning potential.

In a recent study from our laboratory, Palincsar and Brown (1984) demonstrated the efficiency of training cognitive skills by a procedure that mimicked the "ideal" internalization mode suggested by Vygotsky and showed the importance of aiming instruction beyond the child's existing level of competence. The subjects were seventh-graders, not officially diagnosed as learning-disabled but referred by their teachers as children with severe reading comprehension problems. They were able to decode at grade level, but in spite of this, the major remedial training they had received prior to our intervention was aimed at decoding skills. Because of their supposed incompetence on comprehension tasks, they were rarely exposed to comprehension exercises on which, presumably, they were expected to fail. In the training sessions, the children took part in tutorial dialogues, one-on-one with the experimenter; the tutor and the child engaged in an interactive learning game that involved taking turns in leading a dialogue concerning small segments of texts. Both the tutor and the child would read a text segment, and then the dialogue leader would engage in a variety of comprehension-fostering activities such as paraphrasing the main idea, questioning any ambiguities, predicting the possible questions that might be asked about the segment, and hypothesizing about the content of the remaining passage segments. The dialogue leader would then ask the other a question on the segment. In the next segment the roles were reversed.

Initially, the tutor modeled these activities, and the child had great difficulty assuming the role of dialogue leader when her turn came. The tutor was forced to resort to constructing paraphrases and questions for the tutee to mimic. In this initial phase, the tutor was modeling effective comprehension-fostering strategies, but the child was a relatively passive observer.

In the intermediate phase, the tutee became much more capable of playing her role as dialogue leader, and by the end of 10 sessions she was providing paraphrases and questions of some sophistication. For example, in the initial sessions 55% of questions produced by the tutees were judged to be nonquestions or questions needing clarification, but by the end of the session only 4% of questions were so judged. And at the beginning of the sessions only 11% of the questions were aimed at main ideas, but by the end of the sessions 64% of all questions probed comprehension of salient gist. Similar progress was made in producing paraphrases of the main ideas of the text segment. At the beginning of the sessions only 11% of summary statements captured main ideas, whereas at the end 60% of the statements were so classified. The comprehension-monitoring activities of the tutees certainly improved, becoming more and more like those modeled by the tutor. With repeated interactive experiences, with the tutor and child mutually constructing a cohesive representation of the text, the tutees became able to employ these monitoring functions for themselves.

This improvement was revealed not just in the interactive sessions but on privately read passages where the students were required to answer comprehension questions on their own. In the laboratory, such tests of comprehension were given throughout the experiment. On these independent tests, performance improved from 10% to 85% correct. And in the classroom, the students moved from the 7th to the 40th percentile compared with all other seventh-graders in the school. Not only did the students learn to perform comprehension-fostering activities in interaction with their tutor, they were also able to *internalize* these procedures as part of their own cognitive processes for reading. Via the intervention of a supportive, knowledgeable other, the child is led to the limits of her own understanding. The tutor did *not*, however, tell the child what to do; she entered into an interaction where the child and the tutor were mutually responsible for getting the task done. As the child adopts more of the essential skills initially undertaken by the adult, the adult relinquishes control. Transference of power is gradually and mutually agreed upon.

Training that mimics naturally occurring teaching styles does seem to be very successful. Palincsar, in her Ph.D. thesis, is investigating the feasibility of classroom teachers conducting similar training procedures in group settings. Her initial data are encouraging. An important side benefit she noticed is that the teachers' "theory of the child" changed dramatically after experiencing the reciprocal questioning sessions. Teachers claim that they had "no idea" that these children (poor comprehenders) were capable of asking such ingenious questions. By testing the limits of a child's abilities, by aiming instruction at the upper rather than the lower bound of a child's zone, a quite different picture of competence is revealed. As the teacher's "theory of the child" changes, so does the level and type of performance she demands. The teacher is in fact functioning in the child's "region of sensitivity to instruction" (Wood and Middleton, 1975) or zone of proximal development (Vygotsky, 1978). As the child advances so does the level of collaboration demanded by the teacher. The teacher systematically shapes their joint experiences in such a way that the child will be drawn into taking more and more responsibility for the dyad's work. In so doing the teacher not only provides an optimal learning environment, she also models appropriate comprehension-fostering activities; these crucial regulatory activities are thereby made *overt* and *explicit*.

Conclusion

We have described two important educational implications of Vygotsky's theory of a zone of proximal development that we are pursuing in our laboratory. First, there is the potential application of the idea to the design of dynamic measures of learning potential within a domain. Learning profiles such as context-bound or reflective, appear to be stable and have potential for adding significantly to the diagnostic and remedial sensitivity of testing procedures over and above existing static IQ and achievement measures. This potential is particularly promising for the early identification of mild learning problems.

The second educational implication of Vygotsky's theory is the importance of aiming instruction at the upper bound of a child's zone. By concentrating on the level a student can reach with aid, the student is led to levels of success previously not envisaged by either the student or the teacher. If educational practices are geared only to the student's level of unaided competence, that student may be denied the very experience necessary to increase her zone of proximal development. We believe that both of these ideas have important implications for contemporary educational practice.

NOTES

Preparation of this manuscript and portions of the research reported therein have been supported by PHS Grants HD-05951 and HD-00111 from the National Institute of Child Health and Human Development, as well as fellowships awarded to the second author by the University of Illinois at Urbana–Champaign. Thanks are also due to Joseph C. Campione for helpful criticisms regarding portions of the manuscript.

1   It should come as no surprise that significant IQ-related differences in learning performance occurred only when the task was of an appropriate level of difficulty for the child. In other words, it appears that the item types learned were too simple for the fifth-graders, and thus IQ effects were not manifested here as they were in the case of the younger children. The various transfer items were apparently more challenging for all of the children, however; and thus IQ-related differences in transfer ability appeared in both age groups.

REFERENCES

Au, K. 1980. A test of the social organizational hypothesis: Relationships between participation structures and learning to read. Doctoral dissertation, University of Illinois.

Baker, L., and Brown, A. L. 1984a. Metacognition and the reading process. In P. D. Pearson (Ed.), *A handbook of reading research*. New York: Longman.

Baker, L., and Brown, A. L. 1984b. Cognitive monitoring in reading. In J. Flood (Ed.), *Understanding reading comprehension*. Newark, Del.: International Reading Association.

Binet, A. 1909. *Les idées modernes sur les infants*. Paris: Ernest Flamarion.

Bransford, J. D., Stein, B. S., Arbitman-Smith, R., and Vye, N.J. In press. Three approaches to improving thinking and learning skills. In S. Chipman, J. Segal, and R. Glaser (Eds.), *Thinking and learning skills: Current research and open questions* (Vol. 2) Hillsdale, N.J.: Erlbaum.

Brown, A. L. 1975. The development of memory: Knowing, knowing about knowing, and knowing how to know. In H. W. Reese (Ed.), *Advances in child development and behavior* (Vol. 10). New York: Academic Press.

Brown, A. L. 1978. Knowing when, where, and how to remember: A problem of metacognition, In R. Glaser (Ed.), *Advances in instructional psychology* (Vol. 1). Hillsdale, N.J.: Erlbaum.

Brown, A. L. 1980. Metacognitive development and reading. In R. J. Spiro, B. Bruce, and W. Brewer (Eds.), *Theoretical issues in reading comprehensions: Perspectives from cognitive psychology, linguistics, artificial intelligence, and education*. Hillsdale, N.J.: Erlbaum.

Brown, A. L. 1982a. Learning and development: The problems of compatibility, access, and induction. *Human development*, *25*, 89–115.

Brown, A. L. 1982b. Metacognition, executive control, self-regulation and other even more mysterious mechanisms. In F. E. Weinert and R. H. Kluwe (Eds.), *Learning by thinking*. West Germany: Kuhlhammer.

Brown, A. L., Bransford, J. D., Ferrara, R. A., and Campione, J. C. 1983. Learning, remembering, and understanding. In J. H. Flavell and E. M. Markman (Eds.), *Carmichael's manual of child psychology* (Vol. 1). New York: Wiley.

Brown, A. L., and Campione, J. C. 1978. Memory strategies in learning: Training children to study strategically. In H. L. Pick, H. W. Leibowitz, J. E. Singer, A. Steinschneider, and H. W. Stevenson (Eds.), *Psychology from research to practice*. New York: Plenum Press.

Brown, A. L., and Campione, J. C. 1981. Inducing flexible thinking: A problem of access. In M. Friedman, J. P. Das, and N. O'Connor (Eds.), *Intelligence and learning*. New York: Plenum Press.

Brown, A. L., and French, L. A. 1979. The zone of potential development: Implications for intelligence testing in the year 2000. *Intelligence*, *3*, 255–277.

Brown, A. L. Palincsar, A. S., and Armbruster, B. B. In press. Inducing comprehension-fostering activities in interactive learning situations. In H. Mandl, N. Stein, and T. Trabasso (Eds.), *Learning and comprehension of texts*. Hillsdale, N.J.: Erlbaum.

Brożek, J. 1972. To test or not to test: Trends in the Soviet views. *Journal of the History of the Behavioral Sciences*, *8*, 243–248.

Bryant, N. Brown, A. L., and Campione, J. C. 1983. Preschool children's learning and transfer of matrices problems: A study of proximal development. Manuscript, University of Illinois.

Budoff, M. 1974. *Learning potential and educability among the educable mentally retarded*. Final report, Project No. 312312, OEG-0-8-080506-4597. Department of Health, Education, and Welfare. December.

Campione, J. C., and Brown, A. L. 1977. Memory and metamemory development in educable retarded children. In R. V. Kail, Jr., and J. W. Hagen (Eds.), *Perspectives on the development of memory and cognition*. Hillsdale, N.J.: Erlbaum.

Campione, J. C., and Brown, A. L. 1978. Toward a theory of intelligence: Contributions from research with retarded children. *Intelligence*, *2*, 279–304.

Campione, J. C., and Brown, A. L., and Ferrara, R. A. 1982. Mental retardation and intelligence. In R. J. Sternberg (Ed.), *Handbook of human intelligence*. Cambridge: Cambridge University Press.

Cole, M., and Traupmann, K. 1980. Comparative cognitive research: Learning from a learning disabled child. In A. Collins (Ed.), *Minnesota symposium on child psychology*. Hillsdale, N.J.: Erlbaum.

Collins, J. 1980. Differential treatment in reading groups. In J. Cook-Gumperz (Ed.), *Educational discourse*. London: Heinneman.

Egorova, T. V. 1973. *Pecularities of memory and thinking in developmentally backward school children*. Moscow: Moscow University Press.

Fattu, N. A., Mech, E., and Kapos, E. 1954. Some statistical relationships between selected response dimensions and problem-solving proficiency. *Psychological Monographs*, *68*, (Whole No. 377).

Ferrara, R. A., Brown, A. L., and Campione, J. C. 1983. Children's learning and transfer of inductive reasoning rules: A study of proximal development. Manuscript, University of Illinois.

Feuerstein, R. 1969. The instrumental enrichment method: An outline of theory and technique. Manuscript, Hadassah-Wiza-Canada Research Institute, Jerusalem.

Feuerstein, R. 1979. *The dynamic assessment of retarded performers: The learning potential assessment device, theory, instruments, and techniques*. Baltimore: University Park Press.

Feuerstein, R. 1980. *Instrumental enrichment: An intervention program for cognitive modifiability*. Baltimore: University Park Press.

Feuerstein, R., Rand, Y., Hoffman, M., Hoffman, M., and Miller, R. 1979. Cognitive modifiability in retarded adolescents: Effects of instrumental enrichment. *American Journal of Mental Deficiency*, *83*, 539–550.

Gagné, R. M. 1970. *The conditions of learning* (2nd ed.). New York: Holt, Rinehart and Winston.

Gelman, R. 1978. Cognitive development. *Annual Review of Psychology*, *29*, 297–332.

Gumperz, J. J. 1980. *Ethnography and controlled experimentation in the study of reading*. Paper presented at the Reading Comprehension Conference, Center for the Study of Reading, University of Illinois, Champaign, May.

Haywood, H. C., Filler, J. W., Jr., Shifman, M. A., and Chatelanat, G. 1975. Behavioral assessment in mental retardation. In P. McReynolds (Ed.), *Advances in psychological assessment* (Vol. 3). Palo Alto, Calif.: Science and Behavior Books.

Haywood, H. C., and Smith, R. A. 1979. *Modifications of cognitive functions in slow learning adolescents*. Paper presented at the International Association of Mental Deficiency meetings, Jerusalem, August.

Höffding, H. 1982. *Outlines of psychology*. Translated by M. E. Lowndes. London: Macmillan.

Jacobs, P. I., and Vandeventer, M. 1972. Evaluating the teaching of intelligence. *Educational and Psychological Measurement*, *32*, 235–248.

Kotovsky, K. and Simon, H. A. 1973. Empirical tests of a theory of human acquisition of concepts for sequential patterns. *Cognitive Psychology*, *4*, 399–424.

Laboratory of Comparative Human Cognition. 1983. Culture and cognitive development. In W. Kessen (Ed.), *Handbook of child psychology* (Vol. 1). *History, theory and method*. New York: Wiley.

McDermott, R. D. 1978. Some reasons for focusing on classrooms in reading research. In P. D. Pearson and J. Hansen (Eds.), *Reading: Disciplined inquiry in process and practice*. Twenty-seventh yearbook of the National Reading Conference. Clemson, S.C.: National Reading Conference.

Mehan, H. 1973. Assessing children's language using abilities: Methodological and cross-cultural implications. In M. Armer and A. D. Grimshaw (Eds.), *Comparative social research: Methodological problems and strategies*. New York: Wiley.

Narrol, H., and Bachor, D. G. 1975. An introduction to Feuerstein's approach to assessing and developing cognitive potential. *Interchange*, *6*, 2–16.

Palincsar, A. S., and Brown, A. L. 1984. Reciprocal teaching of comprehension-fostering and monitoring activities. *Cognition and instruction*. Hillsdale, N.J.: Erlbaum.

Resnick, L. B., and Glaser, R. 1976. Problem solving and intelligence. In L. B. Resnick (Ed.), *The nature of intelligence*. Hillsdale, N.J.: Erlbaum.

Thorndike, E. L. 1926. *The measurement of intelligence*. New York: Teacher's College, Columbia University.

Thorndike, E. L., and Woodworth, R. S. 1901. The influence of improvements in one mental function upon the efficiency of other functions. *Psychological Review*, *8*, 247–261, 384–395, 553–564.

Vlasova, T. A. 1972. New advances in Soviet defectology. *Soviet Education*. *14* (1–3), 20–39.

Vlasova, T. A., and Pevzner, M. S. (Eds.). 1971. *Deti s vremennymi zaderzhkami razvitiya* [Children with temporary retardation in development]. Moscow: Pedagogika.

Vygotsky, L. S. 1978. *Mind in society: The development of higher psychological processes*. Cambridge: Harvard University Press.

Wertsch, J. V. 1978. Adult–child interaction and the roots of metacognition. *Quarterly Newsletter of the Institute for Comparative Human Development*, *1*, 15–18.

Wood, D., and Middleton, D. 1975. A study of assisted problem-solving. *British Journal of Psychology*, *66*, 181–191.

Wozniak, R. H. 1975. Psychology and education of the learning disabled child in the Soviet Union. In W. Cruikshank and D. P. Hallahan (Eds.), *Perceptual and learning disabilities in children*, Vol. 1, *Psychoeducational practices*. Syracuse: Syracuse University Press.

Zabramna, S. D. (Ed.). 1971. *Otbor detei vo vspomogatel'nye shkoly*. [The selection of children for schools for the mentally retarded.] Moscow: Prosveshchenie.

13

The tacit background of children's judgments

KARSTEN HUNDEIDE

Interpretive background and recurrent episodes

For most people life is organized in terms of routines and recurrent episodes: We get up in the morning, have breakfast, travel to work, and so on – the same thing day after day, year after year. There may be slight variations, and some routines are more variable than others, but the basic feature of recurrence is preponderant.

This certainly has advantages in the sense that we can *predict both forward and backward*. When some new situation comes up, we can reconstruct its past because most events are tied into routines, and we can anticipate its future – after B comes C and then D and then the goal. Most of our life is organized in such routines with a typical, recurrent structure, and this makes it easier for us to understand both our fellow human beings and maybe also ourselves. With just a short look out the window we see our neighbor passing, and we conclude, "He is going early to work today." We do not see physical movements, not even actions, *we see human beings carrying out goal-directed projects within the tracks of well-established routines*. Both the tracks and the projects are well known to us, so we do not need to ponder inductively about the meaning of the movements we see (e.g., our neighbor passing). It is rather the other way around, from above to below. We project the tracks of a routine and project from *a repertoire of typical episodes* relevant and likely in such situations. Just a short look out the window is sufficient to conclude firmly, "He was going to. . . ." In other words, we understand and attribute meaning to other people's behavior by *assimilating it into a structure of typical recurrent episodes with definite goals*.

It is this repertoire of recurrent episodes and routines from everyday life that constitutes what I would like to call our *interpretive background*. This is basically a shared collective structure organized as episodes that reflects the regularities of life within a society with a particular social structure, culture, language, history, and ecology. In fact, in order to experience anything as ordered and meaningful, there must be some *recurrence* in our

306

experience. A world of unique experiences is impossible because unique-ness presupposes a basis of ordinary, recurrent experience. The atypical is only possible with reference to the typical. Any meaningful and ordered experience – "It is *this* – not *that*" and presupposes recurrence. It must have happened before.

The basis of all meaningful and ordered experience is therefore re-currence and typification. Any meaningful experience must be recognized as a variant of a typical, recurrent episode, and it is this *recognition* that is usually described as "assimilation" or "construction of meaning." The point I wish to convey is that we do not interpret the world around us in terms of isolated units of things, actions, or even utterances. Rather, these are always embedded in contexts, or more specifically, in typical social episodes (Forgas, 1979; Harre and Secord, 1972), "settings" (Barker, 1965), "situations" (Thomas and Znanicki, 1923), or "frames" (Goffman, 1974) that regulate "what can go on." It is this *superordinate framework* that conveys "sense" to the discrete units. In most of our external daily actions this is obvious. When we are hungry at midday and go for lunch, we not only obtain food, but also participate in a more or less strictly organized social event where our particular, discrete actions are regulated and take on meaning from being embedded in the total episode. We understand and define ourselves as intentionally participating in particular social episodes, and our understanding or interpretation of other people's behavior and utterances is determined by the particular episode we *assume* they are tak-ing part in. In Norway when a person puts his hand out a car window, this will most probably be interpreted as an episode of greeting a friend, whereas in England the same movement might be interpreted as a signal to cars behind that the person is going to slow down. Thus we see the same movement and two completely different interpretations, depending upon which episode the movement is assimilated into. In fact, it is usually not possible to understand isolated movements or utterances without taking into account the total cultural context or episode in which it is embedded. This is what Geertz (1973) has called "thick description" as opposed to the behaviorists' "thin description."

Episodic definitions and problem solving

When it comes to external actions embedded in social episodes, it is fairly obvious that "thick description" is necessary to get to the "sense" of the act. But what about internal action, problem solving, and reasoning? It seems that like Piaget, we often tend to assume that such operations are regulated by logical structures that are more or less abstracted and dissociated from the sociocultural context. We tend to operate on the basis of this assumption even though Wason and Johnson-Laird (1972) have warned us that most people do not seem to solve even deductive problems by reference to logical models, but by reference to concrete experience. This is of course particularly evident among people "without writing" who are outside Western intellectual influence (Luria, 1976; Cole and Scribner, 1974). However, according to Wason and Johnson-Laird, it also applies to Western thinkers, even those specially trained in logic. This may seem surprising to Piaget, and recently he has in fact modified his theory on this point (see Piaget, 1972). However, it would not be surprising to Vygotsky because, if he was correct in assuming that mental operations have their origin in interactions among people, then the initial *prototypical episode* remains relatively closely associated with what later becomes internalized and abstracted as mental operations. It still concerns operations derived from a cultural context, and it still is not yet clear *how far the dissociation goes* when interaction between people becomes mental operations and internal dialogues. What is clear is that most people seem to think more in concrete, recurrent episodes from daily life than we would expect from Piaget's theory of formal operations.

Let us turn to a concrete example: Boschowitsch (1974, p. 217) has described how children give completely different replies to physics problems depending upon whether they were asked in the classroom by a teacher or were asked informally by a psychologist during recess. When the teacher in the classroom asked questions such as "Why does a piece of wood float?" the children all repeated Archimedes' law that they had learned earlier. When the psychologist asked the same question during recess, most of them gave "preoperational replies" of the type "It floats because it is light." When the psychologist asked them why they answered differently than they had in the classroom with the teacher, they answered, "Oh, do you want me to reply as I did in the classroom?" and then repeated Archimedes' law. Somehow *the correct logical procedure seems to have been embedded in a social episode involving a formal classroom setting with an authoritarian-looking teacher posing the questions*. It is a special game in a special setting.

As a second example consider the following. A student of mine who had taught mathematics to mildly retarded children told me about an experience he had while trying to teach a fourth-grader how to solve equations. This pupil had a long history of school failure, and no matter how my student tried to help him, it was all in vain. The pupil simply repeated that it was too difficult and that he was stupid since he did "not even know how to read properly." Any attempt to help this pupil within a traditional school setting was bound to fail since he immediately assimilated it to previous episodes of failure. This pupil did not even try to solve the problems presented to him; he had predefined the outcome.

On one occasion my student took this pupil into the teacher's room after a class and asked him if he would like to participate in a game that he used to play when he was a boy. The student agreed. My student then asked him: "Think of a number, add 2, what do you get?" The boy answered "6" and my student told the boy that he had been thinking of 4. This astonished the pupil and he wanted to learn the secret. After a few attempts they changed roles and he had no trouble solving such equations in his mind. There was evidently nothing wrong with his mental operations in this new context. However, on the following day when my student tried to explain equations to him in the traditional manner (i.e., in accordance with a textbook in a classroom setting) there was no change. The pupil could not understand. His "mental retardation" seemed to be due more to his definition of the teaching episode and his anticipated role as a failure (Hundeide, 1980) than to any deficiency in mental operations per se.

Mental operations, I suspect, are always embedded in a broader framework of typical episodes and self-definitions, and these may block or facilitate the manifestations of such operations. This conclusion is in fact very much in line with Leont'ev's (1981) analysis of how an "action" may be embedded in different "activities" and thus achieve different "senses":

Let us imagine that a child is trying to solve a particular problem which has been assigned in his homework. She/he of course is conscious of the goal of his/her action. It is to find the required solution and write it down. His/her action is directed towards that goal. But how is this goal consciously understood, i.e., what sense does this action have for the child? In order to answer this, we must know the *activity* in which this action is included or, what amounts to the same thing, what is the motive that energizes this action. Maybe the motive is to master arithmetic, maybe it is to avoid angering the teacher, or finally, maybe it is simply to make it possible to go out and play with one's friends. In all of these cases the goal is objectively the same – to solve the assigned problem. But the sense of this action for the child is different in the various cases. Therefore, the same action will be psychologically different for him/her. (Quoted in Wertsch, 1981b)

This example illustrates very clearly the fact that different actions and operations may have different senses (in this case boring or interesting) depending upon the overall activity in which they are embedded. But there is another and more important aspect of this that is particularly relevant for problem solving since this is a *sequentially organized activity*. If a problem x is assimilated into activity or episodic structure a, the *sequential implications* ($x - y - z$) may be completely different than when it is assimilated into episodic structure b ($x - d - e$). Therefore, if the correct solution presupposes the sequence $x - y - z$, *it depends upon the episodic definition of the problem, that is, in what order and through what sequence of steps it is plausible to proceed*. So solving and understanding a problem is not only a question of executing a sequence of mental operations, it is also a question of *defining the problem* as part of a context or episode *that has sequential implications in which such operations are plausible*. From this point of view, Duncker's (1945) functional fixedness and much of the earlier research on "set" and "direction" (Johnson, 1955) can be interpreted as cases of episodic definitions with relevant or irrelevant sequential implications.

The tacit background

As mentioned earlier, our interpretive background is constituted by recurrent episodes and routines from everyday life that are taken for granted and in this sense unconscious. This background provides a definite direction and *structure to our expectations about what is going to take place*, provided the episodic definition is clear. Now, let us say there is some deviation from the expected pattern. Provided that there is some commitment to the whole episode, then this deviation will stand out. Attention will be aroused and the deviation will appear as *a phenomenon of interest*. We find this reaction to deviations from expectancy at all developmental levels, from infants (Kagan, 1971) and animals to adult human beings (Eckblad, 1981).

When we reflect on this phenomenon or when a disruption in goal-directed activities occurs, then it becomes *a problem to be solved*. But it is important to recognize that this *concerns a background of expectancies that are usually taken for granted*. A single objective event may be experienced as a trivial routine experience by one person, as an unusual phenomenon to be explained by another, and as an obstacle or an adaptive problem requiring procedural solutions by a third. Analyzing the solution or response in terms of correctness is, therefore, to beg the question. What interests us in this context is not correctness, but why this is a problem and in which way it is a problem. That is, we are concerned with identifying the tacit assumptions or expectations that create and define the problem.

We tend to overlook the fact that problems only exist in relation to a background of expectations that are usually taken for granted. For this reason we tend to objectify both problems and "correct replies." An alternative way to proceed is to accept the incorrect reply and try to investigate what could have been the "real question" given this reply. Furthermore, one can go one step further: Given this problem, what could be the tacit background of expectancies?

Such an approach is relevant not only to cognitive and developmental psychology, but also to historical and cross-cultural studies. When we study other cultures with different institutions and episodic structuring of reality, we may find that the definition required for the proper execution of certain mental operations that are of interest to us are *outside the episodic repertoire of that culture*. In such cases, an orthodox Piagetian diagnostician runs the risk of diagnosing an entire culture as "preoperational." Cole and Scribner (1974) provide some illuminating examples of this. In order to prevent this, one needs a framework that takes into account the historical and cultural basis of individual minds: the collective institutionalized knowledge and routines, categorization of reality with its typifications, world view, normative expectations as to how people, situations, and the world are and should be, and so forth. All this is tacit knowledge that has its origin beyond the individual, and it is this sociocultural basis that forms the interpretive background of our individual minds. *It seems to me that this is exactly what the Vygotskian tradition is trying to take into account* (Vygotsky, 1978; Luria, 1976). Leont'ev's theory of activity seems to be particularly relevant in this respect (Leont'ev, 1981; Cole, 1980; Wertsch, 1981a).

Before leaving the subject of the relationship between what is taken for granted and what is problematic, I would like to add a few more points, emphasizing the relativity that is implicit in such a historical–cultural view. What comes into the focus of awareness, what is interesting and problematic is always related to a *standard* of what is taken for granted as typical and normal. Let us call this the "standard of normative expectancies." Our awareness is not engaged by the familiar and the trivial that is in complete agreement with this standard. Rather, it is the *deviations* from this standard that attract our attention. It *must* be so; it would not be possible to experience anything as new if we did not have reference to a standard of what is old and familiar. In other words, our reaction to novelty is a *relational reaction*: It is "this in relation to that." But so are all our other psychological reactions and constructions. What we experience as depressing, uplifting, boring, exciting, pathological, and normal is always based on a standard, and *it is the deviations from that standard that create reactions*. But deviations from a standard can go in two different directions, namely deviation in the *level of intensity or quantity* of a single dimension and deviation in the *category or dimension itself*.

Let us first consider deviations as to levels of intensity. This applies in particular to our affective and perceptual reactions. Feelings of sadness or happiness, perceptions of beauty or ugliness, heat or cold are all based on *comparison with a tacit standard of expectancy about a definite level of intensity* along various dimensions. It is very important to recognize that *if this standard changes, the experience will also change*. Such experiences are therefore always *relative*; they depend on the level of stability of the standard of normative expectancy. As this standard changes, new experiences become habituated and taken for granted. This implies that *there is never a direct relationship between relational experiences and absolute physical stimulus conditions*. The relationship is always based on the established standard of normative expectancy at any time (Helson, 1964; Crosby, 1976). This is important because we sometimes tend to associate affective states (e.g., feelings of unhappiness and despair) directly with physical conditions, but these conditions might not appear to be unusual to people who live in extreme poverty according to our standards. Hence there is no *direct* connection here. It always depends upon a comparison with a standard of normative expectancy. If poverty is someone's only "world," the standard of expectancy will be adjusted to this external condition and feelings of deprivation will not arise. According to this model, such feelings will appear only when the standard is adjusted to a level that is higher than the present condition. The adjustability of the standard of normative expectancy can therefore be considered an important adaptive mechanism that may prevent sustained states of extreme emotional reactions.

When it comes to deviation from a *category* or dimension, we are concerned with the *breadth of experience* or the monotony–variation dimension. In a world that is completely homogeneous in certain aspects – like the fish in the water – there cannot possibly be any awareness of those aspects because such *awareness presupposes a comparison with alternatives*. As is the case with the fish's standard of normative expectancy, which we could call a *recurrent alternative,* there is no deviation, no comparison, and therefore no awareness.

In other words, awareness of an aspect presupposes a comparison with a standard or a contrasting alternative. Even more strongly we might say that *aspects are not inherent in the things themselves, but are construed through a comparison with contrasting alternatives*. This is an insight that according to Rommetveit (Chapter 8, this volume) should be attributed to Wittgenstein (1968).

Let us take another example to see how this can be applied historically to the experience of aspects in music. When we listen to, say, Mozart, the striking quality that completely dominates our experience is the historical style of "Vienna classicism." This is the first thing we recognize. Only gradually do we learn to discern the particular qualities of Mozart compared to Haydn and others. In other words, from our present "position" in the twentieth century, we have available certain typical recurrent style alternatives that were not available to Mozart. He could not possibly experience his historical presuppositions in the same way we do. For him most of what we associate with his music would probably have to be part of his taken-for-granted background. In more general terms, the experience of hearing Mozart's music will depend upon which style alternatives we take for granted as a basis for *comparison*. Therefore, there must necessarily be many possible ways of experiencing his music.

There is thus always a basis of homogeneity and recurrence of typical alternatives that are taken for granted, and it is this "background" that becomes our "interpretive position" from which reality is "seen," "defined," or "construed." Depending on the "interpretive position" of the experiencing person or the recurrent alternatives available to him, the meanings of a piece of music, a sentence, an action, or a situation may be experienced or "construed" differently (Kelly, 1955; Rommetveit, 1979). Relativity is therefore something fundamental in human experience. It is as applicable to the study of affective reactions and perceptual judgments as it is to the study of the construction of meaning, aspects, and "realities." Fortunately, beyond such temporary changes and variations, there is a more stable historical–cultural background, social structure, and ecological environment. These provide a basis for the recurrence and stability used in our construction of reality. Still it is a construction, and it is a construction from a certain position, as we shall see.

Perspectivism, contrasting alternatives, and abstraction

"Knowledge is always from a position," says Mannheim (1936), and the same applies to all cultural manifestations. Not only as individuals, but also as groups and communities *our perspectives are bound by our historical-cultural background of recurrence*, which is our "position" in the broad sense of the word. This is the taken-for-granted interpretative background. The word "position" implies a *pluralism of perspectives*; it implies that our present insight is *never absolute* but *partial* and *relative* and might be *changed when we move into a different position*.

This perspectival–spatial metaphor has been fruitfully applied in the study of ideology, attitudes, and the production of knowledge in general. Mannheim (1936), who was one of the leading proponents of this tradition, expressed the essence of perspectivity in the following way.

It is not a source of error that in a visual picture of an object in space we can. . .get only a perspective view. The problem is not how we might arrive at a nonperspective picture, but how, by juxtaposing the various points of view, each perspective may be recognized as such and thereby a new level of objectivity attained. . .the false ideal of a detached, impersonal point of view must be replaced by the ideal of an essentially human point of view which is within the limits of a human perspective, constantly trying to enlarge itself. . . .Perspectivism refers to the existential determination of knowledge in opposition to the immanent and objectivist determination. (Pp. 266–267)

The essence of perspectivism is therefore the recognition that knowledge and cultural manifestations are never absolute and universally valid, but are always *partial* and *relative*. But this does not mean that there are no criteria for deciding what is right and wrong. Rather it means that such criteria never can be formulated in absolute terms. They can be formulated only in terms of the perspective of a given situation [see Rommetveit (1979) for a similar argument]. This approach to knowledge and other cultural manifestations of the human mind has far-reaching implications for cross-cultural psychology and for the interpretation of any kind of sociocultural deviation. I will return to these issues in the final section of this chapter.

In addition to the general description of perspectivism outlined so far, I would like to add a few more specific points, using Figure 1 as a point of reference.

1. When one is in a definite position such as A, there are certain things one can see directly (i.e., directly ahead or in front). They occupy a *central position in the field of vision* (a_2). Other things are in the *periphery*, and still others again are *outside one's field of vision* or perspective (B alternatives, C, and A).

2. When this spatial model is interpreted metaphorically as applying to issues of thinking and judgment, we can include that when we are in a definite *interpretive position*; there are certain conclusions, judgments, and insights that can be *immediately seen as plausible and evident*. Other insights are impossible, irrelevent or implausible from this position.

3. Although it may seem to be a trivial implication, it is significant to note that in order to arrive at a definite conclusion or insight, one must be in the *right position*, a position from which this conclusion can be seen as evident and plausible. This is completely in agreement with Wertheimer's recommendations for sound thinking (Wertheimer, 1945). It follows that if one is in "*a false position*" in relation to a certain conclusion or insight, there is little point in elaborating alternatives from that position. Instead, one needs to "restructure the field," as the Gestalt psychologists put it; one must redefine the situation (Kelly, 1955; Raaheim, 1978). This means that one must *come to another interpretative position* from which the conclusion can be seen as evident and plausible. This may also have some practical implications. With reference to what was said earlier about episodic definitions and sequential implications, being in the "right position" means defining the problem within an episode with sequential implications that make the "correct solution" plausible. (Rommetveit, 1978; Hundeide, 1981b)

4. It is *not possible to see one's own position*. In order to see it, one *must be outside it*, which means that one is in a new position. In other words, there is always a taken-for-granted background of premises and assumptions that forms a basis. We are always in some position, and a nonperspectivistic view is not possible, at least not for human beings. This does not in any way preclude self-reflection. But even that is from a position that cannot be "seen" at the moment of cognition.

5. On the right side of the figure, there is a representation of a movement from A or B to C. I have called this an *expansion of perspective*. It is an expansion because position C has a wider perspective with more options than the two other positions. This expansion may result from a *confrontation* between

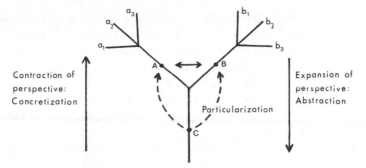

Figure 1. Spatial model of alternative perspectives.

positions, between *the recurrent alternative one takes for granted* and *a contrasting alternative* (A — B). In order to solve this conflict, the person may have to "move back" to the more detached and abstract position C. From this position both conflicting perspectives may be integrated and united. This *may* take place, but there is also the possibility of *uncoordinated alternation* between the two positions and perspectives. It is possible to shift back and forth between the two perspectives without integrating them into a unified solution. We can sometimes see this shifting in conversation experiments with young children. Moving from position B or A to C involves *abstraction* and *particularization*. A and B are no longer absolute alternatives, but they become *particular cases* under C.

6. There is also the opposite movement from C to A or B. I call this the *contraction of perspective*. This term was chosen because it is a movement from a wider more inclusive position to a narrower one with fewer options. Contraction of perspective may take place under conditions of monotony, reduced variation, or the absence of contrasting alternatives. Under such conditions, the focus of awareness will be directed to the more concrete details where there is still some variation and contrasts. But if the monotony persists, even these details become recurrent, and awareness is attracted to even finer nuances and details, while at the same time the more general and abstract aspects of one's background continue to fade away. This contraction and *concretization of perspective* may take place in institutions, prisons, and camps with extremely monotonous routines.

What is described under the terms expansion and contraction of perspective should be viewed not only as momentary reactions to variation, but also as *two general developmental principles*. These principles regulate human cognition in accordance with more or less stabilized cognitive styles corresponding to the level of variation and *breadth of contrasting alternatives* in a form of life. Somehow, when we think about abstraction, we tend to think of a process of finding a common denominator among preexisting attributes. According to a perspectivistic view, abstraction is a more constructive process that cannot be separated from the generation of an aspect. Both presuppose the presence of a contrasting alternative: One cannot abstract without abstracting *something*, and one cannot generate an aspect without presupposing some level of abstraction. Thus in our earlier Wittgensteinian conclusion that "what I perceive in the drawing of an aspect is not a property of the object, but an internal relation between it and other objects" (1968, p. 212), we were concerned not only with a new theory of abstraction and cognitive development. It follows from this that the context of variation and contrast in one's way of life within a community plays an important role in determining which aspects are generated and at what level of abstraction.

Since the context of variation and contrast will vary from one society to another, we should also expect variability with regard to cognitive styles, reality constructions, and what is taken for granted and what is foregrounded. Knowledge has its origins in what is problematic. Therefore, what is problematic has its origins in deviations from what is taken for granted. It follows that knowledge is as variable and relative as the taken-for-granted background, which we know changes from one historical period to another and from one culture to another. It changes as the recurrences of life and the standard of normative expectancies change. In fact, we do not need to look back very far in history to witness such changes. I would argue that since the 1960s there has been a slow, invisible change in most Western countries in recurrences and standards of normative expectancies about the basic values of our existence and tradition. Because these changes take place gradually, we tend to accept them as minor variations from what is normal. But over a period of 10 to 15 years the changes have become substantial. Before we go further, I would like to provide some examples of how this perspectivistic model can be used in concrete experimentation with children.

Overcoming perspectivistic restraints: Piagetian experiments

At a situational level, where numerous interpretative positions within a person's repertoire are available, it is very important to consider the general definition of the situation, the saliency of various situational features, and when and how the situation is parsed. This has important implications for Piagetian experiments, as I will try to show with some examples from the research we have done in Oslo. First, consider a Piagetian class-inclusion experiment that Rommetveit and I replicated. In this study we used drawings of various objects – for example, five flowers: four

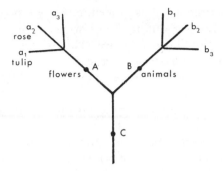

Figure 2. Spatial model of alternative perspectives for "tulips or flowers" question.

tulips and one rose. In the traditional procedure the objects are presented, and the following class-inclusion question is asked: "Can you tell me, are there more tulips or more flowers?"

By means of Figure 2 it is possible to come to a "perspectivistic diagnosis" of the positions that a subject may adopt when asked this kind of question. When presented with the two types of flowers – tulips and a rose – a subject automatically tends to focus on the details and differences between the two subclasses, while taking the superordinate class "flowers" for granted. In accordance with the model above, the subject will be at position A. It is from this position that the subject responds to the class-inclusion question "Are there more flowers than tulips?" But a subject in position A does not see flowers because they are taken for granted. In order to compare flowers with tulips, he must be in position C from which both the superordinate and the subordinate class can be seen simultaneously. Thus we find a conflict here: By presenting the drawing of the two subclasses, tulips and rose, *the experimenter is inviting the person to adopt a particular position from which the correct solution to the problem becomes unlikely*. I would argue that this is the reason for the high level of incorrect responses to this problem. The difficulty encountered in this kind of task is not necessarily the intellectual operation of class inclusion. Rather, it is *the problem of overcoming the perspectivistic restraint of being in a false position*. The child is invited to adopt position A and then asked questions from the perspective of position C.

If this is so, then it should be possible in accordance with our model to suggest to a subject how to adopt a position from which he can "see" the correct solution. There are two ways to do this. We can either *reduce the impact of the two subclasses*, a_1 and a_2, and thereby weaken the "invitation" to adopt position A; or we can *present a contrasting alternative to A*, that is, B, so that position C might be adopted. (See Donaldson, 1977.) The first procedure is in some way similar to "screening procedures" used by Bruner

(1966) in conservation experiments. This procedure was adopted in the study just outlined. Instead of presenting the drawings of the stimulus figures and the questions simultaneously, we changed the sequence slightly by *presenting the question first and the drawings afterward*. In this way the overpowering impact of the two subclasses (a_1 and a_2) was reduced while the question came more into the foreground. That is, temptation to adopt position A was reduced. As we expected, significantly more children were able to answer correctly when we followed this procedure than when we used the traditional one. The slight change in temporal sequence of presentation of stimulus figures and instruction was sufficient to change the perspectivistic restraints, and the task became considerably easier. Thus *solving a class-inclusion task is not only a question of the presence or absence of concrete opinions, it is also a question of overcoming perspectivistic restraints that may vary within the same "operation" or task*.

The next type of study I will mention is also a Piagetian experiment, but in this case the emphasis is on *the power of the question* to induce a perspective and thus to locate a person in a particular interpretive position (Hundeide, 1980, 1981a, 1981b). In this case I tried to bring the children into a false position, thereby *deceiving them to give "incorrect" replies to questions and problems they could easily manage under normal conditions*. Within the Piagetian tradition these experiments would probably be characterized as examples of "countersuggestion" (Smedslund, 1969). Countersuggestion is used to investigate the "real" presence of operative structures. It turns out that those structures prove to be extremely susceptible to countersuggestion, probably more susceptible than a Piagetian framework would allow.

First consider the question. When a person is asked a question, he is invited to share another person's perspective. If he accepts the invitation or the "contract" (Rommetveit and Blakar, 1979), he is committed to operate or reply within the *options of the question*. For example, consider the question "Do you think he should be spanked or just sent to bed early?" The options here are clearly specified and leave little room for further possibilities. A question therefore has a *premise or a fact that is taken for granted*. In the question, "Why are you angry?" the premise that you are angry is taken for granted. In other words a question has both a *premise that is taken for granted* and *options for responding*. The latter presents the speaker with a problem. Because attention is always directed to what is problematic and away from what is taken for granted, *a question becomes a very powerful attention-controlling and directing device*. It can easily be used for deceptive purposes. By introducing an unacceptable premise (A) as the taken-for-granted part of the question and specifying various alternatives that become problematic (a_1, a_2, ...), attention is directed away from the premise itself to the problem of selecting the best alternative (a₁ or a₂). In this way an unacceptable premise is tacitly accepted while attention is directed to the options of the question.

Let us examine how this works in interviews on children's orientation toward moral intentionality versus internal consequence. By the age of 9 or 10 years most children tend to base their moral evaluations on the intention behind an action rather than on the external damage caused by the action. They therefore tend to state that a boy who has broken a small cup while he was in the process of stealing should be more severely punished than a boy who unintentionally broke a large crystal bowl while helping his mother wash dishes (Piaget, 1932).

Instead of presenting the question in the traditional way by beginning with the issue of intentionality versus external damage (A versus B), I *restricted the options of the question to only external damage alternatives* (a₁ or a₂?) by asking, "Do you think he should be spanked or just sent to bed early?" By changing the question to this form, 27 of the 33 children who had already displayed an intention orientation changed to an external damage orientation. A simple perspectivistic manipulation – the *contraction of perspective* – changed the diagnosis of the subjects' moral development.

It is possible to change children's moral judgments by this procedure, it should be possible to change their conservation judgments similarly. We demonstrated this as follows. Instead of asking children the open-ended (number) conservation question "Are there more there, the same amount in both, or more here?" an experimenter pointed to one of the rows of elements as shown below and asked, *"Why are there more (or less) here?"*

```
1.  "Why more here?"  X     X   X   X     X
                         X X X X X
2.  "Why less here?"         X X X X X
                      X     X   X   X     X
```

Despite the fact that about 90% of the children at the highest level (9 to 10 years of age) had previously been diagnosed as having mastered number conservation, about 57% of these children accepted the question and gave nonconservational replies. An average of more than 70% of the children between 5-1/2 and 10 years of age accepted the question (Hundeide, 1981a). An interesting point here is that most children seemed to accept the premise of the question with no reservation. They seemed to be completely unaware of the fact that they had been deceived and that there was any inconsistency with their usual logical reasoning in similar situations.

Some have rejected this interpretation by arguing that the children probably were simply obeying the authoritative experimenter or paying lip service to his hints. In order to test this alternative interpretation another condition was added in which the experimenter first asked the usual conservation question: "Are there more there, an equal amount in both, or more here?" and then he added, "*I believe there are more here!*" (nonconservational hint). To our surprise, *only 1 of 16 children (7 to 8 years of age) obeyed the nonconservational suggestion.* Thirteen children resisted and gave appropriate conservation replies. In contrast, in the first condition where the nonconserving premise was implied in the question, 11 children accepted the nonconserving premise and only 6 resisted and gave appropriate conservation replies. Thus, despite the clearly "authoritative" hint of the experimenter to give a nonconserving reply, almost all the children rejected this suggestion.

It seems to me that the critical factor producing these results is not authority, but the *options of the question* (Hundeide, 1981a). When children are deceived in these experiments, it is not because they surrender to authority, but because *they see only one alternative* as a relevant and plausible reply to *the given* question. We already know that when the options of the question permit an appropriate conservation reply, as in the usual number conservation experiment, most 7- to 8-year-old children give appropriate replies. What we do not know is whether they would give a nonconserving reply in a situation where the options of the question permit only nonconserving replies ("Why are there more here?") and *the experimenter is a nonauthoritative person.*

In order to investigate this, we picked out a rather withdrawn but intelligent girl who was willing to serve as experimenter. She was trained in the rather simple procedure described above. (Children were first asked to match rows of elements to be equal in number, then one row was spread out and the experimenter asked, "Can you tell me, why are there less. . .here?" while pointing to the row that had been spread out. Another experimenter watched the performance through a one-way screen.) Most children reacted first with surprise and then laughter to this new situation of being asked odd questions by one of their friends. Despite the laughter, half of the children gave nonconserving replies as expected on the basis of the option provided by the question. This was less than in the same condition with an adult experimenter (13 of 20). However, there were far more nonconserving replies than in the "open" situation with the usual conservation question (5 of 20). Thus the deceiving effect of presenting a question with only a nonconserving option seems to persist despite the reduced authority (and credibility) of the experimenter.

Children are responding neither to authority nor to Piagetian structures in these experiments. What they are responding to is a nonlogical principle of *plausibility and embeddedness* within an episodic Gestalt. These are usually taken for granted and make certain options more plausible than others. This type of cognition seems to be more akin to aesthetic evaluation than to logical reasoning; it seems to be that it is quite prevalent.

REFERENCES

Barker, R. G. 1965. Explorations in ecological psychology. *American Psychologist, 20*, 1–14.
Boschowitsch, J. L. 1974. *Die Personlichkeit und ihre Entwicklung im Schulalter*. Berlin: Volk und Wissen v. Verlag.
Bruner, J. 1966. *Studies in cognitive growth*. New York: Wiley.
Cole, M. 1980. *Culture and cognitive development*. Manuscript.
Cole, M., and Scribner, S. 1974. *Culture and thought*. New York: Wiley.
Crosby, F. 1976. A model of egotistical relative deprivation. *Psychological Review, 83* (2), 85–113.
Donaldson, M. 1977. *Children's minds*. Glasgow: Fontana Originals.
Duncker, K. 1945. On problem-solving. *Psychological Monographs, 58*(5), 1–112.
Eckblad, G. 1981. *Scheme theory: A conceptual framework for cognitive-motivational processes*. New York: Academic Press.
Forgas, J. P. 1979. *Social episodes: The study of interaction rituals*. New York: Academic Press.
Geertz, C. 1973. *The interpretation of cultures: Selected essays*. New York: Basic Books.
Goffman, E. 1974. *Frame analysis: An essay on the organization of experience*. Cambridge: Harvard University Press.
Harre, R., and Secord, P. F. 1972. *The explanation of social behavior*. Oxford: Blackwell.
Helson, H. 1964. *Adaptation-level theory: An experimental and systematic approach*. New York: Wiley.
Hundeide, K. 1980. The origin of the child's replies in experimental situations. *Quarterly Newsletter of the Laboratory of Comparative Human Cognition, 2*(1), 15–18.
Hundeide, K. 1981a. Contractual congruence and logical consistency. *Quarterly Newsletter of the Laboratory of Comparative Human Cognition, 3*(4), 77–79.
Hundeide, K. 1981b. Experiments on the power of the question. Progress report, University of Oslo.
Johnson, D. M. 1955. *The psychology of thought and judgement*. New York: Harper.
Kagan, J. 1971. *Change and continuity in infancy*. New York: Wiley.
Kelly, G. 1955. *The psychology of personal constructs*. New York: Norton.
Leont'ev, A. N. 1981. The problem of activity in psychology. In J. V. Wertsch (Ed.), *The concept of activity in Soviet psychology*. Armonk, N.Y.: Sharpe.
Luria, A. R. 1976. *Cognitive development: Its cultural and social foundation*. Cambridge: Harvard University Press.
Mannheim, K. 1936. *Ideology and utopia: An introduction to the sociology of knowledge*. Translated by L. Wirth and E. Shils. New York: Harcourt, Brace.
Piaget, J. 1932. *The moral development of the child*. London: Kegan Paul.
Piaget, J. 1972. Intellectual evolution from adolescence to adulthood. *Human Development, 15*, 1–12.

Raaheim, K. 1978. *Problem solving and intelligence*. Oslo: Universitetsforlaget.

Rommetveit, R. 1978. On Piagetian cognitive operations, semantic competence and message-structure in adult–child communication. In I. Markova, *The social context of language*. New York: Wiley.

Rommetveit, R. 1979. Language games, syntactic structure, and hermeneutics: In search of a preface to a conceptual framework for research on language and human communication. In R. Rommetveit and R. Blakar (Eds.), *Studies of language, thought, and verbal communication*. New York: Academic Press.

Rommetviet, R., and Blakar, R. 1979. *Studies of language, thought, and verbal communication*. New York: Academic Press.

Smedslund, J. 1969. Psychological diagnostics. *Psychological Bulletin*, *71*(3), 237–248.

Thomas, W. I., and Znanieki, F. 1923. *The Polish peasant in Europe and America*. New York: Dover.

Vygotsky, L. S. 1978. *Mind in society: The development of higher psychological processes*. Cambridge: Harvard University Press.

Wason, P. C., and Johnson-Laird, P. N. 1972. *Psychology of reasoning*. Cambridge: Harvard University Press.

Wertheimer, M. 1945. *Productive thinking*. New York: Harper.

Wertsch, J. V. 1981a. The concept of activity in Soviet psychology: An introduction. In J. V. Wertsch (Ed.), *The concept of activity in Soviet psychology*. Armonk, N.Y.: Sharpe.

Wertsch, J. V. 1981b. A state of the art review of Soviet research in cognitive psychology. *Storia e Critica Della Psicologia*, *2*(2), 219–295.

Wittgenstein, L. 1968. *Philosophical investigations*. Oxford: Blackwell.

14

Exploring Vygotskian perspectives in education: the cognitive value of peer interaction

ELLICE A. FORMAN and COURTNEY B. CAZDEN

Two important and related themes in Vygotsky's writings are the social foundations of cognition and the importance of instruction in development:

An important point to note about Vygotsky's ideas on the social origins of cognition is that it is at this point that he uses the notion of internalization. He is not simply claiming that social interaction leads to the development of the child's abilities in problem-solving, memory, etc.; rather, he is saying that the very means (especially speech) used in social interaction are taken over by the individual child and internalized. Thus, Vygotsky is making a very strong statement here about internalization and the social foundations of cognition. (Wertsch, 1981, p. 146)

If all the development of a child's mental life takes place in the process of social intercourse, this implies that this intercourse and its most systematized form, the teaching process, forms the development of the child, creates new mental formations, and develops higher processes of mental life. Teaching, which sometimes seems to wait upon development, is in actual fact its decisive motive force. . . .The assimilation of general human experience in the teaching process is the most important specifically human form of mental development in ontogenesis. This deeply significant proposition defines an essentially new approach to the most important theoretical problem of psychology, the challenge of actively developing the mind. It is in this that the main significance of this aspect of Vygotsky's enquiries lies. (Leontiev and Luria, 1968, p. 365)

In all of Vygotsky's writings with which we are familiar, the social relationship referred to as "teaching" is the one-to-one relationship between one adult and one child. When we try to explore Vygotskian perspectives for education, we immediately confront questions about the role of the student peer group. Even if formal education takes place in a group context only for economic reasons, because no society can afford a teacher for each individual child, the presence of peers should not be ignored or relegated only to discussions of issues in classroom management and control.

We see two separate but related issues concerning the group presence. First, there are the problems posed for the teacher in carrying out direct teaching to a group of students; second, there are the questions raised for the teacher's more indirect planning for the social organization of all work related talk in the classroom setting, specifically the contribution that peers can make to each other. We focus on the second set of questions in this chapter. This is not to underestimate the importance of the first. If teaching is conceived as assistance to the child in the child's zone of proximal development, then teaching to a group of children whose "zones" overlap only in part, or not at all, poses obvious problems. But to state the problem thus seems mainly to give new labels to the familiar problem of within-group variation in any group being taught. We focus instead on the less discussed problem of the potential contribution of social interactions among the children themselves.

Understanding this contribution has both practical and theoretical significance. Practically, despite the fact that school classrooms are unusually crowded social environments, group work is rarely encouraged (Galton, Simon, and Croll, 1980), perhaps in part because there has been no clear rationale for its value. [See Sharan (1980) for one review of arguments and evidence.] Theoretically, most developmental research studies in the United States have traditionally focused on the value of peer interactions in the socialization of behavior and personality and have said less about their possible value for cognition and intellectual learning. According to Lawler (1980), until recently the same has been true of most writing on education in the Soviet Union – for example, the work of Makarenko.

Interactions among peers focused on intellectual content can be placed on a continuum, depending on the distribution of knowledge or skill among the children, and therefore on the roles they take toward each other. At one extreme, one child knows more than the others and is expected to act as a peer tutor [or "consultant" in the recent Soviet work of M. D. Vinogradova and I.B. Pervin, summarized in Lawler (1980)]. In the contrasting case, knowledge is equal, or at least not intentionally unequal, and the give and take of equal status collaboration is expected. We present research first on two different forms of peer tutoring and then on collaboration. Because empirical as well as theoretical analysis of peer interactions is at such a beginning stage, we include excerpts from interaction protocols, not only as evidence for our interpretations, but to provide material for alternative interpretations as well.

Peer tutoring

The report of Vygotsky's pupil, Levina, points to possible cognitive benefits to a tutor from the activity of giving verbal instructions to peers:

Vygotsky said that speech does not include within itself the magical power to create intellectual functioning. It acquires this capacity only through being used in its instrumental capacity. (Levina, 1981, p. 296)

To the extent that this is true, then what Levina calls the "intellectualization" as well as the internalization of speech should be promoted by the use of instrumental speech to others. Levina suggests exactly that

what is silently perceived as something unitary and whole is immediately broken up into its component elements in any attempt to make a verbal formulation of it. It is easy to be convinced of this as soon as one tries to introduce the clarity of a verbal characterization into an unconscious impression. What are the motivating forces behind this type of verbal formulation? What is it that compels the child to represent his/her perceptions verbally and to formulate and label his/her actions? In answering this question, Vygotsky laid great stress on factors having to do with the social order. He thought that in labeling an ongoing action, the child initially pays tribute to people in the environment by means of verbal representation. He/she makes this representation accessible to them, as if to clarify it. Vygotsky believed that the very act of labeling arose out of the necessity for giving one's own actions a specialized form comprehensible to others. (Levina, 1981, p. 288–289)

Levina's examples of labeling stimulated by the need to communicate to another, taken from notes and protocols collected under Vygotsky's supervision, contain only child speech that is directed back to the experimenter. Though the need to communicate to peers is not mentioned, it seems consistent with the Levina–Vygotsky perspective that the need to communicate cate to a less knowledgeable other – such as a peer – would motivate the identical process at least as strongly. Instruction of peers could, in this respect, be an intermediate step between receptively being directed by the speech of another and productively and covertly directing one's own mental processes via inner speech.

The first analysis of peer tutoring comes from research in an inner-city multigrade primary classroom in San Diego. Twelve peer tutoring sequences called instructional changes (ICs) were videotaped for analysis (Cazden et al., 1978; Carrasco, Vera, and Cazden, 1981; Mehan and Riel, 1982). Briefly, in each IC the teacher (T) taught a lesson to one child who then taught the same lesson to one or more peers. Leola, a black third-grader, was asked to learn and then teach a language arts task. Here are the first three items on her worksheet in completed form:

1. new   1. Y $\emptyset$ʎo $\emptyset$u   2. t ʎ$\emptyset$o l $\emptyset$d   3. m $\emptyset$ ʎ e
2. no
3. off   Y o u   t o l d   m e

Following is a transcription, minus repetitions, corrections, and so on, of the teacher's (T) directions as she talked Leola (L) through the first two items on the task:

Item 1
T: Okay, now number one here says *new*. What's the opposite of *new*?
L: Old.
T: *Old*. How would you spell old?

L: O-L-D.
T: Okay, in the letters that are on this paper, cross out the letters you just used for spelling *old.*
L: (*L. does it.*)
T: Good. What word is left?
L: Y-O-U.
T: What does it spell?
L: You.
T: Okay, and down here you'll write *you.*

Item 2
T: Okay, now number two there says. . .
L: No.
T: *No.* What's the opposite of *no?*
L: Yes.
T: Okay, how do you spell *yes?*
L: Y-E-S
T: All right. Now what are you going. . .
L: (*L crosses out the letters Y-E-S*) Told.

Note first that the T's questions serve to talk Leola through the task until she can do it herself, as Wertsch (1978) has shown for mothers' help to their preschool children in a puzzle-copying task. That such aid does help Leola work independently is shown by a comparison of T's instructions for the first and second items. The first three questions are repeated, but then a much vaguer and incomplete question, "Now what are you going. . .," is sufficient, and Leola takes off on her own.

The second noteworthy aspect of this IC from the Levina–Vygotsky perspective is the development of increased articulateness and precision in Leola's verbalizations of the task. If one considers the entire instructional chain as a "discourse imitation test," the T's instructions must be recon-structed by the tutor's cognitive, linguistic, and sociolinguistic system. Whereas T taught with questions, Leola teaches with statements, often "You gotta X." [Mehan and Riel (1982) show that this contrast in teaching styles was characteristic of all 12 ICs.]

It was not immediately easy for Leola to put the directions for this task into words. When Leola first tried to explain to T, pretask, what she was going to tell her group, she included explicit reference to only one of the four essential components, the idea of having some letters "left":

T: Tell me what you are going to tell them to do.
L: Spell these letters, and then put out that letter, and then have another letter left.

T goes over the instructions again, this time asking Leola specifically to say the word "opposite." Leola then includes that word, but with the vague verb "do":

T: You want to cross out the opposite of "new." You better say that, because it's going to be really important. They are going to read "new," and then what are they going to do?

L: Do the opposite of it.

Leola achieves the clearest explanation in round 3 (without hesitations and self-repairs):

L: The opposite of *off* is *on,* so on number three, you gotta cross *on* off. O-N. And it is *me* left, M-E.

Overall, one is tempted to argue that the changes in Leola's instructions constitute an example of what Wertsch and Stone (1978), following the Soviet psychologists, call microgenesis – that is, development within an observable time period, and it is a kind of development that Leola seemed to need. In the nine lessons analyzed by Mehan (1979), some three hours of talk in all, she spoke four times, and only twice more than one word. This is not to say she was in any way nonverbal, but is to suggest that she could benefit from challenges to formulate academic content in words, and that the demands of tutoring, including the need for repeated formulation and for corrections of others, provide that challenge well. If there is any validity to the internalization hypothesis, practice in explicit overt formulation should ultimately aid inner speech as well. Vague, inexplicit speech – or a unitary and unformulated perception, in Levina's words – is not the same as predication and "sense" in inner speech.

Finally, there is an interesting reduction of information in Leola's instructions after round 3. With two exceptions, in all the rounds after 3 Leola is talking out loud, head down, while she does her own work. In the reduced rounds 4–5 and 7–10, the reduction in information is more by alternative formulations of the components than by deletion of them altogether. For example, the critical word "opposite" is spoken only in rounds 1 to 3, and then when the first item has to be repeated (1R) and round 6. In the other rounds, Leola says only "out is in" (presupposing that *is* means *is the opposite of*) or, even more briefly, simply places the two words in juxtaposition: "west east." In the two exceptions, 1R and 6, explicitness returns as Leola corrects her tutees and she notices that they have made a mistake.

Two alternative explanations are possible for the decreased explicitness in the reduced rounds. It may be due either to Leola's understanding that the concept of "opposites" can now be assumed or to the decreased explicitness that characterizes speech to oneself. As Wertsch (1979) points out, the decay of old or "given" information is functionally equivalent in dialogue and private speech.

The second analysis of peer tutoring comes from observations by

Kamler (1980) in a second-grade classroom in New Hampshire in which Donald Graves's research team was observing the teaching of writing. The teacher, Egan, held regular conferences with individual children. In addition, she encouraged the children to hold "peer conferences" about their writing with each other. Here is one observer's account of the conferences between two children, Jill and Debbie:

> On March 11, Jill was one of six children scheduled for a writing conference. . . .
> At Egan's direction, Jill and the other conferees went to the language table. Egan had requested that Jill first spend time with seven-year-old Debbie going over the book to be sure it was ready for a conference. . . .
> Jill began by reading each page aloud to Debbie. . . . As Jill listened to her own words, she made changes on pages 1, 2, and 3 without any prompting or comment from Debbie, and on pages 4, 5, and 8 in direct response to questions Debbie asked. . . .
> At the conclusion of this half hour conference, Jill had made six content changes which affected the overall meaning of the piece. She had deleted information which made no sense or which she could not support; she added information to clarify or explain. Debbie's presence was crucial to the content revisions of the draft. Her physical presence forced Jill to reread the book for the first time since composing; Debbie seemed to make the concept of audience visible for Jill. Jill also needed an active reader to ask questions. . . .
> [Later] Debbie claimed her time: "O.K., Jill, you help me now!" They reversed roles, returned to the language table to work on Debbie's book *Ice Follies,* until Mrs. Egan was ready to see Jill twenty minutes later. (Kamler, 1980, pp. 683–685)

Note first that this is a more reciprocal model of peer assistance. The roles of writer and helpful questioner are interchangeable among the children. All the children can learn what to do and say in the questioner role from the teacher's model in the conferences with her, a consistent model of how to ask helpful questions that are focused on the content of writing, not form. The teacher believes that questions focused on content are more helpful than questions about form; they are also the kind of questions that children can understandingly ask of each other. The teacher's model thus makes it possible for the children to take turns performing the teacher's role for each other – to the benefit of each child as author, who can have so many more experiences with a responsive audience; and to the benefit of each child as critic, who can internalize such questions through the process of not only answering them to the teacher, but of asking them of peers as well.

For these benefits to occur, the teacher's model must be learnable by the children. Graves reports (pers. comm.) that the conference structure of another teacher in the same school was not as learnable by the children, and so there was less of a multiplier effect via peer conferences in his classroom. This comparison suggests that the intellectual value of peer interactions in a classroom will be enhanced when the teacher consistently models a kind of interaction in which the children can learn to speak to each other.

As Kamler points out, the child writer benefits in two different ways from the peer's presence. Most obviously, the peer asks questions, following the adult model but with content appropriate to the writing at hand; and some of Jill's changes (pages 4, 5, and 8) were in direct response to Debbie's questions. Less obviously, the peer silently but no less effectively represents the needs of an audience and makes "the concept of audience visible."

We can locate the effect of such a silent audience in the otherwise empty cell created by Wertsch and Stone's (pers. comm.) separation of the interpsychological/intrapsychological and external/internal dimensions in Vygotsky's analysis. Wertsch and Stone separated the two dimensions in order to make a place for egocentric speech. In Vygotsky's words, "Egocentric speech is internal speech in its psychological function and external speech physiologically" (1956, p. 87) – that is, intrapsychological in function but external in form. We suggest that the changes Jill made in response to Debbie's silent presence are exactly the opposite: internal in form (though recorded in writing) and interpsychological in function, to make the writing more informative to another.

Peer collaboration

In comparison with peer tutoring, even less is understood about the intellectual value of peer collaboration. This may be partly due to the fact that collaboration requires a work environment that is even further from traditional classroom organization. Peer tutoring tasks tend to resemble common classroom activities: filling in workbooks, reading aloud, editing written assignments, and so forth. In these activities the tutor helps inform, guide, and/or correct the tutee's work. Collaboration requires a mutual task in which the partners work together to produce something that neither could have produced alone. Given the focus on individual achievement in most Western industrial societies, curricula that promote collaboration are rarely found in schools or studied by educators or psychologists.

Research on peer collaboration has thus been sparse. The major exception to this generalization is a body of research conducted by a group of Genevan psychologists (Doise, Mugny, and Perret-Clermont, 1975, 1976; Mugny and Doise, 1978; Perret-Clermont, 1980). They have conducted a series of experiments to examine the effect of peer collaboration on logical reasoning skills associated with the Piagetian stage of concrete operations: perspective taking, conversation, and so on.

Most of the Genevan research employs a training study design in which subjects are randomly assigned to treatment or control groups in which they are exposed to different social contexts. For example, the subjects in the treatment group may be asked to solve a conservation task in a small peer group composed of conservers and nonconservers, while subjects in the control group are asked to solve the same problem alone. All subjects are individually pretested and posttested on some standard measure of concrete-operational reasoning, and the effect of exposure to peer collaboration is assessed by comparing the pretest-to-posttest gains in concrete-operational reasoning found in each group. The Genevans have employed this same training study design across a number of studies in which the particular reasoning task chosen, the social groups assembled, and the criteria used to evaluate cognitive growth are systematically varied. After reviewing this entire body of research, Perret-Clermont (1980) concludes that peer interaction enhances the development of logical reasoning through a process of active cognitive reorganization induced by cognitive conflict. She claims also that cognitive conflict is most likely to occur in situations where children with moderately discrepant perspectives (e.g., conservers and transitional subjects) are asked to reach a consensus.

Two Russian researchers, Lomov (1978) and Kol'tsova (1978), and two Japanese investigators, Inagaki and Hatano (Inagaki, 1981; Inagaki and Hatano, 1968, 1977) have reached similar conclusions – that peer interaction helps individuals acknowledge and integrate a variety of perspectives on a problem, and that this process of coordination, in turn, produces superior intellectual results. For Kol'tsova, the results are precise, rich, and logically rigorous definitions of a social science concept. For Inagaki and Hatano, the results are generalizable and stable conservation concepts. For Perret-Clermont, the results are increased ability to use concrete operational logic.

In none of these studies were subjects' interactions during collaborative problem solving systematically observed. The studies provide only anecdotal evidence to support the hypothesis that peer interaction is capable of enhancing intellectual performance because it forces individuals to recognize and coordinate conflicting perspectives on a problem. To test this hypothesis, one would need to examine the process of social coordination that occurs during problem solving in order to isolate the social conditions that are the most responsible for cognitive growth. For example, one could observe the interactions that occur while the group is working in order to differentiate those groups in which members work closely together and frequently attempt to coordinate their differing perspectives from those in which members work largely on their own. Then one could examine how these different group interactional patterns affect the problem-solving strategies used. Just this approach is advocated by Perret-Clermont:

We have also shown that, for the task to have educational value, it is not sufficient for it merely to engage children in joint activity; there must also be confrontation between different points of view. Are all the activities described as "cooperation" by research workers such as to induce real inter-individual coordinations which are the source of cognitive conflict? This question can only be answered by the systematic observation which remains to be done. (1980, p. 196)

In further studies of the psychology of intelligence, we should envisage not solely the effect of inter-individual coordination on *judgment* behavior, or on *performance* as an index of development...but also the impact of different types of social interaction, and in particular of partner's strategies, on the *strategy* which the subject adopts in order to carry out the task. (1980, p. 192)

We will describe a recent study (Forman, 1981) in which videotapes of collaborative problem-solving sessions were analyzed for the social interactional patterns used and the problem-solving strategies employed. In addition, individual measures of logical reasoning were collected on this sample of collaborative problem solvers that were compared with similar measures collected on a previous sample of solitary problem solvers.

The research design used by Forman is a modification of the training study design utilized by Perret-Clermont and her colleagues. Instead of providing only one opportunity for children to solve a problem in a collaborative fashion, Forman exposed her subjects to a total of 11 problem-solving sessions. There are several reasons for using a longitudinal design to assess children's problem-solving skills. One can observe the process of cognitive growth directly, rather than having to infer it from pretest-posttest performance; and children can develop stable working relationships. In addition, a longitudinal design was chosen for this study so that the data collected on collaborative problem solving could be compared with similar longitudinal data collected by Kuhn and Ho (1980) on solitary problem solving. [See Kuhn and Phelps (1979) and Forman (1981) for a more detailed explanation of the strengths of this kind of longitudinal design.]

Forman's study thus provides two kinds of information about collaboration: how the reasoning strategies of collaborative problem solvers differ from those of solitary problem solvers and how some collaborative partnerships differ from others in both social interactional patterns and cognitive strategy usage. In the following discussion, we will focus on these two kinds of data: comparisons of collaborators with solitary problem solvers and comparisons among different collaborative partnerships. We will then discuss the findings of Forman's study in light of Perret-Clermont's hypothesis and what seems to us the essential and complementary theory of Vygotsky.

Forman's study

Like Perret-Clermont, Forman asked children to cooperate in the solution of a logical reasoning task. Unlike Perret-Clermont, Forman selected a chemical reaction task that has been used to assess the ability to isolate variables in a multivariate context (Kuhn and Phelps, 1982). In addition, her subjects were older (approximately 9 years of age) than those selected by Perret-Clermont (4–7 years).

In both the study conducted by Forman (1981) and that conducted by Kuhn and Ho (1980) the subjects were fourth- to fifth-grade, middle-class children – 15 singletons (Kuhn and Ho) and 4 pairs (Forman) – who showed no ability to isolate variables in a multivariate task known as the "simple plant problem." In addition to the pretest used for subject selection, all subjects were given an additional pretest: a combinations problem in which subjects were asked to arrange five kinds of snacks in all possible combinations. The singletons and pairs participated in 11 problem-solving sessions, approximately once a week over a three-month period. The two pretest measures were readministered as posttests within a week after the final problem-solving session. All pretests and posttests were administered individually.

The chemical reaction problem consisted of a series of seven chemical problems that were ordered in terms of logical complexity. Problem 1, the simplest, requires that subjects identify the one chemical from a set of five odorless, colorless chemicals that is necessary and sufficient for producing a specified color change when mixed with a reagent. In problems 2 and 3, two or three of the five chemicals are capable of producing the color change, either separately or together. In problem 4, two chemicals are capable of producing the change, but only when *both* of them are present; and so forth.

Problem 1, with a different operative chemical each time, was presented for the first four sessions. This procedure insured that the children were repeatedly exposed to the simplest problem in the series before more difficult problems were introduced. After the fourth session, a new problem in the series was presented whenever the previous problem had been solved once. Thus, progress through the problem series is one measure of the effectiveness of the subjects' problem-solving strategies.

Each of the 11 problem-solving sessions in both studies followed the same format. First, two demonstration experiments were performed by the experimenter. Then, the children were asked a standard set of questions about the demonstration, for example, "What do you think makes a difference in whether it turns purple or not?" Next, the children were invited to set up the experiments they wanted to try in order to determine what chemical(s) were responsible for the change. No mixing of chemicals was permitted during this setting-up phase of the task. After the experiments were set up and some additional questions about them were posed, the children were permitted to mix together the combinations they had selected. In Forman's study, the dyads were encouraged to work together on setting up and mixing the chemical experiments. Finally, after the results from the experiments had been observed, the experimenter repeated the original set of questions in order to assess whether the correct chemical(s) had been identified.

Forman analyzed only the part of the sessions devoted to planning and setting up the experiments. Four sessions for each of three subject pairs (George and Bruce: session 3, 5, 8, 11; Lisa and Linda: sessions 3, 5, 9, 11; Matt and Mitch: sessions 3, 5, 8, 10) – 12 tapes in all – were coded. (The fourth pair had been included only as insurance against illness etc.) The two coding systems used in the analysis consisted of one set of social interactional categories and one set of experimentation categories. In this chapter, we will discuss only one type of social behavior code (procedural interactions) and three types of experimentation strategies (random, variable isolation, and combinatorial).

Procedural interactions occurred during most of the problem-solving sessions coded (a range of 71% to 100% of the available time). They were defined as all activities carried out by one or both children that focus on getting the task accomplished.[1] Examples of procedural interactions were distributing and arranging task materials, choosing chemical experiments, and recording experiments. Three levels of procedural interactions were identified: parallel, associative, and cooperative [adapted from Parten's (1932) study of social interaction]. These three levels represent three qualitatively different approaches to the sharing of ideas and the division of labor. During parallel procedural interactions, children share materials and exchange comments about the task. However, they make few if any attempts to monitor the work of the other or to inform the other of their own thoughts and actions. Associative procedural interactions occur when children try to exchange information about some of the combinations each one has selected. However, at the associative level, no attempt is made to coordinate the roles of the two partners. Cooperative interactions require that both children constantly monitor each other's work and play coordinated roles in performing task procedures.

The experimentation strategy codes were adapted from Kuhn and Phelps (1982). Three basic types of experimentation strategies were observed: a random or trial-and-error strategy; an isolation-of-variables strategy; and a combinatorial strategy. The random experiments strategy represents a relatively ineffective, unsystematic approach to experimentation. The variable isolation strategy is effective for solving the first three problems only. The more advanced problems, 4 through 7, require both experimental isolation and combinatorial strategies. Thus, this experimentation coding system was devised to identify when or if this strategy shift (from only variable isolation to both variable isolation and combinatorial) occurred.

Experimental strategy codes were assigned to a dyad based solely on the type of chemical experiments set up. Neither the type of social organization used to select these experiments nor the kinds of conversations that occurred during the setting-up process affected the assignment of an experimentation code. Thus, the coding of experimentation strategies constituted an assessment of each dyad's behavior that was independent of that obtained by coding their social interactions.

For the comparisons of the problem-solving achievements of collaborators versus singletons, two kinds of data are available: the number of chemical problems solved during the 11 sessions and pretest-to-posttest change scores. The first comparison produced striking differences between collaboration and solitary problem solving. While Kuhn and Ho found that only 4 of the 15 singletons solved problems 1 through 3 in the 11 sessions, all 4 of Forman's dyads solved problems 1 through 4 in the same amount of time. In addition, one dyad (George and Bruce) solved problems 1 through 6 during this three-month period, an achievement approached by none of Kuhn and Ho's subjects.

The pretest-posttest comparison between singletons and dyads produced more mixed results. These results are displayed in Tables 1 and 2 (ignoring for now the initials in parentheses). On the simple plant problem (Table 1), the singletons showed greater progress than the pairs between the pretest and posttest. In contrast, subjects who had worked in pairs seemed to show greater progress on the combinations problem (Table 2) than did the subjects who had worked alone.[2] Thus, while the pairs seemed able to master the series of chemical problems at a much faster rate than did the singletons, they did not show consistently greater pretest–posttest gains.

One clear difference between these two comparisons (progress through the problems versus posttest performance) is that both partners were able to contribute to the solution of each chemical problem presented, but on the pretest–posttest measures the partners were on their own. The relatively sophisticated problem-solving strategies that collaborators were able to display when they could assist each other were not as apparent when each partner was asked to work alone on similar problems.

Another reason why collaborators did not always outperform the singletons may lie in difference among the partnerships. Due to the very small number of dyads examined, large differences between dyads may obscure

Table 1. *Pretest and posttest category frequencies on the simple plant problem*

Group	Predominantly concrete	Transitional	Predominantly formal	Total N
Pretest				
Singletons	15	0	0	15
Pairs	8	0	0	8
Posttest				
Singletons	4	5	6	15
Pairs	6 M1, L2, M2, G, K1, K2	1 (B)	1 (L1)	8

Table 2. *Pretest and posttest category frequencies on the combination problem*

Group	Predominantly concrete	Transitional	Predominantly formal	Total N
Pretest				
Singletons	15	0	0	15
Pairs	8	0	0	8
Posttest				
Singletons	12	3	0	15
Pairs	5 K2, L1, M1, K1, G	1 L2, M2, B	0	8

all but massive differences between dyads and singletons. Therefore, we turn to the second set of comparisons: those among dyads. First, we will discuss the types of social interactions that occurred over time in the three collaborative partnerships examined. Second, we will look at the experimentation strategies used by those same dyads. Third, we will reexamine their pretest–posttest data.

The most obvious difference among the social behaviors of the three dyads concerned the development of procedural interaction patterns. All procedural interactions were classified as either parallel, associative, or cooperative. Table 3 shows that all three dyads engaged in predominantly parallel and associative interactions during the first session coded (session 3 for all three dyads). Only Lisa and Linda showed any degree of cooperative behavior during this session. However, by sessions 5, 8, and 11 George and Bruce were entirely cooperative. Lisa and Linda retained some associative interaction patterns in session 5, but by sessions 9 and 11 they too were engaging in cooperative interactions. In contrast, Matt and Mitch never cooperated throughout the three-month period. The interaction pattern that Matt and Mitch seemed to prefer was either predominantly or entirely parallel in nature.

Table 3. *Percentage of procedural time spent in parallel, associative, and coopera-tive activities*

	Type of procedural activity (%)		
Subject pair	Parallel	Associate	Cooperative
George and Bruce			
Session 3	61	39	0
Session 5	0	0	100
Session 8	0	0	100
Session 11	0	0	100
Lisa and Linda			
Session 3	42	26	32
Session 5	0	44	55
Session 9	0	0	100
Session 11	0	0	100
Matt and Mitch			
Session 3	90	10	0
Session 5	85	15	0
Session 8	100	0	0
Session 10	100	0	0

Table 4 summarizes the differences in experimentation strategies used in each pair's last two sessions. All three pairs used similar kinds of experimentation strategies during the earlier sessions. George and Bruce, the dyad who solved the greatest number of problems, used both an isolation of variables and a combinatorial strategy in the two later sessions. Lisa and Linda used only the variable isolation strategy in session 9 but both strategies by session 11. In contrast, Matt and Mitch produced either random experiments or experiments capable of isolating single variables throughout the study, despite the fact that neither of these strategies was sufficient for solving the advanced problems that were presented to them during sessions 8 and 10.

Returning to the pretest–posttest measures, we find that George and Bruce, who worked so well together, did not maintain this high degree of performance when they were tested individually. The initials on Tables 1 and 2 show the posttest status of the six children whose tapes were analyzed: George (G), Bruce (B), Lisa (L1), Linda (L2), Matt (M1), Mitch (M2), plus the remaining unanalyzed fourth pair (K1 and K2). On the simple plant problem (Table 1), the children receiving the highest scores were Bruce and Lisa; on the combinations problem (Table 2), Bruce, Linda, and Mitch exhibited the most advanced/reasoning skills. Thus, the clear differences

Table 4. *Experimentation strategies used in chemical problems 4–7*

Subject pair	Random combinations	Isolation-of-variables strategy	Systematic combinatorial strategy
George and Bruce			
Session 8		X	X
Session 11		X	X
Lisa and Linda			
Session 9		X	
Session 11		X	X
Matt and Mitch			
Session 8	X	X	
Session 10		X	

among dyads that were apparent on the videotapes of collaborative problem-solving sessions were not reflected in the posttest results.

In summary, when pairs were compared with singletons, the pairs solved the chemical combination problems at a much faster rate. However, the pairs did not do better than the singletons on all of the posttest measures. Singletons appeared to outperform the pairs on the simple plant problem, a test of a subject's ability to isolate variables, whereas the pairs seemed to do better on the combinations problem.

When comparisons were made between the pairs, it was found that George and Bruce solved more chemical combination problems than did the other pairs. In addition, George and Bruce were the first pair to switch to an entirely cooperative interaction pattern and to use a combinatorial experimentation strategy. On some of these variables, that is, the degree of cooperation shown and the use of a combinatorial strategy, Lisa and Linda appeared to hold an intermediate position between the two pairs of boys. However, these fairly consistent differences in interactional style and problem-solving strategy use were not reflected in the posttest performance of these children. In general, George and Bruce did not exhibit consistently higher levels of reasoning on their individual posttests than did the other subjects.

Discussion

What can these results tell us about the hypothesis proposed by Perret-Clermont that peer interaction can induce cognitive conflict that, in turn, results in cognitive restructuring and growth? Forman did find an association between high levels of social coordination (cooperative procedural interactions) and the use of certain experimentation strategies (combinatorial strategies). However, she did not devise a measure of cognitive conflict for her study, and her findings thus cannot establish that social coordination results in cognitive conflict, which then affects problem-solving skills.

One reason why cognitive conflict was not assessed was that overt indices of conflict, that is, arguments, were relatively rare during the portion of the problem-solving session examined – the setting-up phase of the task during which experimentation strategies were most apparent. In this portion of the session, hypotheses concerning the experiments could be proposed but not tested. During most of the setting-up time, children were busy working, separetely or together, on laying out and sharing task materials and on planning and choosing experiments. Among the children who interacted at a cooperative level, a great deal of mutual support, encouragement, correction, and guidance was exchanged. For example, one child would select chemical combinations while the other checked for duplicates. Instead of conflicting points of view, one saw two people attempting to construct and implement a joint experimentation plan to be tested later on in the task.

Conflicting points of view were apparent later in the problem-solving session, when most or all of the results of the experiments were visible. At that time, one could observe children forming distinct and sometimes opposing conclusions about the problem solution. Just such a conflict occurred in problem-solving session 3 between George and Bruce: Here is a summary of their interaction taken from a videotape record.

In this session, chemical C alone was the solution to the chemical problem. The two boys set up and mixed the following set of experiments: B, C, BE, CD, CE, DE, BDE, CDF, DEF. In addition, they could examine the results of the two demonstration experiments: BCE, DEF. All experiments containing chemical C turned purple, the rest remained clear.

After all the experiments were mixed, the experimenter asked both children, "What makes a difference in whether it turns purple?" Bruce initially concluded that the answer was C and E. George expressed his surprise that a single element, for example, C, produced the desired color change. In response to the standard prompt from the experimenter, "Can you be sure it's C and E?" Bruce reexamined some experiments and found one that contained E (and not C) that did not change color. Bruce, however, did not conclude at this point that C was the only operative chemical. George then asked Bruce whether all the experiments containing C produced the desired color change. Bruce scanned each experiment containing C and announced that each did change color.

Based on the experimental evidence and some information remembered from previous sessions, George concluded that C was the solution to the problem. Bruce, however, contradicted George by asserting it was F. At this point, they both reexamined the experiments. Afterward, George still concluded it was C and Bruce concluded it was C and F.

Th experimenter asked whether they could be sure of their answers. George replied that he was sure of C but not of F. Once again, the evidence was examined. This time, Bruce identified the experiment CDF as indicating the F was an operative chemical. George countered this argument by comparing it with experiment DEF that did not produce the desired reaction. Bruce responded that D and E were more powerful liquids than F and therefore prevented F from working. George then tried another approach by asking Bruce how he could tell it was F and not C that made the mixture CDF turn purple. Bruce replied by asking George how he could tell it wasn't both C and F that made CDF turn purple. George's concluding remark was an assertion that he just knew it was C alone.

This interchange shows the kinds of activities that conflicting solutions to the problem seemed to induce. The children returned repeatedly to the experimental evidence for supporting data. Because their conclusions differed, they were forced to acknowledge information that refuted their own inferences as well as data that supported them. These data then had to be integrated into a convincing argument in support of their own point of view. Counterarguments to their partner's position also had to be constructed. Bruce, in particular, was forced to revise his conclusions based on the evidence George brought to his attention. Despite his efforts, George was unable to convince Bruce to accept his conclusion. Unfortunately, they had not provided themselves with enough of the appropriate experimental evidence in session 3 to enable them to reach a consensus about the solution.

Collaboration on the chemical reaction task thus seems to involve two different types of social interactive processes. The first process, which occurs during the setting-up or planning stage of the task, involves either separate (parallel) working patterns or closely coordinated cooperative patterns. Cooperation during the setting-up stage consists of mutual guidance, encouragement, and support. Often during this phase of the task, complementary problem-solving roles are assumed.

Later on in the task, when experimental evidence is being examined, the second kind of interactive process occurs. At this time, each child seems to be reaching independent conclusions about the solution of the task that are based on all or only some of the available experimental evidence. After each child comes to a conclusion, he or she may find that his or her partner does not agree. In this circumstance, overt conflicting perspectives on the experimental evidence are expressed in the form of an argument. Arguments capable of producing a consensus seemed to be those that made use of appropriate supporting evidence.

It appears that Perret-Clermont's notion that cognitive conflict is the mediator between peer interaction and cognitive reorganization can be tested best in contexts where overt manifestations of conflict are likely. These contexts seem to occur when children have access to a wealth of empirical evidence, when this evidence is capable of suggesting at least two distinct solutions to the problem, and when a consensual solution is solicited.

Perret-Clermont's hypothesis about the importance of cognitive conflict comes from Piaget's theory concerning the role of social factors in development. Most of the past research on the topic of peer collaboration has been based upon Piaget's ideas. Piaget placed more importance on peer interaction than upon adult–child interaction, so it is not surprising that the bulk of research on collaboration has shared a Piagetian perspective.

In order to understand the limitations as well as the strengths of this perspective on collaboration, one needs to appreciate the role that peer interaction plays in Piaget's theory. Piaget (1970) identified four factors that he believed are necessary for a theory of cognitive development: maturation, experience with the physical environment, social experiences, and equilibration or self-regulation. In addition, Piaget claimed that equilibration is the most fundamental of the four factors. Peer interaction, and social experiences in general, derive their importance from the influence they can exert on equilibration through the introduction of cognitive conflict. Perret-Clermont shares this view of development when she writes:

Of course, cognitive conflict of this kind does not create the *forms* of operations, but it brings about the disequilibriums which make cognitive elaboration necessary, and in this way cognitive conflict confers a special role on the social factor as one among other factors leading to mental growth. Social–cognitive conflict may be figuratively likened to the catalyst in a chemical reaction: it is not present at all in the final product, but it is nevertheless indispensable if the reaction is to take place. (Perret-Clermont, 1980, p. 178)

When Piaget looks at peer interaction, therefore, he looks for evidence of disequilibrium, that is, cognitive conflict. He is not interested in describing or explaining social interactional processes as a whole. Piaget's theory is most helpful in explaining those situations where cognitive conflict is clearly and overtly expressed in external social behaviors, for example, arguments. However, in situations where overt conflict is not apparent and where mutual guidance and support are evident, his theory provides few clues concerning the role of social factors in development. Fortunately, Vygotsky's writings on adult–child interaction offer insights into the intellectual value of these kinds of peer interactions.

To illustrate how Vygotsky's ideas shed light on some of the processes involved in peer collaboration, we will discuss another set of observations of George and Bruce. One of the most puzzling findings from Forman's study was the discrepancy between how a dyad functions as a unit and how the partners function separately. George and Bruce were clearly the most successful collaborators, yet they did not show the same consistently high level of functioning when they were posttested separately. This discrepancy between dyadic and individual performance levels was also apparent when subjects who collaborated were compared with those who worked alone. On the posttest measures, which were individually administered, collaborative problem solvers did not do better than solitary problem solvers. Nevertheless, collaborative partners were able to solve many more chemical problems than could solitary problem solvers during the same period of time.

Vygotsky acknowledged that a discrepancy might exist between solitary and social problem solving when he developed his notion of the zone of proximal development. He defined this zone as *"the distance between the actual developmental level as determined by independent problem solving and the level of potential development as determined through problem solving under adult guidance or in collaboration with more capable peers"* (1978, p. 86). Thus, Vygotsky hypothesized that children would be able to solve problems with assistance from an adult or more capable peer before they could solve them alone. This seemingly obvious observation was then used to reach several original conclusions. One conclusion was that the zone of proximal development could be used to identify those skills most amenable to instruction. Another was that learning consists of the internalization of social interactional processes. According to Vygotsky, development proceeds when interpsychological regulation is transformed into intrapsychological regulation.

Returning to Forman's data, it appears that a similar process of interpsychological to intrapsychological regulation may also occur in collaborative contexts where neither partner can be seen as objectively "more capable," but where the partners may assume separate but complementary social roles. One child may perform an observing, guiding, and correcting role while the other performs the task procedures. This observing partner seems to provide some of the same kinds of assistance that has been called scaffolding by Wood, Bruner, and Ross (1976). Such support from an observing partner seems to enable the two collaborators to solve problems together before they are capable of solving the same problems alone. When collaborators assume complementary roles, they begin to resemble the peer tutors described earlier. For example, the observer/performer roles are functionally similar to the critic/author roles observed in Egan's New Hampshire classroom.

In addition, one can see in Forman's data instances where problem-solving strategies first appear as social interactional procedures and are later internalized. Remember that a combinatorial problem was administered to each child individually at three different times (as a pretest, as an immediate posttest and as a delayed posttest). In addition, these same children were presented with a similar combinatorial problem in each problem-solving session when they were asked to decide jointly which chemical mixtures to set up. Therefore, a comparison can be made between the combinations generated by each child when he or she worked alone or in pairs.

Both George and Bruce used an empirical strategy to generate combinations during their pretest – for example, selecting a combination at random and then basing the next combination on the first by adding, subtracting, or substituting one of its elements. The third combination would then be produced by copying, with another minor revision, the second combination. Pairwise checking of each new combination with each previous combination was the empirical procedure used for guarding against duplications.

In their early collaborative problem-solving sessions, George and Bruce worked in parallel and each used an empirical strategy similar to the one used on the pretest to generate combinations. After about a month of working together, they devised a social procedure for generating combinations empirically by assuming complementary problem-solving roles: One selected chemicals and the other checked their uniqueness.

After two months, they had begun to organize their combinations into groups based on their number of elements. In addition, they had devised a deductive system for generating two-element combinations. This deductive procedure enabled the child who had previously done the checking to prompt, correct, and reinforce the selections of his partner. Higher-order combinations were produced empirically using the familiar social procedure.

At the last session, the boys continued to assume complementary roles but now used the blackboard as a recording device. They produced combinations in a highly organized fashion – singles, two-element combinations, three-element combinations, and so on – and were able to generate almost all of the 31 possible combinations. They used a deductive procedure for generating the two-element combinations but still relied on their empirical procedure for the higher-order combinations.

At the first posttest one week after the last collaborative session, the degree to which each boy had internalized a deductive combinatorial system was assessed by asking them to generate combinations independently. Bruce was able to generate all 10 two-element combinations deductively on his own, but George was not. George used an empirical system to generate combinations. On the second posttest four months later, however, both boys had internalized a deductive procedure for producing two-element combinations.

It appears that these two boys were able to apply a preexisting intra-psychological rule, an empirical combinatorial procedure, to a collaborative context by dividing the procedure into complementary problem-solving roles.With repeated exposure to the problem, these boys were able to progress to a deductive procedure for generating simple, two-element combinations. At first, deductive reasoning was clearly a social activity for George and Bruce. Each time one partner selected a series of combinations, the other guided, prompted, and corrected his selections. Later, one partner was able to demonstrate that he had internalized this deductive procedure by using it to generate all possible two-element combinations on his own. Four months later, both partners were able to generate all possible pairs of five objects deductively by themselves. Thus, for these two boys, deductive combinatorial reasoning first appeared in a collaborative context. Only one of the two boys was initially able to show that he had internalized this procedure when he generated combinations alone. Months later, however, both boys had internalized this deductive process.

In summary, a Piagetian perspective on the role of social factors in development can be useful in understanding situations where overt indices of cognitive conflict are present. However, if one wants to understand the cognitive consequences of other social interactional contexts, Vygotsky's ideas may be more helpful. In tasks where experimental evidence was being generated and where managerial skills were required, by assuming complementary problem-solving roles, peers could perform tasks together before they could perform them alone. The peer observer seemed to provide some of the same kinds of "scaffolding" assistance that others have attributed to the adult in teaching contexts.

Thus, the Vygotskian perspective enables us to see that collaborative tasks requiring data generation, planning, and management can provide another set of valuable experiences for children. In these tasks, a common set of assumptions, procedures, and information needs to be constructed. These tasks require children to integrate their conflicting task conceptions into a mutual plan. One way to achieve a shared task perspective is to assume complementary problem-solving roles. Then each child learns to use speech to guide the actions of her or his partner and, in turn, to be guided by the partner's speech. Exposure to this form of social regulation can enable children to master difficult problems together before they are capable of solving them alone. More importantly, experience with social forms of regulation can provide children with just the tools they need to master problems on their own. It enables them to observe and reflect on the problem-solving process as a whole and to select those procedures that are the most effective. When they can apply this social understanding to themselves, they can then solve, independently, those tasks that they had previously been able to solve only with assistance.

Thus, collaborative problem solving seems to offer some of the same experiences for children that peer tutoring provides: the need to give verbal instructions to peers, the impetus for self-reflection encouraged by a visible audience, and the need to respond to peer questions and challenges. The reciprocal model of peer assistance that characterized the children in Egan's classroom is even more apparent in collaborative problem-solving contexts, similar to those observed by Forman.

Conclusion

In conclusion, in these analyses we are not talking about a children's culture separate from adults. What Leont'ev and Luria discuss as the "most important specifically human form of mental development" – namely, "the assimilation of general human experience in the teaching process" – must ultimately be grounded in adult–child interactions. But peer (and cross-age) relationships can function as intermediate transforming contexts between social and external adult–child interactions and the individual child's inner speech.

Although such peer interactions take place in home and community as well as at school, they may be especially important in school because of limitations and rigidities characteristic of adult–child interactions in that institutional setting. Cazden (1983) argues for the value to child development of a category of parent–child interactions of which the peek-a-boo game and picture book reading are familiar examples. In interactions such as these, there is a predictable structure in which the mother initially enacts the entire script herself and then the child takes an increasingly active role, eventually speaking all the parts initially spoken by the mother. The contrast between such learning environments and the classroom is striking. In school lessons, teachers give directions and children nonverbally carry them out; teachers ask questions and children answer them, frequently with only a word or a phrase. Most importantly, these roles are not reversible, at least not within the context of teacher–child interactions. Children never give directions to teachers, and questions addressed to teachers are rare except for asking permission. The only context in which children can reverse interactional roles with the same intellectual content, giving directions as well as following them, and asking questions as well as answering them, is with their peers.

NOTES

Forman's research was supported, in part, by a grant from Radcliffe College; by a grant to Deanna Kuhn from the Milton Fund, Harvard University; and by NIMH Grant No. 5 T32 MH15786 to the Department of Psychology, Northwestern

University. We would like to thank the students, faculty, and principle of the Stratton Elementary School, Arlington, Massachusetts for their generous participation in this research; and Leonard Scinto, Addison Stone, and Jim Wertsch for their helpful comments on earlier drafts of this chapter.

1 Other social interactional codes were used to identify conversations that served to plan, reflect upon, or organize these procedural activities (metaprocedural interactions), task-focused jokes (playful interactions), task-focused observations (shared observations), and off-task behavior.

2 A second set of posttests was administered to both samples four months after the first posttest. The pairs constantly outperformed the singletons on both second posttest measures. However, the interpretation of these findings is problematic due to the fact that this four-month period occurred during the school year for the pairs but during the summer for the singletons.

REFERENCES

Carrasco, R. L., Vera, A., and Cazden, C. B. 1981. Aspects of bilingual students communicative competence in the classroom: A case study. In R. Duran (Ed.), *Latino language and communicative behavior. Discourse processes: Advances in research and theory,* (Vol. 6). Norwood, N.J.: Ablex.

Cazden, C. B. 1983. Peekaboo as an instructional model: Discourse development at school and at home. In B. Bain (Ed.), *The sociogenesis of language and human conduct: A multi-disciplinary book of readings.* N.Y.: Plenum, pp. 33–58.

Cazden, C. B., Cox, M., Dickinson, D. Steinberg, Z., and Stone, C. 1978. "You all gonna hafta listen": Peer teaching in a primary classroom. In W. A. Collins (Ed.), *Children's language and communication.* 12th Annual Minnesota Symposium on Child Development. Hillsdale, N.J.: Erlbaum, pp. 183–231.

Doise, W., Mugny, G., and Perret-Clermont, A. N. 1975. Social interaction and the development of cognitive operations. *European Journal of Social Psychology,* 5(3), 367–383.

Doise, W., Mugny, G., and Perret-Clermont, A. N. 1976. Social interaction and cognitive development: Further evidence. *European Journal of Social Psychology,* 6, 245–247.

Forman, E. A. 1981. The role of collaboration in problem-solving in children. Doctoral dissertation, Harvard University.

Galton, M., Simon, B., and Croll, P. 1980. *Inside the primary classroom.* Boston: Routledge & Kegan Paul.

Inagaki, K. 1981. Facilitation of knowledge integration through classroom discussion. *Quarterly Newsletter of the Laboratory of Comparative Human Cognition,* 3(3), 26–28.

Inagaki, K., and Hatano, G. 1968. Motivational influences on epistemic observation. *Japanese Journal of Educational Psychology,* 6, 191–202.

Inagaki, K., and Hatano, G. 1977. Amplification of cognitive motivation and its effects on epistemic observation. *American Educational Research Journal, 14,* 485–491.

Inhelder, B., and Piaget, J. 1958. *The growth of logical thinking from childhood to adolescence.* New York: Basic Books.

Kamler, B. 1980. One child, one teacher, one classroom: The story of one piece of writing. *Language Arts*, 57, 680–693.

Kol'tsova, V. A. 1978. Experimental study of cognitive activity in communication (with specific reference to concept formation). *Soviet Psychology*, 17, 23–38.

Kuhn, D., and Ho, V. 1980. Self-directed activity and cognitive development. *Journal of Applied Developmental Psychology*, 1(2), 119–133.

Kuhn, D., and Phelps, E. 1979. A methodology for observing development of a formal reasoning strategy. *New Directions for Child Development*, 5, 45–58.

Kuhn, D., and Phelps, E. 1982. The development of problem-solving strategies. In H. Reese (Ed.), *Advances in child development* (Vol. 17). New York: Academic Press.

Lawler, J. 1980. Collectivity and individuality in Soviet educational theory. *Contemporary Educational Psychology*, 5, 163–174.

Leont'ev, A. N. 1981. The problem of activity in psychology. In J. V. Wertsch (Ed.), *The concept of activity in Soviet psychology*. Armonk, N.Y.: Sharpe, pp. 37–71.

Leont'ev, A. N., and Luria, A. R. 1968. The psychological ideas of L. S. Vygotsky. In B. B. Wolman (Ed.), *Historical roots of contemporary psychology*. New York: Harper and Row.

Levina, R. E. 1981. L. S. Vygotsky's ideas about the planning function of speech in children. In J. V. Wertsch (Ed.), *The concept of activity in Soviet psychology*. Armont, N.Y.: Sharpe, pp. 279–299.

Lomov, B. F. 1978. Psychological processes and communication. *Soviet Psychology*, 17, 3–22.

Mehan, H. 1979. *Learning lessons*. Cambridge: Harvard University Press.

Mehan, H., and Riel, M. M. 1982. Teachers' and students' instructional strategies. In L. Adler (Ed.), *Cross-cultural research at issue*. New York: Academic Press.

Mugny, G., and Doise, W. 1978. Socio-cognitive conflict and structure of individual and collective performances. *European Journal of Social Psychology*, 8, 181–192.

Parten, M. 1932. Social participation among preschool children. *Journal of Abnormal and Social Psychology*, 27, 243–269.

Perret-Clermont, A. N. 1980. *Social interaction and cognitive development in children*. New York: Academic Press.

Piaget, J. 1970. Piaget's theory. In P. H. Mussen (Ed.), *Carmichael's manual of child psychology* (3rd ed., Vol. 1). New York: Wiley, pp. 703–732.

Sharan, S. 1980. Cooperative learning in small groups: Recent methods and effects on achievement, attitudes, and ethnic relations. *Review of Educational Research*, 50, 241–271.

Simon, B. (Ed.), 1957. *Psychology in the Soviet Union*. Stanford, Calif.: Stanford University Press.

Simon, B., and Simon, J. (Eds.). 1963. *Educational psychology in the USSR*. Stanford, Calif.: Stanford University Press.

Slavina, L. S. 1957. Specific features of the intellectual work of unsuccessful pupils. In B. Simon (Ed.), *Psychology in the Soviet Union*. Stanford, Calif.: Stanford University Press, pp. 205–212.

Vygotsky, L. S. 1956. *Izbrannye psikhologicheskie issledovaniya*. [Selected psychological research.] Moscow: Izdatel'stzo Akademii Pedagogicheskikh Nauk RFSFR.

Vygotsky, L. S. 1978. *Mind in society*. Edited by M. Cole, V. John-Steiner, S. Scribner, and E. Souberman. Cambridge: Harvard University Press.

Vygotsky, L. S. 1981. The genesis of higher mental functions. In J. V. Wertsch (Ed.), *The concept of activity in Soviet psychology*. Armonk, N.Y.: Sharpe.

Wertsch, J. V. 1978. Adult–child interaction and the roots of metacognition. *Quarterly Newsletter of the Institute for Comparative Human Development*, *2*(1), 15–18.

Wertsch, J. V. 1979. The regulation of human action and the given-new organization of private speech. In G. Zivin (Ed.), *The development of self-regulation through private speech*. New York: Wiley, pp. 79–98.

Wertsch, J. V. (Ed.). 1981. *The concept of activity in Soviet Psychology*. Armonk, N.Y.: Sharpe.

Wertsch, J. V., and Stone, C. A. 1978. Microgenesis as a tool for developmental analysis. *Quarterly Newsletter of the Laboratory of Comparative Human Development*, *1*(1), 8–10.

Wood, D., Bruner, J. S., and Ross, G. 1976. The role of tutoring in problem-solving. *Journal of Child Psychology and Psychiatry*, *17*, 89–100.

15

The road to competence in an alien land: a Vygotskian perspective on bilingualism

VERA JOHN-STEINER

"The psychologist's most vital challenge is that of uncovering and bringing to light the hidden mechanisms underlying complex human psychology," wrote Vygotsky (1960). This orientation characterized most of the scientific work of this great Russian psychologist, including his analysis of the varied forms of language. He delineated the role of transformations and the unification of diverse processes in the course of cognitive development. In his analysis of writing, for instance, he emphasized that it is not just a simple extension or translation of spoken language into written symbols, "it is language without sound; it is language in idea form; it is monologue language, a conversation with a white piece of paper"[1] (n.d., pp 2–3).

In acquiring the written form of language, he wrote, children do not "simply retrace the history of spoken language." Vygotsky suggests, in comparing these different processes, that "development is never completed in all areas according to a single schema, its paths are myriad in their forms" (n.d., p. 46). In order to learn to write, the child joins the early, unconsciously acquired processes of speech with the more arbitrary intellectual activities of middle childhood, which entail conscious intention and realization.

A comparison between native- and second-language acquisition reveals a similar distinction according to Vygotsky. The issues of bilingualism concerned him; he saw these as important in his country "where many nationalities are intertwined in geographic, economic and socio-cultural relationships" (p. 1). The use of two or more languages interested him theoretically as well, as he recognized in the study of bilingualism an important context for the examination of the role of language in thought.

In his paper "The Question of Multilingualism in Childhood" (1935), Vygotsky criticized the associationist model of bilingual acquisition put forth by Epstein. In its stead he proposed a different approach that stressed the unification of diverse processes characterizing the acquisition of first and second languages:

Different paths of development which take place under different conditions cannot lead to completely identical results. It would be a miracle if the acquisition of a

348

foreign language through school instruction repeated, or reproduced that which was done earlier, under different conditions, for the development of the native language. These differences, no matter how different they are, should not distract us from the fact that both of the processes of the native and foreign language have between them a great deal in common. . . .*they are internally united.* (1935, p. 26)

The similarities and the differences between the acquisition of a first versus a second language have been the subject of much recent controversy among psycholinguists. Some researchers have emphasized a basically common process: Dulay and Burt (1978) ascribe what they see as a shared development "to universal innate mechanisms which cause them to formulate certain hypotheses about the language system being acquired" (p. 348). The evidence they cite is that young Chinese and Spanish learners acquired 11 English morphemes in virtually the same order. Although these findings have been replicated by other investigators, some of them differ in their interpretations from those offered by Dulay and Burt. Larsen-Freeman (1978) attributes the similarity of this grammatical development across learners from different speech communities to the language input they hear. These are the features that occur at the greatest frequency in the speech of adults addressing children.

A somewhat different approach is taken by Susan Ervin-Tripp (1974) in an article entitled "Is Second Language Learning Like the First?" In this paper she reports on her research with children learning a second language in a "natural" (nonschool) environment. Young Anglophone children living in Geneva, Switzerland were her subjects to whom she administered comprehension, imitation, and translation tests. These children learning French exhibited similar skills and strategies to those used by children acquiring a first language. "Second language learners, like children, remember best the items they can interpret," she wrote (p. 116). Children in both situations both use word order strategies and display lexical overgeneralizations. She concluded her study as follows:

In broad outlines, then the conclusion is tenable that first and second language learning is similar in natural situations. However, if children come to the task with some knowledge available, there may be very accelerated progress in some respects, so that the rate of development will not look the same for all details. In every respect we found that in the age range of four through nine, older children had an advantage and learned faster. (P. 126)

Increasingly, the advantage of older children and adolescents is documented, particularly in the areas of syntax and morphology. These results lead one to ask: Do older children just learn faster, or do they rely on different approaches than do younger learners?

Vygotsky supports the latter position; he views the acquisition of a second language as represented by a different line of development than the first, particularly if the learner is literate in his or her first language:

The child assimilates his/her native language unconsciously and unintentionally but acquires a forgeign language with conscious realization and intention. . . .A child never begins the acquisition of his native language with studying the alphabet, with reading and writing, with conscious and deliberate construction of phrases, with word definitions, with the study of grammar. But all of this usually takes place at the beginning of acquiring a foreign language. (n.d., pp. 2–3)

And he writes further that

if the development of the native language begins with free, spontaneous use of speech and is culminated in the conscious realization of linguistic forms and their mastery, then development of a foreign language begins with conscious realization of language and arbitrary command of it and culminates in spontaneous, free speech. But, between those opposing paths of development, there exists a mutual dependency just as between the development of scientific and spontaneous concepts. This kind of conscious and deliberate acquisition of a foreign language obviously depends on a known level of development of the native language. . . . (P. 48)

In this discussion of first- and second-language acquisition, Vygotsky's emphasis upon the role of conscious learning in the mastery of a new tongue may be an exaggerated one. His view is probably due to his placing such learning exclusively in a school context. In spite of possible differences in methods of second-language acquisition in varying contexts of learning, which he did not take into account, his general conclusion is well supported by recent research – *namely that acquisition of a second language is indeed dependent upon the level of development of the native language*.

Evidence supporting such a position is presented by Skutnabb-Kangas and Toukomaa (1976) in their large-scale study of Finnish immigrant students enrolled in Swedish schools. They found that students who had moved from Finland to Sweden at an average age of 10 years knew their first language and learned Swedish much better than their younger siblings. Worst off were pupils who were 7–8 years old during their parents' immigration: "The verbal development of these students," wrote the authors, "who moved just after school was beginning [children begin school at 7 in Sweden] underwent serious disturbances after the move. This also had a detrimental effect on their learning Swedish" (p. 75).

Contemporary investigators (e.g., Paulston, 1978) emphasize the better memory storage and the more fully developed conceptual system of older children and adolscents as part of their advantage over the highly imitative younger children learning a second language. It is also likely that more experienced learners make more *conscious* use of cognitive and linguistic strategies that they first developed while acquiring their native language. Vygotsky (1935) commented that "the child acquiring a foreign language is already in command of a system of meaning in the native language which she/he transfers to the sphere of another language" (p. 48). There may be other aspects of this metalinguistic process which have not been sufficiently emphasized to date. One of these is the role of native language literacy in the acquisition of a second language. Very young children need to interpret and analyze a new language as part of a rapid on-line processing of the flow of speech, particularly if they are learning in a noninstructional context. But the learning of writing contributes to a deeper, more conscious aware- ness of one's own speech, a notion that Vygotsky has so effectively de- scribed. Does this kind of an analysis contribute to second-language acquisition?

The findings reported by Skutnabb-Kangas and Toukomaa indicate such a possibility. They discussed the particular vulnerability of 7- and 8- year-old children in terms of both rapid language loss and the difficulties these children experienced in learning a second language when compared with their older siblings. This is not only the age when most children start to learn to read and write; it is also the developmental period when the dif- ferentiation of social, private, and inner speech first begins. This is a slow but crucial process: It is dependent upon the finely tuned communicative exchanges between children and their caretakers. Wells (1981) reported that the way in which meaning is negotiated between generations in the preschool period affects the acquisition of reading. Fuson (1979) found in her survey of the development of self-regulating speech the facilitating effects of verbalizations upon memory, attention, and representational activities. It is quite likely that these important uses of language may not develop well when children find themselves under severe pressure to acquire a second language.

The language-learning advantages of older children in Sweden as well as in Canada and Holland are of interest in this regard. Swain (1980) reported results of a large-scale study in Ontario of Anglophone students who were placed into French immersion programs. Students who first entered such a program in seventh grade, and who were tested while in tenth grade, per- formed better on a French reading task than students who first attended immersion classes in kindergarten and consequently had spent many more hours in such a program. Swain commented on these findings as follows:

These results, then, suggest that in school settings, at least, older learners are more efficient in some aspects of language learning than young learners. It has been sug- gested that this is so because older learners are cognitively more mature. Their ability to abstract, classify and generalize may aid in the task of consciously for- mulating and applying second language rules. (Pp. 5–6)

The advantages of older learners in acquiring the rule-governed aspects of a second language were also found by Snow and Hoefnagel-Höhle (1978) in their studies of native English speakers living in Holland.

Vygotsky proposed that the attainment of literacy itself contributes to linguistic–cognitive development, as it requires "the conscious realization of one's linguistic processes." In addition, work within the Vygotskian tradition reveals that there is a powerful linkage between *inter*personal uses of language (particularly in tutorial exchanges) and the development of the cognitive *intra*personal functions of speech. This position is further elaborated by John-Steiner and Tatter (1983) and by several of the authors included in the present volume: Wertsch and Stone's (chapter 7) microgenetic studies demonstrate the role of task-relevant dialogue shaping children's problem-solving behavior. Their work also points to the lengthy development that leads to the full use of cognitive–representational functions of speech. Similarly, effective strategies used in solving memory tasks also have long developmental growth spans. Flavell (1977) described some of these strategies as follows: "It is possible that this age trend [the use of verbal and imaginal elaboration techniques] is part of a more general trend toward the use of active, elaborative and inferential (constructive) comprehension strategies in the service of memory goals" (p. 12).

There is as yet a paucity of studies focusing on strategies used in second-language learning in contrast to those examining memory and problem-solving approaches. The few studies that do exist in this area highlight the importance of the second-language learner's active participation in his or her learning, both in immersion situations and in classroom settings.

Learning to learn: strategies of second-language acquisition

Whereas the baby and the toddler have to learn what to talk about and what categories words represent, "the second-language learner could be said to be learning new forms for old conversational uses and ideas," wrote Susan Ervin-Tripp (1981, p. 2). Some of the conversational routines Ervin-Tripp has identified among young learners serve to attract the attention of their partners at play. These kindergarten children who find themselves in a linguistically novel situation are able to plan, ask for information, announce their intentions, and engage in joking as well. Formal linguistic development is slow among these 5-year-olds, but they are resourceful in maximizing their communicative means.

The same conclusion emerges from Lilly Wong Fillmore's study (1979) that dealt with Spanish-speaking children newly arrived from Mexico. The investigator paired these children with Anglo friends and taped their interactions over the period of a school year. The taping sessions were held in a playroom full of toys and school materials. The results indicate the importance of social and cognitive strategies in second-language acquisition. Nora, the most successful of Fillmore's subjects, was adept at placing herself in interactional situations where she received maximum exposure to the new language. Her choice of activities also supported her language growth, while some of the boys in this study who preferred motoric games lacked similar opportunities for language practice.

Fillmore (1979) formulated the strategies children used in simple terms: (1) "Assume that what people are saying is directly relevant to the situation at hand, or to what they or you are experiencing. Metastrategy: Guess" (p. 210). There are many opportunities within the daily experiences of children at play or in the classroom where the situation provides cues for figuring out what others are saying. (2) "Get some expressions you understand and start talking" (p. 211). A reliance upon formulaic expressions, such as "You wanna play?" is useful in initiating conversations. These expressions also provide data for the learner's more analytical efforts aimed at figuring out the structure of the new language. (3) "Look for recurring parts in the formulas you know" (p. 212). Even 5-year-olds have some experience in generalizing from situation to situation and in using certain sentence frames productively. Nora's speech behavior offered many such examples: "How do you do dese September por manana?" "How do you do dese tortillas?" and "How do you do dese in English?" A related strategy that Ervin-Tripp had also stressed in her analysis is (4) "Make the most of what you got" (p. 215). The young children in these studies stretched their limited repertoires of forms and structures using them in many diverse situations. At times these extensions were barely adequate to convey their intentions, but the children's classmates cooperated in decoding these messages. "C'mon me you house, " or "C'mon me to the shoe" are examples of such early efforts at making use of their limited means. (5) "Work on big things: save the details for later" (p. 218). The children tended to use English word order, but while they worked on the major constituents of the language, they frequently neglected grammatical morphemes and auxiliaries, leaving these for the later stages of their acquisition of the new language.

These strategies identified by Fillmore were particularly effective in a situation where the children had varied opportunities to learn informally in the context of play. One of the ways in which the English-speaking friends of these five Mexican children modified their language was to limit their talk to the activities at hand. They did not avoid distant topics, however, when they addressed the experimenter.

Immigrant children who are first exposed to a target language in a highly structured classroom do not find adequate contextual support for their language-learning efforts. In these first- and second-grade classrooms, activities are of a pencil-and-paper kind, and the teacher does most of the talking. Thus, in such settings, there are limited opportunities for second-language learners to connect familiar activities with new expressions. This may account for the fact the Finnish immigrant children who entered Swedish schools as first-graders experienced the most severe difficulties in their academic and linguistic development. They were too old to learn their second language through play as did Fillmore's kindergarten-age subjects. At the same time they were too young to have developed literacy and cognitive strategies, which were available to their older siblings who had had a few years of education in their native language.

As yet there are few detailed studies dealing with the processes of second-language learning in middle childhood. Consequently, the cognitive strategies used by school-age children have to be inferred from classroom achievement studies and from experimental research in this area. In one study of elicited imitation of native Arabic speakers who were learning English as a second language, Hamayan, Saegart, and Larudee (1975) found that older subjects performed much better on imitation tasks than did younger learners. The advantage of the former group was attributed by the authors to the greater attention span of preadolescents and to their memory heuristics. The longer memory span of older second-language learners was noticed by Evelyn Hatch (1977) as well, who found their ability to repeat long sequences, including a series of idiomatic expressions, important in their acquisition patterns.

It is important, however, not to assume that older learners will make rapid language learning progress in all situations. In one case study of a 13-year-old middle-class adolescent boy from Colombia, the investigators observed little progress in the development of their subject, Ricardo, over a three-month period. Butterworth and Hatch (1978) noted that he did not inflect his verbs; he simply added a rising intonation to his utterances when forming a question and placed WH-words within a sentence, as in "You watch television what?" In contrast with these elementary aspects of his syntax, the length of Ricardo's utterances doubled during the study period. His vocabulary increased as well, though some of his expressions were idiosyncratic as he used a pattern of nominalization – for example, "He for selling" when he meant "He's a salesman."

The authors ascribe the slow progress of their subject to a heavily burdened language-learning process. Whereas young children can insert their simplified messages into the shared context of activities, the adolescent has many more interests and frequently suffers from the pressure of unmet communicative needs. In addition, it is important in the early stages of both first- and second-language learning to have some control over the rate and complexity of language input to which one is exposed. [The fine-tuning of exchanges between young learners and their caretakers contributes to an accelerated rate of language development. See Cross (1977).]

The language-learning conditions facing the young adolescent Ricardo provided him with few opportunities to control his input. His progress was linked to his own efforts at trying to unravel the varied levels of his target language. Lacking formal instruction in English, he adopted a simplification strategy, and in this way some of his utterances resembled that of Fillmore's young subjects.

In a case study of an adult learner, Schumann (1978) similarly found little linguistic progress in the development of an untutored 33-year-old adult. Alberto was able to convey simple communicative messages, but his language stabilized at a pidginized form of English at the end of the 10-month research period. Schumann proposed that this learner was severely affected by the large social and psychological distance that existed between the speakers of the target language and himself. Thus, it is likely that the active, elaborative, and inferential strategies that support cognitive mastery are easily interfered with when second-language learners find themselves in socially discriminating settings.

The critical role of the social environment in learning a second language was stressed by Vygotsky. He criticized a purely psychometric interpretation of low IQ scores of Chinese-American children in San Francisco who were tested in English. This investigation was an example of many others "where the concrete conditions in which the children's development took place" were neglected. Instead, Vygotsky suggested that "the entire problem of bilingualism should be viewed dynamically, not statistically" (1935, p. 21). Such a view includes an understanding of the social and educational factors that shape the increasingly competent use of second language as well as its arrested development.

One of the issues raised by these case studies is that of formal instruction. A number of scholars have proposed that the combination of classroom lessons with varied exposure to noninstructional interactions profit the older learner. In contrast with young children who learn in highly contextualized settings, the older learner needs assistance in breaking the code. In an influential theory of second-language acquisition, Krashen (1980) suggests that formal knowledge is of little use to adults unless it is linked to many opportunities to practice one's weaker language in personally rewarding situations. The role of comprehensible input is stressed by Krashen, as is the learner's role in generating actively such a language resource.

In a study of strategies used by high-school students in a second-language classroom situation, Bialystok (1978) found that their own activities outside of school, such as going to foreign-language movies, reading books, and talking to speakers, proved to be a determining factor in their learning. Those students who relied heavily on these forms of "functional practicing" performed best on written and oral tasks in their target language. Bialystok reminds us that it is those students who are highly motivated (regardless of their aptitude) who engage in these highly effective strategies. This finding may explain the immobilizing effect of the social and psychological distance upon learning which was documented by Schumann's (1978) case study of Alberto. A related finding was reported by Seliger (1977) in his classroom study of adult second-language learners. He found that those who practice "by initiating interactions, and thereby cause a concomitant input from others" (p. 265) outperformed the more passive learners. The effectiveness of generating one's own input, of exposing oneself to many diverse, verbally rich interactional situations was also shown in Fillmore's study. Nora, her most efficient young learner, exemplified a "functional practicing" strategy at the kindergarten level.

In addition to these *communicative* strategies that are already in use by very young second-language learners, adults also rely on *analytical* approaches. One of these is "monitoring," where language learners use their formal knowledge to modify their oral or written productions. Krashen and Pon (1975) describe the self-correcting behavior of a native speaker of Chinese, a woman in her 40s whose informal interactions in English they had taped. The speaker was able to correct close to 95% of her errors, which led the investigators to conclude that "the fact that the vast majority of errors were correctable by the subject suggests that she had a conscious knowledge of the rules. . .[but] that such conscious knowledge is applied only when sufficient processing time is available" (p. 126).

These studies illustrate a new trend in second-language research, a focus on *process approaches*. This contrasts with earlier work that was primarily product-oriented, that is, that used achievement measures and teachers' ratings in assessing second-language proficiencies. An exclusive reliance on output measures can be misleading, as shown in the Skutnabb-Kangas and Toukomaa research described above. Swedish teachers of Finnish children, impressed by their pupils' good pronunciation, failed to realize that these children had difficulties with the more complex cognitive uses of their second language.

A study of Ghanaian children is of great interest in this regard. G. Omani Collison (1974) examined the development of concept formation using Lansdown's colloquium approach to science instruction. The method consisted of groups of children manipulating materials and then describing their observations to each other and to their teachers: "Each child has the opportunity to organize her or his learning into a meaningful system. As they speak and think together, their perceptions are further sharpened by the concrete effort to synthesize their observations" (p. 447). Collison relied on Vygotsky's scheme of concept development in assessing the level of complexity of the childrens' observations and compared these when made in their vernacular languages (Ga and Twi) and in English. The findings indicate that when the children used their native languages as opposed to their school language, "they made more statements, their statements were more often at the complex and preconceptual level, they reported more relationships based on non-obvious linkages, and they used models more frequently" (p. 454). This researcher's conclusion that education in a foreign language may interfere with childrens' conceptual development is similar to that of Skutnabb-Kangas and Toukomaa. It is also supported by Cummins's (1980) analysis of the cognitive academic aspects of language proficiency (CALP).

Cummins has reported a number of statistical studies that led him to the conclusion that the level of CALP in the native tongue is related to the mastery of the second language: "Because L_1 and L_2 CALP are manifestations of the same underlying dimension, previous learning of literacy-related functions of language (in L_1) will predict future learning of these functions (in L_2)." (L_1 refers to the first language and L_2 to the second language acquired by learner in the literature of applied linguistics.) Cummins further proposes that these relationships do not develop in an "affective vacuum" (p. 179). If a student has little (or conflicting) motivation to learn a second language, as in some of the cases described above, these cognitive skills may not be adequately mobilized for the task at hand. The notion of CALP has been criticized (see Edelsky et al., 1980 pp. 11–12), particularly as Cummins has based it upon traditional measures of language proficiency. But the argument for a strong cognitive component of language proficiency does not rest on his analysis alone, as both product- and process-oriented studies support such a notion.

Similarly, there is strong support for the thesis presented in this chapter, which was first proposed by Vygotsky a half-century ago, namely that the acquisition of a second language is dependent upon the level of development of the native language. But the Vygotskian perspective reaches beyond this important statement, as it places the issues of bilingualism into the broader framework of the psychology of language and thought. In this way, it is possible to leave the "surface" of these studies and to explore, according to his suggestions, the internal structures involved in the speech development of bilinguals.

The relationship of language to thought is not one of static connections; it changes with the shifting lines of development of the two languages. Central to the examination of bilingualism is the question: How do speakers of two or more languages achieve a separation of them at the production level while uniting them internally at the level of verbal meaning and thought? It is the exploration of these seemingly contradictory processes that motivates my preliminary work on second-language acquisition in immersion situations.

Some aspects and stages of second-language development: a pilot study

Most researchers focus on observable processes of classroom interactions and on tested measures of achievement in their studies of second-language acquisition. An additional source of information consists of learners' self-reports. This is of particular value when one attempts to answer the question just posed concerning seemingly contradictory processes of development in dual language acquisition. The observations of sophisticated adult learners clarifies issues that cannot be approached through external observations alone. For instance, what are the strategies learners use to obtain comprehensible input? How can the beginning second-language speaker initiate conversations with native speakers? How do adults utilize their generalized knowledge of language structures and avoid interference errors due to an inappropriate transfer? In brief, what are some of the ways of linking old and new knowledge in the course of acquiring a target language?

These are some of the concerns that governed my approach to this pilot study, which was first initiated during the 1980 Summer Institute of the Linguistic Society of America. Five of the subjects were foreign scholars in attendance at the institute. Additional participants were native speakers of English who had worked and studied abroad (e.g., an American linguist who had studied child language acquisition in Hungary) and speakers of French, German, Czech, Japanese, and Spanish whose work or studies brought them to this country,[2] including a Hungarian graduate student in anthropology who was interviewed several times during his first four months in the United States.

The specific questions asked of the participants covered learner strategies dealing with exposure to comprehensible input (source, speed, modality); processing strategies (including comprehension, memory, and representational activities); production strategies (translation, covert rehearsal, monitoring); as well as the choice of topic and setting that influence speech in a weaker language. Lastly, the exploration of some affective sociolinguistic issues that have been reported by Schumann (1978) and others as significant in the acquisition of a second language were included. In addition to eliciting learners' self-reports concerning previously identified strategies and affective issues, these interviews were aimed at gathering information relevant to issues Vygotsky had delineated, such as the role of verbal thinking in bilinguals.

Stage I: leaning on the known

All participants in this pilot study had studied their target language before arriving in this country, where they underwent an "immersion" experience. Some of the subjects lived with relatives and spoke their native language with them at home; others found themselves in a totally foreign environment day and night. During the first stage of their second-language learning through immersion, the participants described as their primary concern the need to exercise control over the rate and content of the input language.

Input strategies. Conversations were very difficult for these individuals; they preferred to speak to one person at a time and to try to find a mutually agreeable topic of conversation. In these highly personal settings the learner would frequently lean forward and signal through eye contact and gesture his or her ability to comprehend or failure to do so.

One of the participants, an American woman who had studied in Mexico for a summer, kept a language-learning diary during her stay. She had recorded her use of questions as a means of restricting the topics of conversations with her hosts. She realized that it was easier to follow what was said in response to her questions. Or when a subject initiated by others dealt with an abstract topic, English cognates were included that aided in her efforts at comprehension.

In spite of these strategies, most second-language learners in this study tended to avoid conversational situations during these early weeks. Some of the learners put off appointments with doctors or dentists, as they felt unsure of themselves and were embarrassed by their lack of comprehension and fluency in the target language. The participants also complained that most people lack know-how in "foreign-talk"; there is frequently a lack of awareness of how to best adapt one's language to help adult nonnative speakers. Many individuals reported that when they asked for clarification, people tended to raise their voices instead of slowing their speech or paraphrasing their utterances.

Stephen Krashen (1980) has proposed that language is acquired by containing structures slightly above the second-language learner's level of competence. "This is done with the help of context or extralinguistic information" (p. 4). The availability of such comprehensible input may not be quite as widespread as Krashen suggests, however. It is for this reason that the combination of classroom lessons with informal opportunities to hear and practice a target language are found helpful in the early stages of the acquisition process. Language instructors are specialists in effective "foreigner talk"; they know how to simplify their syntax or to adjust the rate of their speech to the level of their listeners' comprehension abilities. Tutorial situations are particularly valuable in assisting the second-language learner's efforts toward the immediacy of comprehension required by "on-line" processing.

The difference between children and adults acquiring a target language in "natural" situations is that the former are supplied with many contextual cues through their shared activities with native-speaking peers. The conversation among adults lacks such contextual cues. It is for this reason that motivated adult learners seek a multiplicity of language input. Written materials are particularly important to them: "I made sure that I checked every word that I came in contact with. I spent a lot of time looking at store signs, the back labels of things, announcements. This is all I did, I think, the first two months of my stay," recalled an American linguist of the beginning of his field trip to Hungary.

An immigrant woman who spoke three languages before she came to America recalled the following: "I learned my English mostly at home, reading books (understanding ten to fifteen words only at the beginning). Later I read plays with which I had been familiar in translation. " Other participants reported that children's books and newspaper stories (particularly those of the human interest kind) were among their resources in acquiring their target language.

The mass media were another important source for second-language input where the learner did not need to respond. Many of those interviewed liked television best – it offered a lot of nonverbal information with which to interpret the language they heard. Linguists, on the other hand, preferred the radio, as they found it a good setting for testing some of their grammatical hypotheses.

The participants who were studying in their weaker language and who had to attend demanding classes found advanced reading to be important. The graduate student who was repeatedly interviewed by me during the first four months of his stay read extensively in preparation for the lectures he attended. When he studied relevant technical vocabulary in this manner, he was able to comprehend much of what he heard. But even after months of exposure to English, he found multiple conversations too difficult to handle.

These reports concerning the role of *written* sources in second-language acquisition support Vygotsky's analysis of the central role of literacy among adult learners.

Processing strategies. During the first few months most learners had difficulty in going directly from form to meaning in their weaker language. Generally, they relied on translation into their native language or on guessing when they were familiar with the domain of discourse. One participant reported that when she "leaned" on her first language as the means of representing the meaning of L_2 utterances, she failed to rehearse or remember what she had heard, as if a translated item would be erased from her mental tape. Several of the adult immigrants spoke of years of reliance upon translation: A German woman recalled her first successful efforts in going directly from the surface forms to the meaning of the language she was studying once she started to read in English. Written materials provided her with the opportunity to isolate a grammatical form or lexical item by examining the text repeatedly. A similar strategy was described by Janet R. Binkley in her letter to the *Linguistic Reporter* (1980): "I would read a paragraph out loud working solely on sounds. . . .then I reread it to get the meaning."

An alternation between what Bialystok (1978) has called "functional" and "formal" practicing characterized the strategies of a number of participants. They would immerse themselves in reading or listening to the radio in order to test areas of weakness in their language only to find that, following such a period of focusing on language structure and vocabulary, their exchanges with native speakers improved.

The European immigrants liked to use dictionaries and to memorize words and texts: "We Europeans learn long poems and history by heart; therefore, we tend to learn English by a lot of memorizing, too," recalled one middle-aged woman. The preparation of domain-specific vocabularies, anthropology in this case, was described by another participant as a helpful method of grouping, classifying, and actively manipulating the language in which he was studying.

The availability of technology also affects certain learning strategies in acquiring and learning when an individual is studying in a weaker language. One student tape-recorded all the lectures he had heard. While repeatedly listening to them he analyzed the material according to semantic and structural schemes, relying on abstracting skills he had developed through his first language.

The diverse ways in which learners approach the complex tasks of comprehending and processing a target language reflects, in part, culturally and educationally specific experiences. Learners' strategies illustrate the notion of *functional learning systems* first proposed by Vygotsky. Cole and Scribner (1974) described functional systems as "flexible and variable organizations of cognitive processes" (p. 193) and suggest that "sociocultural factors play a role in influencing which of possible alternative processes [visual or verbal representation for example] are evoked in a given situation and what role they play in total performance" (p. 193).

Production strategies. Although the participants in this study reported many complex and effective strategies in analyzing and remembering their new language, they often complained about difficulties in engaging in spontaneous talk. One participant reported being frustrated as she was unable to talk about sights that she and her new friend had seen during a leisurely walk to the bakery. There were not enough opportunities to practice new words and phrases, so instead she chose to rely heavily upon verbal routines. Such a strategy, however, made for short conversations. In order to enhance her possibilities for talk, this learner started to include English words in her sentences when conversing with her Mexican hosts. In this way, she thought, they might furnish her with the Spanish equivalents. Thus she could learn them more rapidly and in context.

Another approach that relied upon eliciting comprehensible input and using it as an immediate model to follow was described by a Japanese woman living in the United States. She was eager to talk to her American acquaintances about her involvement with women's issues in her native country. But the theme was beyond her skills at the time. In order to gain some vocabulary and discourse skills, this learner asked her American companions questions dealing with women's issues in this country. The discussion helped her to verbalize her own experience, and in this way she avoided the necessity of item-by-item translation from her native to the target language.

Eliciting a model to follow in one's weaker language is an excellent though infrequently used approach. Most students tend to rely on translation in their early months of study, which can become quite cumbersome. When asked to make presentations in class, students usually prepare themselves by reading. In most instances the written material is available in English (or another target language), and when once read is summarized by the learner in his or her native language. As a result, the learner writes a report in the first language, which then is translated into the target language. Nevertheless, some of the participants reported that a reliance upon translation persisted for a very long time. This characterized the learning of those who were not involved in language classes, but acquired the new tongue solely through immersion.

Sociolinguistic and affective issues. At early stages of second-language learning, criticism is very hard on learners. They feel that individuals who pay close attention to their mistakes in grammar and pronunciation neglect the communicative content of their messages. One woman reported that she started to avoid one of her professors who was only interested in correcting her mistakes "and sort of overlooked my production." A somewhat older woman expressed her feelings more strongly: "Some days when

I am being criticized I feel lonely, hurt, and discouraged. On other days it motivates me to learn faster."

This same student compared children's language learning and production to that of adults:

Children speak in simple sentences but they make fewer mistakes. This is the way they learn to communicate from their playmates. Adults, on the other hand, have their individual ways of expressing themselves as they have stronger needs to present their personalities through words. This makes it harder to understand them if you are a foreigner. It also makes it harder for us to start talking.

The problem of superficiality of contact with speakers of the target community was mentioned repeatedly: "We will say hello, how are you today? It is never like conversations at home." Many foreign students rely on friends and relatives for intimacy, as they are unable to express the complex web of feelings that living in an alien land gives rise to. "When I cannot express my ideas I get very upset," reported a young man from Venezuela. He was echoed by others. Individuals who live alone in this country found their emotional muteness particularly disturbing; they frequently wrote long letters or kept journals in their native tongue recording their reactions to their demanding new life.

In summary, these interviews illustrated the many active and systematic strategies adults used during the first few months of their learning to control their input, to maximize their productions, and to remember features of the new language that they were acquiring. The role of written materials was particularly striking among those learners who received little professional assistance while acquiring a target language in immersion situations.

Vygotsky's analysis was further confirmed by looking at the way in which both linguistic and cognitive knowledge was incorporated into the learning strategies of these individuals. They relied upon their native languages as the internal structure – a system of conceptual hooks and networks – through which they analyzed and ordered their verbal and nonverbal experience.

Stage II: an uneasy alliance of two languages

The major feature of this second phase of language learning is the struggle of many to break their dependence upon their first language. This determination is essential to overcome what some researchers have called "fossilization" in second-language learning.

Input strategies. During the third month of his stay, the Hungarian student no longer needed to tape all of the lectures he attended. Instead, he was able to take notes by writing full sentences in English. In order to check the accuracy of his notes, he borrowed notebooks from his fellow students. In some classes, his attention span lasted only 10–15 minutes, after which he needed a short rest. The signal that he had lost the trend of the lecture was his reverting back to translation into Hungarian. The exhaustive effort involved in listening to and trying to comprehend highly technical material in one's weak language was recalled by other participants as well. The importance of advanced reading as preparation for the skilled processing necessary in these situations was pointed out to them. Others spoke of frequent symptoms of overload: "At times when I am in a big group of people and they all speak English, I get tired. At that moment it is like it is going to be closed, and I don't hear anything anymore." A strategy reported by the young woman who had studied in Mexico when faced with symptoms of overload was to focus on one channel at a time: On certain days she did a great deal of listening, on others she did only reading, resisting her still very strong tendency to translate, word by word, into English.

A more careful analysis of the language input characterized many of the approaches reported at this stage of second-thought language acquisition. Some students relied on multiple readings of texts to analyze form and message; other subjects decomposed sentences and engaged in grammatical analysis, paying close attention to morphology and word order; those particularly eager to expand their vocabulary looked for association and recurrent usage in addition to memorizing word lists. In general, these learners were searching for ways to process their second language without having to translate it into their first.

Processing strategies. Speakers draw upon an internal meaning system while comprehending or producing language. However, as little is known of how the meaning or content of cognitive, linguistic, and affective processes is stored in the brain, it is widely assumed that internal representation is always coded in a specific language. When a native speaker of Spanish says in great frustration, "I cannot think in English," he refers to those planning processes that immediately precede an utterance and that are frequently subvocal in nature.

Similarly, Stephen Krashen (1980) wrote of a "silent period" in second-language acquistion when children do not produce "creative constructions" but repeat whole phrases they had memorized. He further suggested that

adults and children in formal language classes are not allowed a Silent Period. They are asked to produce right away. . . .[thus] performers "fall back" on the first language when they have not yet acquired enough of the second language to initiate the utterance they want. . . . *Performers simply think in the first language*, add vocabulary from the second language to "fill the slots" and make [some] corrections using the conscious monitor. (p. 7)

The task of internalizing a second language and weaving it together with the existing fabric of verbal thought is a complex one. The relationship of language and thought changes with the shifting lines of development of the two languages. In the early stages of second-language acquisition, there is a strong dependence upon the native language as the primary processor for both comprehension and production. But the assumption that competent bilinguals "think in English" while they speak in English and "think in Spanish" when they speak in Spanish is based on a simplified notion of thought. The shift in internal processes referred to in these comments is one of subvocal processes of planning an utterance; it is the increasing ability to plan in one's weaker language that corresponds to the notion of "thinking" in it.

Our investigations are prompted by an alternative hypothesis, an extension of Vygotsky's approach that was described above. We see a dual process at work in the development competencies of the bilingual, namely the separation of two or more languages at the production level, with a concomitant process of unification at the level of verbal meaning and thought. One illustration of the sequences of this development can be found in the note-taking behaviors of adults studying in their weaker language. The participants in this study have developed these skills in their native language – they have learned how to hold incoming information in their active memory while reorganizing it for later storage and classification.

At first, when taking notes in their second language, many try to write down what they hear in translation. Others either tape these lectures or use both their native and target language as a mixture: "In an art technique class, I was writing notes both in German and English," recalled a young immigrant artist. "Sometimes, I found it easier to write in English as I could not think of some technical terms in German. . .it was really a problem; no one could read my notes."

The next, more efficient strategy, consists of taking notes in the language of the lecturer, writing as rapidly as possible, even if the note taker does not comprehend all that is said. Lastly, these well-educated participants are able to use strategies in their target language that they had developed earlier: These consist of listening carefully and writing down only those central themes and ideas that constitute the conceptual core of a lecture. Thus, as learners are increasingly able to comprehend, condense, and store information in their weaker language, they start the process of weaving two meaning systems together.

However, during periods of intensive exposure to a new tongue and the necessity of separating the dominant and weaker language productively, individuals become aware of temporary losses as well as other features of language inhibition in their behavior. A period of great difficulty is frequently noted by students of second-language acquisition, who write of young boys and girls who are unwilling to communicate in *either one* of their languages. A similar process was described by some adults in this study; they did not become totally silent, but spoke of language loss in their native tongue at a time when they were not yet secure in their ability to communicate in their second language. "I find myself searching for words in English, but not translating them from German. I must have thought on a nonlinguistic level. I can't think of it in any language, but I want to say something" was the description given by one of the participants who was trying to capture thoughts that were not easily accessible in either one of the two languages.

Both internalization and externalization of verbal thought require multiple transformations into "syntactically articulated speech intelligible to others" (Vygotsky, 1962, p. 148).

Eventually, the integration of two languages in thinking is powerful enough so that the movements from thought to expression are possible regardless of the topic or domain of discourse. This level of balanced, successful bilingualism is not reached easily. Some learners persist in relying on comprehension and production strategies that protect them from "silent periods" and periods of language inhibition that are common during the long course of dual language acquisition. It is only by working through language loss and periods of inhibition that accompany the separation of two languages at the production level that individuals can reach true proficiency.[3] This loss of fear also results in the unification of old and new knowledge that characterizes the conceptual structure of the successful bilingual: "It is interesting, now that I speak some English as well as Hungarian, I am no longer sure which language I am thinking in."

Stage III: toward unity of thought and diversity of expressions

The fully developed and balanced bilingual is exemplified by the interpreter. The cognitive and linguistic processes of translators and conference interpreters offers a fascinating resource for examining hypotheses concerning dual language proficiencies. Central to the thesis presented in this chapter is that of a largely unified meaning system[4] that emerges in the course of the full mastery of a second language; such an internal system supports the varied and flexible uses of multiple codes among bilinguals. It is difficult to test such a hypothesis as there is no direct access to the internal semantic organization of bilinguals. Interpreter Lynn Visson has suggested,[5] however, that the note taking of consecutive interpreters offers an excellent illustration of this largely hidden process. Theirs is a condensed and personalized method of representing meaning that frees the interpreter from overdependence on either the source or the target language.

In consecutive interpretation the translator waits either until the speaker has finished or until a break is possible (usually 15–20 minutes) to deliver his or her version of the speech in the target language. Whereas simultaneous interpretation requires closely linked listening and speaking skills in two languages, consecutive interpretation relies heavily upon a highly organized semantic memory.

The work of interpreters illustrates the complex relationship of language and thought. Seleskovitch (1978) described the challenge they face as follows: "It is not enough for the interpreter to understand the semantics of individual words, phrases and sentences. . . .it is necessary for him to get the ideas beyond the words and convey those ideas and not the word content of the original language" (p. 333).

In consecutive translation, the interpreter develops an individualized notation system to capture meaning prototypes. These "sign nests" resemble Chinese characters. The use of a graphic shorthand minimizes the possibility of source-language interference in the interpreter's rendition of the speech. As the interpreters shuttle between thought and words, their efforts at transforming meaning into speech are akin to Vygotsky's (1962) description of this process: "A speaker often takes several minutes to disclose one thought. In his mind the whole thought is present at once, but in speech it has to be developed successively. . . .Precisely because thought does not have its automatic counterpart in words, the transition from thought to words leads through meaning" (p. 150).

The mastery of means that make such an enormously complex linguistic and cognitive task possible is barely understood. In this chapter I have tried to propose some possible mechanisms that enhance or interfere with the course of development toward the unity of thought and the diversity of expressions that characterize these virtuosos of bilingualism.

Summary

Second-language acquisition from a Vygotskian perspective as presented in this analysis was aimed at delineating some of the complex and opposing lines of first- versus second-language acquisition.

A review of experimental and psychometric studies was presented showing that age differences in the efficacy of second-language acquisition are linked to the use of linguistic and cognitive strategies. These are developed to a greater extent in older children and adolescents than in younger children. The active participation of learners is central to the task of dual language acquisition: In cases when young immigrants experience a great social and emotional distance between themselves and speakers of a target language, their learning is likely to be inhibited by a sense of passivity or alienation.

The description of learning strategies in immersion situations was elicited from educated adults at different stages of their acquisition process. Whereas conversational exchanges are effective sources for young children learning a second language, adults may need a broader set of learning contexts. The reliance upon written materials among older learners supports Vygotsky's analysis of the central role of literacy in the interaction of first- and second-language development. In the first stage of learning a new language, adults lean heavily on their native tongue. For them it serves as an internal scaffold that is dismantled slowly and painfully as these learners try to reach beyond what they know.

Subsequently, a dual process is at work in the developing competencies of speakers of two languages at the production level; the two languages are increasingly separated into autonomous systems of sound and structure, while at the level of verbal meaning and thought the two languages are increasingly unified. These complex and opposing interrelationships were noted by Vygotsky, who had suggested a two-way interaction between a first and second language. A period of strong dependence upon the native tongue – particularly upon its semantic system – is frequently followed by a reverse effect, a deepened knowledge of the first language. Thus, the effective mastery of two languages. Vygotsky argued, contributes to a more conscious understanding and use of linguistic phenomena in general. He quoted Goethe's comment on the importance of learning more than one language: "He who does not know a single foreign language does not know his own completely."

The realization of such knowledge is best reached by professional bi-linguals – interpreters and translators – whose work is aimed at rendering message meanings across languages. The notation system used in consecutive interpretation is of great interest in this discussion of the meaning level of language organization of bilinguals. And the graphic shorthand developed by these professional bilinguals is effective because it allows them to focus upon the conceptual core of the presentation without being unduly affected by the source or the target language.

One recurrent theme in this analysis is the role of language in thought and the role of thinking in speech that expresses the shifting organization of form and meaning in dual- and second-language acquisition. The analysis of these interactions may yield new insight into the largely hidden workings of the human mind.

Deeper understanding of bilingualism – effective, additive, joyful, and competent use of two or more languages – is increasingly important today as growing numbers of children and adults find themselves in alien lands with little knowledge of the languages spoken around them. A sustained and systematic inquiry into adult second-language acquisition is needed if we are to prevent the cultural inhibition of language and the social costs of alienation so prevalent under these circumstances. It is my belief that the Vygotskian perspective offers significant, though as yet untested opportunities for educational innovations that can help achieve communicative competence for millions of people in many lands.

NOTES

In the fall of 1979, I was the recipient of an IREX fellowship to study bilingualism and second-language acquisition in Budapest, Hungary. The work was started there. The assistance of my collaborator, Dr. Alexszander Javonszkij, was crucial to the conceptualization of some of the issues developed in this chapter; he and his colleagues from the Psychology Institute of the Hungarian Academy of Sciences were most gracious. Javonszkij's knowledge of Vygotsky's work in Russian led us to a small paper of his, entitled "On the Problems of Multilingualism in Childhood."

This analysis of cognitive strategies in second-language acquisition is based on some of Vygotsky's notions; it is also an extension of research and intellectual exchange in Hungary that was made possible by my hosts Drs. J. Patoky, I. Barkoczi, and C. Pleh, members of the Department of General Psychology, Eotvos Lorand University. Drs. G. Szepe and Z. Reger of the Linguistic Institute of the Hungarian Academy of Sciences shared with me their knowledge of the minority-language situation in Hungary. I wish to thank all of my colleagues in Hungary for their hospitality, assistance, and friendship.

1   I wish to thank James Wertsch for making an untitled paper by L. S. Vygotsky on language acquisition available to me. This paper served as an important additional source for the presentation of Vygotsky's thoughts on first- and second-language acquisition as presented in this chapter.

2   Mrs. Sophis Polgar conducted some of these interviews and shared her knowledge with me of the teaching–learning process accumulated throughout her lifetime. But can one ever fully thank one's mother?

3   In the study "Discourse Performance in Russian: A Study of Third-Language Acquisition" by John-Steiner and Jarovinsky (1981) we found an interesting pattern of interference errors. High-school-age bilinguals (speakers of Hungarian and Serbo-Croatian) were given a test for retelling both Russian and Hungarian. The analysis of interference errors revealed a very low rate of mistakes (less than 5%), and none of these was based on Hungarian morphology or syntax. The errors were all transfers from Serbo-Croatian. We interpreted this study as evidence that these students *inhibited* successfully their knowledge of Hungarian while performing in Russian and that their heavy and in general positive reliance upon Serbo-Croatian resulted in their rapid

acquisition of Russian. (The excellence of these students' performance was striking in comparison with the retellings of German-Hungarian adolescent bilinguals.)

4 The notioin "of a largely unified meaning system" needs to be expanded. Briefly, I refer to the integration of semantic domains across languages although I recognize that many lexical items, particularly those linked to childhood experiences, may retain specific connotations in one language that are not shared by corresponding items in a second or third language.

5 Dr. Lynn Visson was one of the intepreters at the 1980 Vygotsky conference held in Chicago. At the end of my presentation she showed me the system of notation that she used for consecutive intepretation. To her I owe this important theoretical insight concerning ways of monitoring meaning representation in the work of interpreters and translators.

REFERENCES

Bialystok, E. 1978. The role of conscious strategies in second language proficiency. Manuscript, Ontario Institute for Studies in Education.

Binkley, J. 1980. Letter. *Linguistic Reporter*, *22*(8), 2.

Butterworth, G., and Hatch, E. 1978. A Spanish-speaking adolescent's acquisition of English syntax. In E. Hatch (Ed.), *Second language acquisition: A book of readings*. Rowley, Mass.: Newbury House.

Cole, M., and Scribner, S. 1974. *Culture and thought*. New York: Wiley.

Collison, G. O. 1974. Concept formation in a second language: A study of Ghanian school children. *Harvard Educational Review 44*(3), 441–457.

Cross, T. 1977. Mother's speech adjustments: The contributions of selected child listener variables. In C. Snow and C. Ferguson (Eds.), *Talking to children*. Cambridge: Cambridge University Press.

Cummins, J. 1980. The cross-lingual dimensions of language proficiency: Implications for bilingual education and the optimal age issue. *TESOL Quarterly 14*(2), 174–187.

Dulay, H. C., and Burt, M. K. 1978. Natural sequences in child second language acquisition. In E. Hatch (Ed.), *Second language acquisition: A book of readings*. Rowley, Mass.: Newbury House.

Edelsky, C., Hudelson, S., Flores, B., Altwerger, B., and Jilbert, K. 1980. A language deficit theory for the 80's: CALP, BICS, and semilingualism. Manuscript, Arizona State University.

Ervin-Tripp, S. 1974. Is second language acquisition like the first? *TESOL Quarterly 8*(2), 111–127.

Ervin-Tripp, S. 1981. Social process in first and second language learning. In H. Winitz (Ed.), *Native language and foreign acquisition*. New York: New York Academy of Science.

Fillmore, C. J. 1976. Frame semantics and the nature of language. In S. R. Harnad, H. D. Steklis, and J. Lancaster (Eds.), *Origins and evolution of language and speech*. New York: New York Academy of Science.

Fillmore, L. W. 1979. Individual differences in second language acquisition. In C. J. Fillmore, D. Kempler, and W. S-Y Wang (Eds.), *Individual differences in language ability and language behavior*. New York: Academic Press.

Flavell, J. 1977. Metacognitive development. Paper presented at the NATO Advanced Study Institute on Structural Process Theories of Complex Human Behavior, Banff, Alberta.

Fuson, C. K. 1979. The development of self-regulating aspects of speech: A review. In G. Zivin (Ed.), *The development of self-regulation through private speech*. New York: Wiley.

Hamayan, E., Saegert, J., and Larudee, P. 1975. Elicited limitation in second language learners. *Working Papers on Bilingualism*, 6, 45–67.

Hatch, E. 1977. Viewpoints: Second language learning. In *Bilingual education: Current perspectives*. Arlington, Va.: Center for Applied Linguistics.

John-Steiner, V., and Tatter, P. 1983. An interactionist model of language acquisition. In B. Bain (Ed.), *The sociogenesis of language and human conduct*. New York: Plenum Press.

Krashen, S. 1980. The input hypothesis. Paper presented at Georgetown Roundtable in Language and Linguistics, Washington, D. C.

Krashen, S., and Pon, P. 1975. An error analysis of an advanced learner of ESL. *Working papers on bilingualism*, 7, 125–129.

Larsen-Freeman, D. E. 1978. An explanation for the morpheme accuracy order of learners of English as a second language. In E. Hatch (Ed.), *Second language acquisition. A book of readings*. Rowley, Mass.: Newbury House.

Paulston, C. 1978. Research. *Bilingual education: Current perspectives* (Vol. 2). Washington, D.C.: Center for Applied Linguistics.

Schumann, J. H. 1978. Second language acquisition: The pidginization hypothesis. In E. Hatch (Ed.), *Second language acquisition: A book of readings*. Rowley, Mass.: Newbury House.

Seleskovitch, D. 1978. Language and cognition. In D. Gerver and H. C. Sinaiko (Eds.), *Language interpretation and communication*. New York: Plenum Press.

Seliger, H. W. 1977. Does practice make perfect? A study of interaction patterns and L_2 competence. *Language Learning* 27(2), 263–278.

Skutnabb-Kangas, P., and Toukomaa, O. 1976. *Teaching migrant children, mother tongue, and learning the language of the host country in the context of the socio-cultural situation of the migrant family*. Tutkimuksia Research Reports. Tampere, Finland: University of Tampere.

Snow, C., and Hoefnagel-Höhle, M. 1978. Age differences in second language acquisition. In E. Hatch (Ed.), *Second language acquisition: A book of readings*. Rowley, Mass.: Newbury House.

Swain, M. 1980. Time and timing in bilingual education. Paper presented to Forum Lecture Series, LSA/TESOL, Summer Institute, Albuquerque.

Vygotsky, L. S. (n.d.) On language acquisition. Manuscript.

Vygotsky, L. S. 1935. The question of multilingualism in childhood. *Children's mental development in the instruction process*. Moscow–Leningrad: State Publishing House.

Vygotsky, L. S. 1960. *The development of higher mental processes*. Moscow: Academy of Pedagogical Sciences, RSFSR.

Vygotsky, L. S. 1962. *Thought and language*. Cambridge: MIT Press.

Wells, G. 1981. *Learning through interaction: The study of language development*. Cambridge: Cambridge University Press.

Name index

Subject Index

378